# The
# Whole Heart
# Book

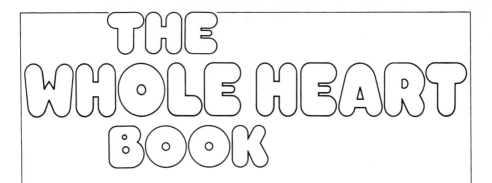

# THE WHOLE HEART BOOK

## James Jackson Nora, M.D., M.P.H.

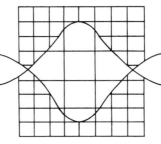

HOLT, RINEHART AND WINSTON
New York

Published by Holt, Rinehart and Winston, 383 Madison Avenue, New York, New York 10017.

Published simultaneously in Canada by Holt, Rinehart and Winston of Canada, Limited.

Library of Congress Cataloging in Publication Data

Nora, James J.
The whole heart book.
Includes index.
    1. Heart—Diseases—Prevention.    I. Title.
RC672.N67    616.1'205    80-387
ISBN Hardbound: 0-03-048251-8
ISBN Paperback: 0-03-048246-1

First Edition

Designer: Lana Giganti
Printed in the United States of America
10  9  8  7  6  5  4  3  2  1

"Nutritional Analyses of Fast Foods reprinted from Public Health Currents, Volume 19, Number 1 C 1979, Ross Laboratories, Columbus, Ohio 43216 with thanks to its authors, Eleanor A. Young, Ph.D., R.D., Ellen H. Brennan, M.S., R.D., and Gaynell L. Irving, R.D."

To May Jackson Nora
and David Bjorn Nora
In Memory

# Acknowledgments

To Peter Collier for showing how the book could be done—and to 143C.

To Joy Ingram for immense help in putting together the tables.

To our patients.

To colleagues, trainees, and staff involved in various aspects of the program: Dr. Randall Lortscher, Dr. Richard Spangler, Dr. Thomas Okin, Dr. Gerald Thurman, Dr. Robin Winkler, Dr. Richard Karsh, Louise Nora, Rose Ann Taylor, Helen Leschnik, and volunteers from the Junior League of Denver.

For fiscal support through research and training grants relevant to the program: The Helen K. and Arthur E. Johnson Foundation; The National Institutes of Health (The National Heart, Lung, and Blood Institute and The National Institute of Child Health and Development); The Colorado Heart Association; and the Junior League of Denver.

And especially to Dr. Audrey Hart Nora.

# CONTENTS

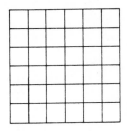

# LIST OF TABLES

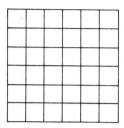

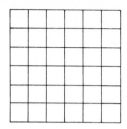

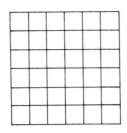

The
Whole Heart
Book

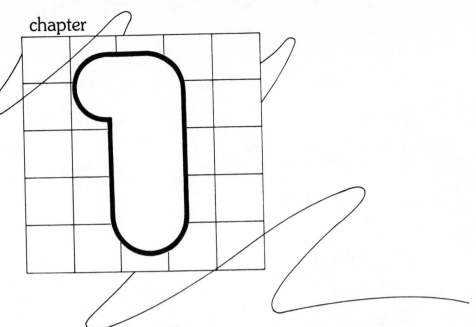

# The Purpose and the Problem

The immodest purpose of this book is to help save your life and make the life you live more livable. Presumptuous? Definitely. But preposterous? Not necessarily. Cardiovascular disease accounts for more deaths in the United States than all other causes combined. That includes cancer, infection, accidents—everything. Yet most people are not even aware of the extent to which it is now possible to discover who is a potential victim of a heart attack or stroke and how cardiovascular disease may be prevented.

Who's to blame for the lack of awareness? Don't worry, there's plenty of guilt to go around. First you should know that up to a few decades ago doctors really couldn't do much for patients. So when the means became available to treat and actually cure disease, you can imagine the enthusiasm and joy within the profession. Good-bye ineffectual sugar pills and dangerous arsenicum; hello penicillin. Western medicine went through an incredible growth phase. Anything was possible as long as there was enough money, and there always seemed to be enough money in the wells of ever-expanding economies.

Then, in the late 1960s, something happened. It happened in many places and in many guises. We became aware that there were limits. The spindle-legged fantasy of the invincibility of science and technology bent and broke under the weight of a reality that we could no longer ignore. For me the intruding reality came from my experience with heart transplantation. Can you imagine a more irrelevant and profligate approach to heart disease? And yet, there I was, one of those on a medical-surgical ego trip, pursuing a therapeutic vapor that could benefit only a few hundred people annually, while one million Americans were dying of cardiovascular diseases every year.

But I owe a debt to heart transplantation, because it started me thinking in what I believe is the right direction. Instead of trying to treat, patch up, or replace hopelessly damaged hearts, why not prevent the hearts from getting damaged in the first place? After all, heart attacks are not the birthright of every American. In fact, there are many places in the world where heart attacks are very rarely encountered. If a Black had a heart attack in South Africa it would be such a medical curiosity that a hospital conference would be convened to study it. Even in highly industrialized Japan the mortality rate from heart disease is less than one-fourth the rate in the United States.

Now let's get back to blame and guilt. How about accusing biomedical research, the medical profession in general, and government policies that continue to pursue curative rather than preventive approaches to disease? The reckless extravagance of the curative strategy is becoming clear only at this late stage, when it's beginning to hit everyone in the pocketbook. Do you know what the bill is? Currently we're paying $206 billion a year for medical care. In five years, at the present rate, it will be $320 billion a year. About 42 percent of this enormous bill comes from your tax dollar. And the average annual medical bill for each man, woman, and child in America is $960. For what? For superior individual and national health? Sorry. We're paying for superior health, but we're getting inferior results.

A few more scapegoats? Corporate greed and irresponsibility are always good ones—how to turn the gossamer dream of the good life into a crushing nightmare. And of course Madison Avenue is there to sell people a life-style that will kill them. But let's stop skimming over the surface of the pond of health and look down into it. Who do you see in there? Who's ultimately to blame? I'm sorry to have to say this, but many of you are. In subsequent pages you'll have an opportunity to evaluate what you've been doing to promote your personal health, the health of your family, and the national health. And if you've been failing, you'll have to accept a generous slice of the pie of blame.

But for some of you there is more credit than blame, because it appears that the disastrous epidemic of heart disease may, even now, be coming under control through preventive medicine. Here is where the concerned and informed layman has actually taken the lead, leaving behind the physicians who continue to be hung up on curative medicine. While cardiologists and epidemiologists have been asking what, if anything, could be done to slow the epidemic of cardiovascular disease, many Americans have been instituting the very changes in their lives that the experts continue to debate. Diet, smoking, exercise, life-style—when you look at these factors in epidemiologic studies, there's always a flaw in the study. And Research Group A can exploit this flaw to attack Research Group B to conclude that Factor C doesn't contribute to heart attacks. After all, if Factor C really turned out to be important, it would deplete the ego investment of Research Group A, not to mention undermining their other investments in grants and contracts.

Well, many of you have seen through the chicanery and have begun resorting to something that in the not-too-remote past was considered an American virtue: common sense. You've been instituting changes in your lives in ways that were intuitively reasonable. You've reached your own conclusions on the debated evidence. And what's been the result? *The epidemic of heart attacks is starting to recede.* Recently I heard one cardiovascular epidemiologist remark in a less than facetious tone: "We'd better hurry up and decide what causes heart attacks before they're all gone."

Let's stop right here. I've given you some good news. I've told you there's hope. Now let's get back to the bad news: Cardiovascular disease isn't gone. *The problem is still very much with us.* To put it in perspective, three times as many people still die of cardiovascular disease (most often heart attacks) as die of cancer. And there are nine cardiovascular deaths for every death by accident. Now, you may argue that people have to die of something, and heart disease is as good as anything. But the problem doesn't have to do with dying—which is as natural as living. The problem with which this book concerns itself is sudden death in the prime of life, when an individual should be at the peak of his productivity. The problem has to do with families deprived of the companionship, guidance, and support of a parent and mate when there are mortgages to be paid and children to be educated. And the problem has to do with human nature: our unwillingness to make a change before being confronted by a crisis. Most people are quite receptive to changing their life-styles *after* sustaining a heart attack, but too few people are willing to make significant changes when no such event is apparently imminent.

No one wants to keep every American alive and on the job until he is 125 years old. Yet surely something can be done about the relatively young and vigorous portion of the one million people who die each year of heart and blood vessel diseases. For 20 to 30 percent of heart attack victims, the first clue about the presence of heart disease is sudden or acute death. *The first clue: death.* Is there no early warning system? What's biomedical science doing about this? What's that multibillion-dollar health bill paying for?

During the past decade we have seen some dramatic accomplishments (and nonaccomplishments) from cardiology and cardiovascular surgery. Even relatively small hospitals now have shiny coronary care units replete with monitors blinking and beeping and presumably helping to sustain life. Coronary bypass surgery is being performed in numbers that boggle the mind and strangle the pocketbook (over a billion dollars worth per year). And, as I mentioned earlier, we have even gone to such extremes as transplanting hearts and are still seeking functional plastic replacements. The rewards for the researchers may be headlines, prizes, and prestige. The rewards for the clinical physicians and surgeons may be incredible incomes. But what about the rewards for the potential victims of heart attacks and other cardiovascular disease? Negligible. We'll discuss some of this later.

## Victims, Potential Victims, and Heredity

Who gets cardiovascular disease? In Chapter 2 we'll pursue this question in more detail. And in many chapters you'll be given tests to determine what specific risk factors you may have, together with programs to combat these risks. But for now, a general (and oversimplified) answer will get us started.

Please refer to Figure 1–1 as you read the next two paragraphs. You're looking at those statistical favorites, normal distribution curves. The small curve on the left represents the fortunate ones. These people *probably* exist—I'd guess maybe 10 percent of Americans—people who are so genetically favored that they simply cannot become victims of heart disease or stroke. That's the *yang* of cardiovascular disease. The *yin* is the small curve on the right—the approximately 10 percent of our population with a dangerously high risk of cardiovascular disease.

These are the ones who are most likely to have heart attacks at *early* ages. You see, heart attacks don't really fit the conception many of you may have: that they strike indiscriminately and without warning. Rather, heart attacks tend to run in families, and *there is warning* but only if you know what the signals are. You should know that the majority of heart attacks—especially those that occur at early ages—cluster in a small percentage of families. These genetically burdened people *do exist.* And if they are to have a chance for a normal life, they must be identified and must become dedicated participants in a lifelong program of cardiovascular health. Such a program can literally mean the difference between early death or disability and a full and active life. To be sure that the numbers are not escaping anyone, we're talking about more than 20 million Americans. I and members of my family are in that high-risk, genetically burdened group. While I don't wish that you join us in this not-too-exclusive club, in the chapters that follow you will have an opportunity to fill out the application forms to see if you qualify.

The rest of you belong in the big curve in the middle. Under very unfavorable circumstances, you can become a victim. However, your risk is much lower, and if you were to have a heart attack it would be likely to occur at a later age. I should also point out that I know of no way to distinguish the 80 percent in the middle curve from the postulated fortunate 10 percent in the curve at the left. Therefore we must arrive at a concept opposing high risk to lower levels of risk, ignoring the possibility that there are those who have no risk at all.

In the next chapter, we'll get into some genetic concepts. Single genes, polygenes, thresholds, and other ideas will be explained in a nonintimidating way. The main genetic idea is that most heart disease results from the interaction of our heredity with our environment. And since we can't do anything about our heredity, we must concentrate on what we do with our environment—the way we live. (But someone with a highest-risk hereditary form of heart disease can decide whether he or she wishes to continue to transmit the disease through future generations.)

*Figure* **1–1:** Hypothetical curves representing how the risk of heart attack may be distributed in the American population.

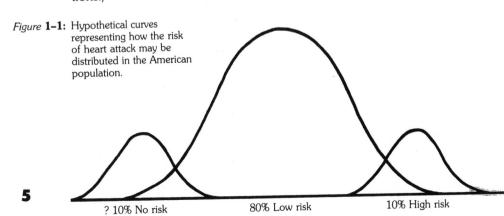

? 10% No risk          80% Low risk          10% High risk

# Introduction to Prevention

For preventing cardiovascular disease, we're going to concentrate on finding out who is at risk, how great the risk is, and what specific changes need to be made for individuals and families. If you are joining us in the high-risk 10 percent of our population, you may face some fairly drastic changes (although you may also find you've already made most of the necessary accommodations). If you're in the lower-risk 90 percent of Americans and are following anything resembling prudent living, you may have to do little or nothing more than you're now doing. Your diet may not need to exclude entirely those tasty omelets and tangy cheeses. And you may not require more than the minimal basic exercise program. This is because we believe that we can now distinguish those at high risk from those at lower risk. And what is good preventive medicine for one person may be totally unnecessary for another.

We started the Whole Heart Program about six years ago as a research effort into the causes of cardiovascular diseases, heart attacks, congenital heart diseases, strokes, and high blood pressure. The Junior League of Denver provided us with many volunteers, allowing us to gather data as we reached out into the community. We collaborated with a number of groups to screen patients and identify families with high risk of early heart attacks. Many of these patients had physicians, but surprisingly, almost half did not. And many physicians requested consultation in developing preventive programs for their patients.

It became immediately evident that our role had expanded far beyond merely finding patients at risk and studying their risk factors. We developed a sense of responsibility toward those who were initially discovered to be at risk—and toward those other family members who were eventually discovered to be at risk as a result of our family studies.

Our evaluation included the usual risk factors: smoking, blood pressure, cholesterol, diabetes, weight, diet, and so on. Beyond the usual approach, we added a thorough genetic history of heart attacks, strokes, and diabetes *in the family,* and the study of new genetic factors. We'll discuss risk-factor evaluation further in later chapters.

Having found the patients at risk—many of whom had no previous clue to an underlying problem—we assumed the responsibility for helping the patient attack the specific risks that he or she had and develop an overall life-style that would be most compatible with cardiovascular health. The major components of a life-style that will reduce the most critical risk factors are covered in the chapters that follow. These elements include cholesterol and lipoprotein management, smoking cessation, blood pressure and stress control, weight reduction, and aerobic exercise. The earlier these risk factors are controlled, the more likely the benefit, so our program has stressed the identification and management of children at risk.

Several recurring themes regarding successful preventive programs will be introduced immediately and repeated often. One theme is that the various elements of the program work together, supplementing, complementing, and lightening the load of the other elements. This is just the opposite of what the initial impression may be—that each prescription is a separate and additional burden. Take diet and exercise, for example. Diet without exercise is not only less effective but is counterproductive, permitting muscle to be wasted with fat, and actually adversely influencing the fat content of the blood. On the other hand, an overweight individual who exercises without a thought to diet will usually increase his caloric intake to meet his increased needs, and little or no weight will be lost. It's equally important that when you're exercising, dieting is simply easier to do. There is a synergistic effect.

The third major element in healthful living is the belief system, the support system. We need all the help we can get. From our family. From our friends. From our church. From our orientation to life. Experience with patients and in my own family has convinced me of this. For healthful living there has to be a deep commitment—almost a religious zeal. But let me add quickly that there are few things I find more abhorrent than pop religious self-improvement. "Lose ten ugly pounds for Jesus." "Christ is my Royal Canadian Air Force co-exerciser." But as far as I know, no successful human culture has existed, and no human being can long exist, without some form of religious orientation. (That sounds awfully pompous. I apologize.) What I'm doing is using the term religion in the sense that Erich Fromm does: "any group-shared system of thought and action that offers an individual a frame of orientation and an object of devotion." A person's religion may indeed be one of the traditional forms, such as Christianity, Judaism, or Buddhism. It may be one of the modern secular (but no less "religious") orientations such as humanism, communism, ethnic pride, or the women's movement. It may even be the pursuit of money or power.

While most of us would find it offensive to become a Christian (Buddhist, humanist) to lose ten ugly pounds, we should also be prepared for failure if we do not make a program of health an important, indeed an integral, part of our lives. The techniques of behavior modification that we will follow are road signs to help us get where we want to go. The road map for the trip is your personal frame of orientation or religion. Make no mistake, it's not easy to change a lifetime of bad habits, nor is it easy to change good habits once they are firmly established. To make changes you will need to call on all of the resources you can muster. The programs will be relatively easy for your younger children. They don't have as many years of bad habits to undo. But the children are not likely to accept a program without your example of participation.

In the Great Learning, attributed to Tseng Tsu (c. fifth century B.C.), it is written that to achieve virtue man must first cultivate himself; then he can cultivate his family, his state, and the world. The program begins with you. And to be successful it must involve everyone in your household.

Throughout this presentation, recommendations for prevention will be geared to ages and stages. Some readers will conclude from looking at themselves and their families that they have little risk, and that they are doing just about what they should be doing to prevent heart attacks. Others may find that their personal and familial risks are so great that nothing less than a complete reorganization of their lives will improve their chances of preventing a cardiovascular disaster.

There is no guarantee that even the most conscientious efforts to prevent cardiovascular disease will always be successful. Although our current knowledge is imperfect, it clearly indicates that a systematic program aimed at achieving optimal cardiovascular health can be highly beneficial. The earlier the program is started, the better. We are just beginning to appreciate that what you do for your children will have more preventive impact than what you do for yourself. Yet at any time in your life, including the period following a heart attack, there can be a program designed to improve cardiovascular function.

This book will emphasize the prevention of heart attacks, which are the most common and dramatic manifestations of atherosclerosis, or hardening of the arteries. Heart attacks are usually caused by a plugging up of the blood vessels that nourish the heart (coronary arteries), causing a segment of heart muscle to die and scar. If the plugging up is gradual and much of the heart muscle stays alive (but receives poor circulation), congestive heart failure may occur without the more dramatic event of a heart attack. This latter category of disease appears in vital statistics as chronic ischemic heart disease. A plugging up of blood vessels to the brain by atherosclerotic disease, if sudden, causes a stroke. Blood vessels in the legs may also plug up—or the major blood vessel to the body, the aorta, may become very narrow because of deposits of cholesterol and scarring over the sites of the deposit. Therefore, much of what is said regarding the prevention of heart attacks applies to the prevention of strokes, chronic ischemic heart disease, and other problems produced by hardening of the arteries. As a bonus, a program for cardiovascular health is unavoidably a program for general good health. Cigarette smoking provides one example. If you kick the smoking habit (or influence your children never to start) in order to improve cardiovascular health, you'll also be doing a great deal to reduce risks from the second leading cause of death, cancer; the fourth leading cause of death, accidents; and the ninth leading cause of death, chronic pulmonary disease.

The key to prevention of any disease is understanding the cause. It has been clear for many decades that heart attacks and strokes tend to run in families. If your family is large enough and close enough for you to know with confidence what diseases have been present and what the causes of death have been, you are a long way toward knowing if you are at risk of a heart attack. The presence or absence of *early-onset coronary heart disease* is what you really need to know about. A close relative dying at 42 with a heart attack is much more significant than a distant relative dying at 80 of the same cause.

But maybe you can't get a good reliable history about heart disease in your family. And just because there is heart disease in the family doesn't mean that everybody, including you, has to get it. So there are some tests in common use that help to tell you about risks. You'll be given a chance to take a test that our research group has developed to help you determine if you are at risk—and how great the risk is. Furthermore, it should be possible within the next few years to develop even more accurate formulas for any patient, which will predict (on the basis of family history, traditional risk factors, and new risk factors now being explored) what the chances are for developing coronary heart disease at a given age. Of course, it's assumed that if someone finds out he has a risk he will take immediate steps to prevent the risk prediction from being realized.

The cause of heart attacks is complicated. Typically, the geneticist looks at coronary heart disease and is impressed with how the cases cluster in families. But after deeper analysis of data, some despair of defining the genetic components. So much of the disease seems to be related to contributions from the environment. This is where the epidemiologist comes in. He looks at the disease and tries to find important risk factors, such as elevated cholesterol, high blood pressure, and smoking. But, as we mentioned earlier, a competent epidemiologist can always find flaws in someone else's epidemiologic study. Subjected to critical analysis, the individual risk factors—the environmental components—may not appear to contribute very much to coronary heart disease. So the epidemiologist gets the discouraging feeling that the disease is primarily genetic.

Although the problem is a difficult one, the first step in its solution is to recognize clearly that both heredity and environment are involved.

What is a safe diet for a person of one genetic makeup may not be safe for another. The complexity of the genetic-environmental interaction is discussed in more detail in the next chapter, and is visually depicted in Figure 2–1.

The chapters that follow will take you up the first steps toward prevention. If you already have symptoms and signs of cardiovascular disease, you should be under a physician's care right now. In a book of this type it would be extremely poor medicine to discuss preventive measures to be used *after* the onset of heart disease. The measures exist, but they should be directed by a physician. Therefore, the recommendation in such a circumstance would be to *seek immediate personal medical supervision.* This book is not intended to replace your physician, but may help you and your physician in evaluating your risk and directing your personal program of cardiovascular health. It may also help you to become a more discriminating medical consumer.

You might ask why it should be accepted that a book designed for medical consumers should have an impact on health. This question requires me to share some information with you that does no credit to the American medical establishment. Recently at a distinguished school of public health, it was reported that Americans are now relying almost as much on books and magazines for health information as they are on their physicians. I must also add that in the chapters that follow it will be quickly appreciated that the amount of information needed for family prevention of cardiovascular disease is surprisingly small. The programs are anything but complicated. The difficulty is in making the commitment to a change in life-style and staying with behavior modification until the new patterns are firmly established.

It is assumed that a physician writing about programs of health has experience with these programs in his patients. What may not be assumed is that the physician has personal experience with what he advocates. In this case, however, the programs discussed not only are for our patients, but are those with which my family lives. You have trouble with diets? We know all about that. And you hate to exercise? We know about that, too. We've been through all the struggles ourselves, and we've concluded that if we can do it—anyone can.

Even you.

This is your invitation to take charge of your own life and health. And for parents, this is a call to be responsive to the health needs of your children.

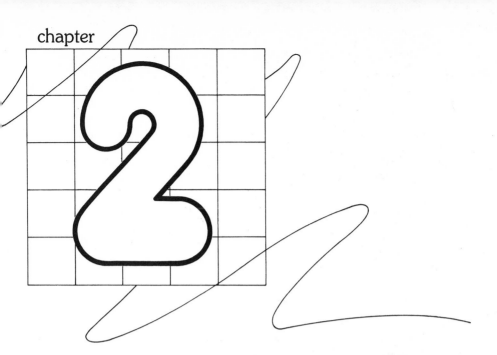

# Know Thyself (And Thy Family)

This is where it all begins—knowing yourself. Through the thousands of years from Delphi to pop psychology the admonition has been: Know thyself. A little later in the chapter you'll be asked to take certain steps along that tortuous and unending path to self-knowledge. But first, for disease prevention, it's important to know not only a lot about yourself, but a lot about your family. It's unfair for a person or family to be subject to heart attacks at early ages when another person or family has little risk of having a heart attack at any age. It's equally unfair for a person or family to have cancer or various other diseases when other people are apparently relatively free of these threats.

Unfair or not, heart attacks and strokes occur in families. This is the concept of *genetic risk,* which is the cornerstone in our thinking about prevention. Some people can smoke two packs of cigarettes a day and get neither heart disease nor cancer. Some cannot. Some people can eat 15 eggs a week, fatty meat every day, and pounds and pounds of butter—and still have a low cholesterol content in their blood. Others who may crave a good omelet or a rich sauce, but religiously avoid these delicacies, are only rewarded by still having a cholesterol level that is too high.

Who are you? What is your risk (if any) of having a heart attack or stroke? One way to find out is to determine whether or not you possess certain risk factors that are often familial. For example, what is your serum cholesterol level? What is your blood pressure? You should also find out as much as possible about the presence or absence of cardiovascular disease and risk factors in other members of your family. Has anyone had a heart attack before 55 years of age? Does anyone have high blood pressure? People often have cholesterol determinations performed during routine physical examination. Does anyone have a high cholesterol level?

The book and television series *Roots* has sent many Americans off to try to trace their families and perhaps come up with some renowned progenitor. It would be less entertaining but much more useful if our search for roots would emphasize the causes and ages of death of our relatives. In this chapter we'll introduce you to the basic ideas about genetic pedigrees. And in this chapter as well as in the Appendix of this book model pedigrees will be provided for you to use to record your

*Figure* **2-1:** Heredity interacting with environment to produce coronary disease.  Areas for study. (From J. J. Nora, and A. H. Nora, *Genetics and Counseling in Cardiovascular Diseases,* [Springfield: Charles C. Thomas, 1978].)

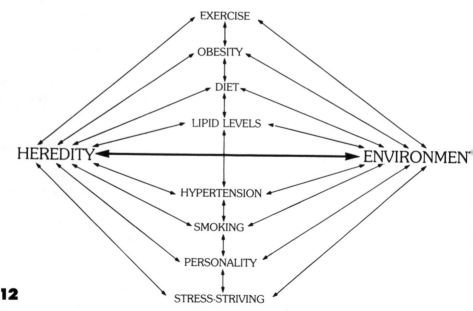

own family history. The accompanying instructions will enable you to be the cardiovascular geneticist for your family.

We've all heard many times that each of us is the product of our heredity and environment. In a very complex manner, both play important roles in heart and blood vessel disease caused by hardening of the arteries. Figure 2–1, as complicated as it may appear, is a greatly oversimplified way to look at how heredity and environment interact to cause coronary heart disease. If your family history, your genetic risk factors, tells us that you are subject to early-onset coronary heart disease, you can't change your parents. But you can change your environmental risk factors, and you must, if you wish to survive. On the other hand, if you don't have genetic risk factors, it may not be necessary for you to impose rigid dietary and other restrictions on yourself. A more moderate program designed to promote good cardiovascular health should be sufficient. What is important at the outset is to know as much as possible about yourself, your family, and your risks.

Certain risk factors are more important than others and will command a longer presentation. In rating the most important risk factors, as I understand them from our studies, I have placed hereditary predisposition first on the list. High cholesterol (and associated blood elements), high blood pressure, and smoking are the three most important factors to emerge from many epidemiologic studies. Stress and striving have received considerable attention, in descriptions of the so-called Type A personality. And the interaction of diet, obesity, and exercise is relatively easy to visualize. There are many other potential factors currently being explored. Some of these may eventually prove to be even more important than those depicted in Figure 2–1. A brief mention of such factors will be made in Chapter 12, but it would be premature to incorporate tentative findings into clinical diagnosis and treatment.

Although Hippocrates, the father of medicine, was probably the first physician to discuss the familial nature of disease, he did not specifically comment on familial heart disease. Very likely, heart attacks were not a common occurrence twenty-five hundred years ago. Actually, one of the first individuals to appreciate that heart attacks run in families was not a physician at all, but the poet and essayist, Matthew Arnold. While traveling in America, Arnold began to experience chest pain that he perceived to be "the sign of a malady which had suddenly struck down in the middle life . . . my father and my grandfather." Matthew Arnold lived with chest pain for less than a year before dying of his familial "malady." One of his biographers must be faulted for disclosing surprisingly deficient scholarship when he described the cause of Arnold's death as "heart failure . . . sudden and quite unexpected." Unexpected to others, perhaps, but not to Matthew Arnold.

To stay with the Arnold family a little longer, Matthew's grandfather, William Arnold, was a collector of customs who died when his son, Thomas, was only 6 years old. Thomas Arnold, Matthew's father, died when he was 46 years old. Although *Encyclopaedia Britannica* devotes only three paragraphs to Thomas Arnold, it seemed important enough in such brief space to point out: "What gave him his power . . . was . . . his severe and lofty estimate of duty." This is a particularly apt description of Type A behavior. And a particularly apt illustration of the interaction of a genetic predisposition to coronary heart disease with a harmful environmental trigger: Type A behavior.

We are indebted to Sir William Osler, the consummate physician-scholar, for bringing the Arnold family to the attention of the medical profession. In the widely used textbook, *Clinical Heart Disease,* Samuel Levine followed Osler's lead when he wrote that heredity was "the most important etiologic factor" in heart attacks. Then, for a period of years, perhaps because of the increasing emphasis on environmental risk factors, the hereditary nature of heart disease received less research attention.

However, with the development of new research techniques in the fifties by Donald Fredrickson and his co-workers at the National Institutes of Health, the inheritance of an important group of risk factors in heart disease came into the spotlight. These risk factors have to do with cholesterol and blood fats (lipids) and their attachment to proteins (lipoproteins). It became evident that certain individuals and families at risk could be identified by a relatively simple screening procedure on a sample of blood, looking at cholesterol, triglycerides, and the patient's serum or plasma after the blood cells have been allowed to settle. Techniques called ultracentrifugation and lipoprotein electrophoresis permit more precise identification and are reserved for those suspected of having an abnormality on the basis of the screening test. These ideas will be discussed in more detail in Chapter 5.

Now let's get back to heart attacks running in families. Long before I came to recognize that our own family was at high risk, I had learned the concept of familial heart disease from my patients. I hadn't been in my practice as a family physician in rural Wisconsin for more than a few weeks when I was called on to care for a 39-year-old farmer who used the same matter-of-fact tone of Matthew Arnold to tell me that the "family malady" was beginning to afflict him. He was having chest pain with exertion. One brother had died at age 38, another at 42, and his father at 40.

Country doctors have the opportunity to get to know their patients well—and their families. Soon I identified several such families, and using the state of the art of 20 years ago, I tried to develop programs for them that would prevent or forestall the heart attacks. I was sufficiently pleased with my efforts to report my study to the *Journal of the American Medical Association,* and to decide that I could work more effectively in this area if I undertook specialty training. But while I was still in cardiology training I began to get unsettling reports on the patients in my former family practice. Although their heart attacks had been delayed, the simple techniques I'd been using were not sufficient to have the long-term impact I'd been hoping for. There was a lot more to preventing heart attacks than a country doctor of 20 years ago could devise. During my training and afterwards, I drifted inexorably into the traditional curative mainstream of cardiologic thought, which eventually reached its high point (or low point) in heart transplantation.

I maintained my interest in the genetics of cardiovascular disease, but for years concentrated more on congenital heart disease (such as holes in the heart present at birth). But what about coronary heart disease in my own family? It came as a complete surprise to me! I found out about my high risk from a free screening test offered at the annual meeting of the American College of Cardiology. Here I was, trained and experienced in both cardiology and genetics—and I first understood about my own familial heart disease as the result of a free screening test. Of course I knew my mother had died in her fifties of "heart disease." We knew she had had rheumatic fever, but starting in her forties she became subject to angina, the chest pain of coronary heart disease. Our thinking about her heart condition had been muddied by her coexisting rheumatic disease. My father had also died of a heart attack. And assorted uncles had succumbed to heart disease. The free screening test informed me that my cholesterol, triglycerides, and lipoproteins were distinctly abnormal. Now the whole family picture came together.

My wife and I began to talk about this problem and discovered immediately that her family also suffered from early-onset coronary heart disease. What a legacy for our children! So we studied them in our laboratory and found that they too had abnormalities in their blood lipids. Needless to say, my interest in preventing heart attacks took on a personal and urgent character. In fact, the original intent of the program in this book was to protect my children—and the children of others—who through no fault of their own were born into a family with a high risk of having heart attacks. As I began to develop what has evolved into the Whole Heart Program, it became obvious that preventive measures are a family affair. You can't devise prudent diets, exercise programs, and commitment to nonsmoking for the child and exclude the parents. Kids are too smart to accept such nonsense.

If commitment to health—physical and emotional well-being—is important, it's important for *all* members of the family, and all ages. As our program has evolved, it is certainly not just for kids. Although infancy and childhood are theoretically better ages for starting preventive measures, patients at risk at any age or stage of their disease process need not be abandoned. While we're trying to insure that our children will have full lives and life-spans, my wife and I certainly haven't given up on ourselves.

According to one epidemiologic study (because of my blood lipid profile), I should have had the onset of coronary heart disease seven years ago. That was just about the time I became interested in looking out for my personal cardiovascular health, not just the health of my patients. That same study predicted that two years ago I had a greater than fifty-fifty chance of having a heart attack. I intend to continue to prove the prediction wrong, and I see no reason why my personal Whole Heart Program should not provide me with many more active years. I'm convinced that there's a suitable program for every age and stage of coronary heart disease. I refer to this system as age- and stage-specific prevention.

## Who Are You? And What Kind of Condition Are You In?

Your response to the first question will tell you a lot about yourself. Don't ruminate over it. Just answer it with whatever comes to mind first. Who are you?

Answer it now.

All right, what did you say? Positive things? Things that indicate pride and satisfaction with yourself. Neutral things—like your name? Or negative things, like: *just* a working stiff; *just* a housewife. Maybe something worse?

If your answer was anything less than positive, you must know that changes will have to be made in the way you think about yourself. That doesn't mean that after years of running yourself down you'll change in one glorious moment. The *decision* to change can come in a "glorious moment," but the change in your attitude toward yourself will be gradual.

Now let's get right into some basics about your physical condition. We'll start with a watch, a yardstick, a tape measure, and a scale.

Just as you sit here, take your pulse. If you have trouble finding your pulse, the two most convenient arteries to use are the carotid and the radial. The carotid artery is in the neck. Find your Adam's apple and slide your finger along either side of it toward the back of your neck until you feel a pulse. Feel it on just one side of your neck (I don't want anyone passing out from massaging both carotid arteries at the same time). This is the pulse you'll probably most often want to check during exercise. The radial pulse is the one you're used to having doctors and nurses check—the one on the inside of your wrist, back from the thumb.

Once you're confident you can feel your pulse, begin to count it while following the sweep second hand of your watch for 15 seconds. Multiply the number by 4. This is your pulse (or heart) rate per minute. You may feel free to count for more than 15 seconds at rest, but when you're testing your response to exercise, you should limit the count to 15 seconds. Because the heart rate begins to slow when exercise is terminated, 15 seconds is probably the maximum period for determining a valid rate. Record your heart (pulse) rate in the appropriate blank space in Table 2–1. (Actually, I've provided room for six family members to record their initial findings. Just put your initials at the tops of the columns.)

If the heart rate of any male family member over 15 years of age is above 80 beats per minute (85 for females), that individual is likely to be even less fit than the average American. And the average American, until recently, has been anything but fit. If your heart rate is under 60 at any age (and you don't have some rare heart block), you're likely to be more fit than the average (unfit) American. There'll be more tests on heart rate and fitness in chapters that follow.

Now for the yardstick. Why don't you see honestly how tall you are? Average-to-short men usually add an inch or two to their reported height. Tall women often shave an inch or two. After you've reported your wish-fulfillment height enough times, you begin to accept the false value as correct. Maybe you've been referring to charts of what you should weigh for 5 feet 10 inches and it turns out you're only 5 feet 8 inches. Obviously you've been kidding yourself about how many pounds overweight you are. So take off your shoes, stand to your full height on a hard surface with your back against a wall, put the yardstick on your head, being sure it's parallel to the floor (you can judge that reasonably well), and put a mark on the wall to record where the undersurface of the yardstick touches the wall. This measurement can be done a little more easily, and perhaps slightly more accurately, if someone helps you.

Next the tape measure. For men, the chest at the nipple line and the waist at the belly button are the measures to make. For women, waist, bust, and hips are the appropriate general measures. For both, stand in a natural relaxed comfortable way. Don't suck in your gut or puff out your chest. Get honest careful measurements (by yourself or with the assistance of an objective family member). Record these measurements in Table 2–1.

The next measurement you may wish to postpone until first thing in the morning: your weight. You should have a good, accurate scale, and if it's not a balance scale, it must be placed on a hard surface, not a carpet. If you don't have a good scale, consider investing in one. If you have an inexpensive scale and don't want to buy another one, you'd better know the idiosyncrasies of the scale you have. Does it give the same weight if you get on first with your right foot as it does with your left? Does its position on the floor change the reading? For the ordinary bathroom scale you may wish to weigh yourself a minimum of three times and record the average. The trick in using inexpensive scales is to try to make all the conditions the same each time you weigh. And the trick about when to weigh yourself is similar. You should weigh at the same time of day in the same minimal amount of clothing (or no clothing) under the same general conditions. On arising and before breakfast is usually a convenient time. Record your weight in Table 2–1.

The final measurements acknowledge that there is a difference between muscle and bone weight, and fat weight. A 5-foot 10-inch, 210-pound fullback may be all muscle, but a 5-foot 10-inch, 175-pound desk jockey may be mostly blubber, and at least 30 pounds overweight. If a man's arms and legs are like toothpicks and he has a spare tire around his middle, he could be fat even if his weight is "below normal" for his height. This is where the "pinch test" comes into play.

If you were enrolled in our Whole Heart Program, we'd measure certain skin fold thicknesses with calipers and do some calculations. You can accomplish something like this (with a moderate sacrifice in accuracy) by using your thumb and index finger, pinching a roll of fat, and measuring it against a ruler. Men and women collect fat in different places—and individual men or women may have their own special fat depots. So you may have to check yourself over to find where you're storing unneeded fat. If you can pinch an inch of fat anywhere, you're overweight.

**Men** ○ Let's start with you. Stand up straight. Tighten your belly muscles and dig your opened index finger and thumb right down to the muscle on either side of your belly button. Now pinch, bring the fingers together until you have a roll of fat that won't get any smaller. Have your ruler ready and hold your fingers so they maintain the measurement. More than one inch here means you're fat—no matter what you weigh. Belly fat is probably the most sensitive guide to obesity in males, but try a couple of other places. Rest a hand on your head and pinch the fat on the back of your arm about halfway between the elbow and shoulder. More than three-fourths of an inch? That's too much fat. Now sit down and hold a leg straight out, locking your knee and tightening those thigh muscles. Take a pinch halfway between your hip and knee. If it's more than an inch, it's excess fat. The same goes for the chest halfway between the nipple and the shoulder. Finally the love-handles. Feel along your side down from the bottom rib to the next bone you find. This is the iliac crest (sometimes erroneously called the hipbone). Now follow this bone around to the back for about four inches. Get hold of a pinch of fat between your iliac crest and your bottom rib and measure it.

**Women** ○ Measure the same areas as men for openers. If you pinch an inch in any area, that's excess fat. Women get a small break in that they're allowed up to an inch of pinch on the back of the arm.

The final box to fill in Table 2–1 relates to present physical activity. It's relatively easy. Do you get regular aerobic exercise? If you have to ask what that is, you probably don't. But I'll give you a definition that will help you fill out the table now, rather than waiting for the more detailed explanation that will follow in Chapter 10, "Run for Your Life." If you exercise regularly three to six days a week, with no more than two days between exercise periods, for no less than 60 minutes a week and at least 10 consecutive minutes per workout, at a heart rate of at least 150, you get a plus (+). If you have regular vigorous exercise weekdays as well as weekends, but don't know what heart rate you attain, you get plus-minus (±). If you don't get regular exercise give yourself a minus (−). Heart rate and exercise will be discussed in Chapter 10.

## Know Thy Family

The preceding section was obviously only a small step toward knowing yourself. The second small step will require that you know some things about your family. If such information is unobtainable (due to adoption or other loss of contact), you can still learn a workable amount of information about the genes you inherited from certain genetic tests and from tests of your children.

Figure 2–2 is a genetic pedigree of a family (curiously similar to my family) that has early-onset coronary heart disease. You'll eventually need to draw your own genetic pedigree, and you can see how it's done by following the technique in this example and in the sample pedigree that you may use to record your own family history (Figure 2–3).

Looking at the legend in Figure 2–3 we see that a circle is a female and a square represents a male. You've already been provided with

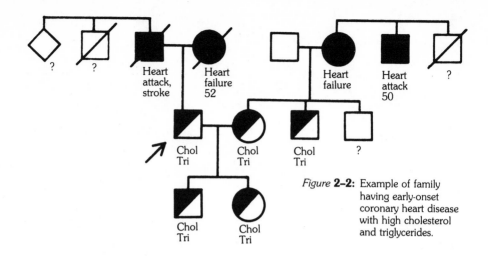

*Figure* **2–2:** Example of family having early-onset coronary heart disease with high cholesterol and triglycerides.

stems on which to hang the circles and squares who are related to you. The person providing the history gets an arrow. He (as in Figure 2–2) is called the proband. Completely darken the circle or square for those in-dividuals who have a clearly established diagnosis of CHD or coronary heart disease (i.e., heart attack or diagnosis by a reputable cardiologist, pathologist, or other physician with necessary skills). If a major risk fac-tor is present, such as high cholesterol (chol), smoking (smoke), triglyc-erides (tri), high blood pressure (hyper, HT, or HBP), fill in half of the circle or square diagonally and specify the risk factor(s). A slash through a circle or square extending outside the borders means that the patient has died, and the number under the circle can be used to specify the age of death or the age of onset of coronary disease.

As you can see in Figure 2–2, there are some gaps in the knowl-edge about this family. There's nothing at all about the grandparents, and there is no knowledge about risk factors in several other family members (depicted by question marks). A diamond may be used to rep-resent one or more persons without specifying the sex. While the pedi-gree in Figure 2–2 would not be entirely satisfactory for research data, it does provide a great deal of information. The average family filling out a genetic pedigree will probably get at least this much and probably more information about heart attacks and risk factors. You can use your own abbreviations for risk factors. It's not necessary to use *diab* for diabetes or HBP for high blood pressure—just make sure you under-stand what your code is.

Table 2–2, which appears on page 33, lists some questions you will want to explore. You should know as much as possible about the presence or absence of these factors in yourself and your family. Some

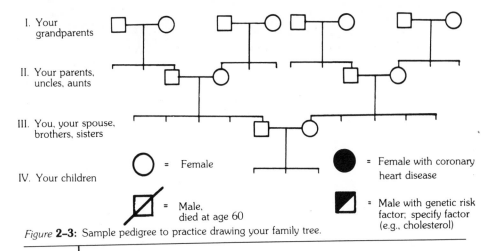

I. Your
grandparents

II. Your parents,
uncles, aunts

III. You, your spouse,
brothers, sisters

IV. Your children

◯ = Female

◻ = Male,
died at age 60

● = Female with coronary
heart disease

◪ = Male with genetic risk
factor; specify factor
(e.g., cholesterol)

*Figure* **2–3:** Sample pedigree to practice drawing your family tree.

This material is repeated for you to fill out in the Tear-Out Appendix

factors will rate full chapters of explanation, and all of them will be discussed at some length in subsequent sections. It will take a while to accumulate all the information you need to fill out the pedigree and to construct your own risk index. For a start, you may be able to draw in only empty circles and squares. If you have an unfortunate family history and have had close relatives die at early ages of heart attacks or strokes, you already know a great deal of the bad news in your family.

Although this has already been said, it will be repeated here and probably once or twice more. Of particular importance in a genetic history are: (1) how closely related a family member with coronary heart disease is, and (2) how young the individual was at the onset of the disease. First-degree relatives are most important—parents, siblings, children—and disease starting before 55 years of age. On a genetic pedigree a first-degree relative is one who relates directly to you without going through another person. A second-degree relative goes through one other person and a third-degree relative through two other persons. If your grandfather (a second-degree relative) or a great-uncle (a third-degree relative) died at 78 of a heart attack, this is much less important than your father or brother dying at 48. And if it's a second cousin who died at 48, that doesn't mean nearly as much as a father or brother dying that early. Another common problem in getting a family history is making sure that the individual who had the disease is actually a blood relative. If Uncle George had a coronary, but it was Aunt Mary who was your father's sister, then Uncle George's coronary has nothing to do with your family risk. He's not genetically related to you.

In obtaining your family history you're going to have to be discriminating and cautious. You will be assuming a role similar to that of a clinical geneticist or even a detective. You are told that an uncle died at 50 of a heart attack. But what was the evidence? You really need to ask how the diagnosis was made. A reputable medical diagnosis? Was he being treated for heart disease? In a hospital? If it was sudden death, was the diagnosis made by autopsy? If Uncle Joe really fell off a barstool and hit his head, you shouldn't make that the basis for getting uptight about heart attacks in your family. It should usually take only a few minutes to ask key questions to confirm the diagnosis.

## Genes and Environment

You're all familiar with the term *gene,* the basic unit of inheritance. Prior to Mendel and his garden peas, it was thought that inheritance was a relatively smooth blending of traits from both parents. Genetic predisposition to heart disease is probably, in most cases, a blending of the small effects of *many* different genes (polygenes) interacting with environmental triggers, such as smoking, diet, exercise, and stress. This is called *multifactorial inheritance.* But there is also the possibility that certain genes may have a large effect, and only one "bad gene" is enough to cause a lot of trouble. About 1 percent of Americans have one of these single genes of large effect—or about one in ten of the 10 percent of our population with high risk of early-onset coronary heart disease has a single-gene or Mendelian disorder. The single-gene disorders seem to have a tendency to be worse than the multifactorial inheritance problems. One particularly unfavorable single-gene problem causes heart attacks even in children. We'll discuss this in Chapter 11.

It follows that, if there are many genes of small effect and some single genes of large effect that produce cardiovascular disease, there are also likely to be some genes that have an effect between large and small. One family may get early-onset coronary heart disease on the basis of a single gene of large effect. Another family may have coronary heart disease due to the cumulative effect of 50 different genes. And a third family may have 3 or 4 genes, each contributing a considerable amount to the problem of coronary disease. From the research point of view, it's useful to try to distinguish these types, because different and specific preventive programs may be required for each family.

## Some Families

In this section we'll look at examples of families to give you more of an idea about how heart disease is transmitted and how we decide what type of inheritance is likely to be involved. We'll also go through a preliminary test—your first mid-term examination—to help you assess your personal and family risks. The final examination and grade come at the end of the book.

In the interest of confidentiality, I've modified a few features in the case histories so that the families will not be immediately identifiable to themselves or to others. But these histories are entirely representative of our families with heart disease. You may find similarities in your own family. And in fact that's the purpose of this exercise. At the end of this chapter you will not yet be required to follow the admonition of Tseng Tsu to extend your sphere of cultivation to your state and your world, but you will be introduced to some more of the forces at work outside your own family.

**Family A** ○ A 28-year-old woman, moderately overweight, came with her three children to see us. "You're the doctor who's doing the study on families with heart disease?" she began. "We've got a problem. My husband died a few weeks ago. Heart attack—29 years old. Perfect health. And he died."

I tried to think of something comforting to say—29-year-old men just don't die that often from heart attacks. "Your doctor told me you'd be coming" was all I could finally offer.

She went on, "His father died when he was 35. Heart attack. There's something wrong in the family. There's got to be. And I'm wondering about my kids."

"And your health?" I asked.

"I'm getting by about as well as you can expect." Her youngest child was in her lap. A 3-year-old girl. The other two children sat quietly. Much more subdued than most kids. Stunned might be a better word. "Doing as much as I can as father and mother."

"You don't have a heart problem?"

"No. Nobody on my side of the family has heart disease. We get cancer. It's the kids' hearts I'm worried about."

Mrs. A, like many lay people, had the concept that diseases run in families. Her husband's family gets heart disease. Her family gets cancer. This is frequently true. Some doubly unfortunate families may get both cancer and heart disease.

Now look at Figure 2–4, the genetic pedigree of Family A. This is a disastrous family history. Deaths in the twenties or thirties with heart attacks usually mean a single gene of large effect. The gene in this case adversely affects receptors on the membrane of the cells so that the machinery for manufacturing cholesterol is not turned off. Two of the children had the disease (cholesterols of 305 and 290), and with it, the

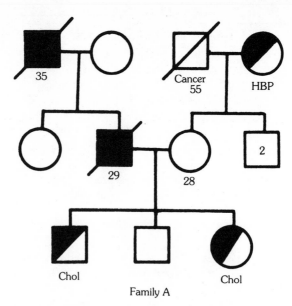

*Figure* **2–4**

Family A

prospects of dying in their twenties, thirties, or forties. But since this is a single gene problem, not a smooth blending, one child can look forward to a normal life, and will require no more than the prudent diet, exercise, and commitment to not smoking that any other low-risk person should have. But the children identified as being at high risk, because they have extremely high cholesterol levels, will require the utmost from present medical resources.

We've started off with the worst possible family situation. The only thing worse would be that some family member would have a double dose of the "bad gene." The probability of that occurring in the North American population is approximately one in one million. But we've had some of these patients, and we'll deal more with this in Chapters 5 and 12.

**Family B** ○  The proband was an attractive, slim young woman, 35 years old. Fashionably dressed. She belonged to a prepaid health plan that provided an annual physical examination and laboratory studies for its subscribers. Her cholesterol was found to be high. Her husband had sustained a nonfatal heart attack the previous year (when he was 44). The husband in this family (Figure 2–5) was thus in the high-risk category, but it was the question of risk in the wife that brought them to our attention. Because prevention is receiving increasing emphasis in prepaid health plans, the two children, aged 6 and 8, had cholesterol studies, which were also abnormally high. Mrs. B held a middle-management executive position in a major corporation in the area. She smoked two packs of cigarettes per day, was on the Pill, and thought of

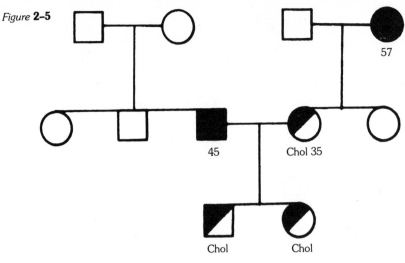

Family B

herself as a gourmet cook who could not consider the substitution of polyunsaturated margarine for real butter.

In this chapter we're interested in the family and the genetics of the disorder. We should also look at Mrs. B as a representative of the leading edge of an epidemic of heart attacks in the sex that is supposed to be spared them. The choice of this family has been made deliberately, to introduce an epidemiologic problem: heart attacks in women. But to be fair, it must be pointed out that heart attacks at early ages still occur much more often in men.

The two children, the mother, and the grandmother (who takes digitalis) all had cholesterol levels well above normal, but not as enormously elevated as was the situation in Family A. The father had a moderate increase in cholesterol and triglycerides and smoked two packs a day, even after his heart attack. We had some uncertainty as to whether this family had a single gene "receptor" defect, a problem caused by more than one gene of large effect, or a problem caused by many genes of small effect. But that's more of a research question. The clinical problem, the matter of interest to this family, is that they are at high risk and should take immediate steps to reduce the risk.

**Family C** ○   This family is more typical in that a man is the index case or proband, a 45-year-old man who was found to have abnormal blood lipids (high cholesterol), high triglycerides, and high beta and pre-beta lipoproteins. These blood abnormalities were found during an extensive screening program, which was offered at no cost to individuals who attended a meeting of a professional society of dentists.

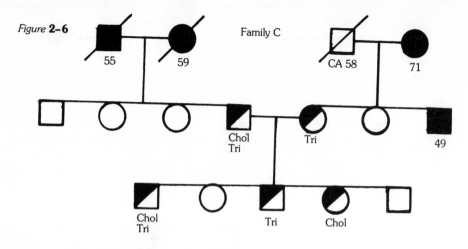

*Figure* **2-6**   Family C

After receiving the report of the abnormality, Dr. C. began thinking about heart attacks. He realized that in both his family and his wife's family there were individuals who had experienced heart attacks in their late forties and early fifties. Arrangements were made to study Dr. C, his wife, and their five children. The genetic pedigree is presented in Figure 2–6. As you can see, both the husband and wife had elevations of blood lipids. They were also moderately overweight. The parents of the husband had both died in their fifties of cardiovascular disease (the father with a heart attack and the mother with a stroke). All of the children had blood fat levels above average, and the three who were overweight had levels higher than we accept as normal. (See Tables 12–1 and 12–2.) There was no large difference between any of the family members in their levels of cholesterol and triglycerides, but those indicated in Figure 2–6 had values above our cut-off points.

Our initial impression was that this family had blood lipid problems that were most likely related to an imprudent diet superimposed on a hereditary predisposition, produced by the small effects of many genes. Families like this should respond well to diet and exercise. When a patient has high blood fat and is overweight, the first step is weight reduction. This takes care of the problem in the majority of cases. If there is high cholesterol in a slim person, this is a more serious matter and is likely to mean a major gene is involved. It also means that a more aggressive preventive program will be indicated.

**Other families** ○   We'll discuss these and other families as we go along. I just wanted you to get an idea about the sort of information you should be getting in your own family history. You should also start getting a feeling for how your family compares with the ones we've selected for discussion throughout this book.

This is an open-book, take-home exam, and you probably will not have all the answers you need today. You'll have to do some homework. For instance, you may not know what your cholesterol, triglycerides, and blood pressure determinations are. However, many of you who are in prepaid medical plans or who have had physical examinations may be able to take the entire examination right now.

The preliminary examination is based on information from a number of published epidemiologic studies, including our own continuing study. We've tried to develop formulas from our own data that will predict precisely an individual's risk. In Chapter 12, after you understand what the data base is, we'll actually have you determine a risk index or formula for you and your family (within the serious limitations of our present knowledge).

A risk formula from an earlier study looked at three major risk factors: high cholesterol ($> 250$ mg), high blood pressure ($> 160$ mm systolic), and smoking ($> 1$ pack/day). If you have one of these risk factors, the chance of having a heart attack is doubled; two factors more than triples the risk, and three risk factors produces a chance of heart attack that is ten times greater than if none of these factors was present.

Our risk index includes both your genetic and environmental risks and is derived from our study of nineteen independent risk factors. Turn your attention to Table 2–2. These are questions you should have answers for, in order to determine your risk or the risk of any other family member. Some of the information requested is standard in many epidemiologic studies. The genetic information and its correlation with epidemiologic findings to build a genetic-epidemiologic risk formula is from our own investigation.

Finally, I'm going to preview certain material that appears in Chapters 11 and 12. Children, in general, have lower levels of serum cholesterol and triglycerides than adults, so we have to shift the threshold of concern to a different point for them. Actually at birth, and for the first two to three months, blood lipids are low and not as predictive of later levels as they are by six months of age. So our current recommendation is to postpone the blood test in infants and children until they are between 1 and 2 years old. After that age, the sooner you find their levels the better for beginning their Whole Heart Program. The levels of presumed abnormality of cholesterol and triglycerides in children appear in Table 12–4.

# The Whole Heart
# Program and the
# Threshold

In Chapter 1, Figure 1–1, you were introduced to the set of distribution curves so dear to geneticists and epidemiologists. By now you may already be able to sense which hypothetical curve your heredity has placed you on—the high-risk or the lower-risk curve. So the time has come to add the concept of threshold. Note that we use the word hypothetical when discussing these curves. Distribution curves of this type are just a way of trying to conceptualize what may be happening in our population.

Let's look at Figure 2–7. Please observe that we've eliminated the "no risk" curve because we don't believe we can be confident about identifying these people. Also note that we've drawn a line through the right side of the curves. This is the threshold of cardiovascular disease. The curves themselves in Figure 2–7 may be taken to represent your heredity. The threshold line is the influence of the environment (diet, exercise, smoking, stress, and so on). On the left side of the threshold you're safe—no cardiovascular disease, no heart attacks. On the right side of the threshold is disease.

So if you don't want a heart attack, stroke, or other cardiovascular disease, what should you do? Change the curve of heredity? Sorry. It's too late for you to do anything about that for your own cardiovascular health. (However, increasing knowledge already indicates how you might influence the genetic load on the next generation.) But back to you. You can't change your own curve of heredity, but you can change your threshold. Move that threshold line as far to the right as you pos-

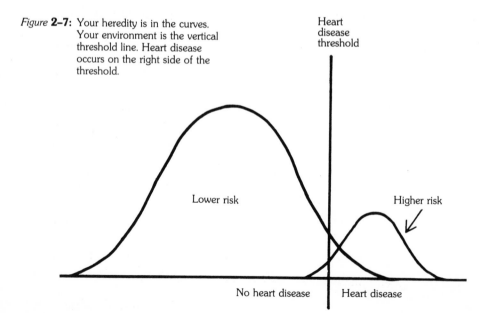

*Figure* **2–7:** Your heredity is in the curves. Your environment is the vertical threshold line. Heart disease occurs on the right side of the threshold.

Heart disease threshold

Lower risk

Higher risk

No heart disease

Heart disease

sibly can. That's what this book is about: helping you find out how to push that threshold to the right.

There is already epidemiologic evidence that the earlier you start to push the threshold to the right the further you can move it. One of the best-known epidemiologic studies into the cause of heart attacks involved the community of Framingham, Massachusetts. The evidence I'm referring to pertains to just one of the many factors you have some control over—the lowering of your cholesterol. The Framingham data revealed a better outcome if you start lowering cholesterol at age 35 than at 45, and also a better result if the cholesterol is lowered at 45 rather than 55. From this same analysis and studies in England and Finland came further evidence that the more deeply you lower your cholesterol—the harder you push on the threshold—the better the outcome. The incidence of heart attacks can be lowered by reducing cholesterol through diet or, in the most resistant cases, through medication. In fact, in a paper written after almost twenty years of operating the Framingham Study, two senior investigators concluded that atherosclerosis should be considered to be a pediatric disease. The most effective prevention should begin in childhood!

Figure 2–8 gives you an idea about what may be accomplished depending on how early you start your Whole Heart Program. For most of you, there is much to be gained, no matter at what age you start. But the greatest rewards are reserved for those who start the earliest. Clearly, an early start on a preventive program is even more important for

*Figure* **2–8:** The earlier you begin a program of cardiovascular health the better your chance to decrease your risk.

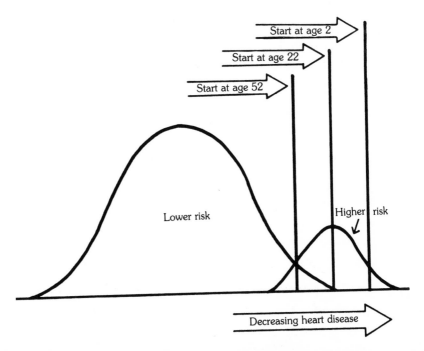

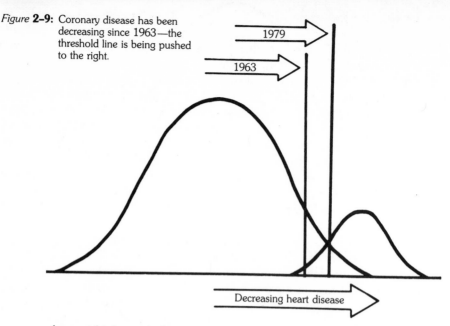

Figure **2-9:** Coronary disease has been decreasing since 1963—the threshold line is being pushed to the right.

1979

1963

Decreasing heart disease

those at higher risk than for those at lower risk. As you can see, by age 52, while even low-risk people may be becoming susceptible to heart disease, the majority of high-risk people are well on their way to serious consequences. One can hope that the more vigorous the preventive measures are, the more successful they may be at any age.

Now let's look at curves and thresholds in a slightly different way—from the point of a view of the population. The peak of deaths from coronary heart disease was reached in 1963—despite the fact that this epidemiologic secret didn't leak out until a couple of years ago. In Figure 2–9 the curves still represent heredity, but now they represent genes in the entire North American population, not just one individual or family. And what's happened? An aroused and concerned public has begun to push the threshold to the right by pursuing a healthier life-style. So for 1979, the threshold for our state—our part of the world—has been pushed a little. The same genes remain in the population, so the curves haven't changed. But the threshold is moving.

In the first chapter I indicated that there are many countries that don't suffer the high incidence rates of heart attacks that we do. Japan and Scandinavia are examples. However, move these Japanese and Scandinavians to the United States and watch their risks climb—watch the threshold *move to the left* as in Figure 2–10. But you now possess enough information to know that the threshold didn't have to move to the left. Our genes haven't changed. It's our environment that has. You also now know the threshold can be pushed back to the right.

And that's the subject of our final illustration for this chapter

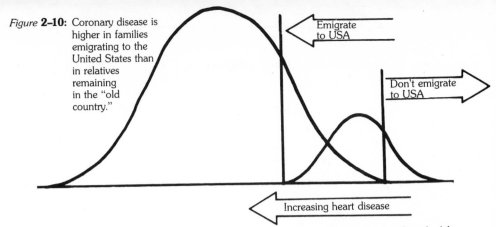

Figure **2-10:** Coronary disease is higher in families emigrating to the United States than in relatives remaining in the "old country."

Emigrate to USA

Don't emigrate to USA

Increasing heart disease

(Figure 2–11). You have the opportunity to push your own threshold. In most cases you can push it hard and far—although in some single gene disorders, your options may be more limited. The biomedical establishment, government, and the business community haven't helped in the past because they couldn't see what was in it for them. Your health and well-being were hardly sufficient motivation. Now the $206 billion medical bill is beginning to bug the bureaucrats. They're beginning to see that there might be something in prevention for them. And business is perceiving some light at the end of the tunnel. Why, personal health could become a whole new growth industry—with megabucks to be made! So business and government get little arrows on your side of the threshold. As I see it, that leaves the medical establishment as the major obstruction.

There's a challenge that might even appeal to Tseng Tsu.

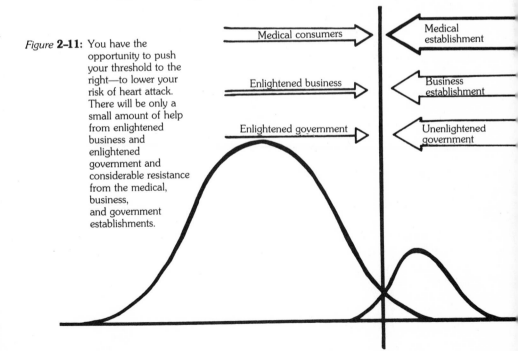

Figure **2-11:** You have the opportunity to push your threshold to the right—to lower your risk of heart attack. There will be only a small amount of help from enlightened business and enlightened government and considerable resistance from the medical, business, and government establishments.

Medical consumers

Medical establishment

Enlightened business

Business establishment

Enlightened government

Unenlightened government

TABLE
**2-1**

# Basic Measurements

| | | | | | | |
|---|---|---|---|---|---|---|
| Pulse rate | | | | | | |
| Height | | | | | | |
| Chest (bust) | | | | | | |
| Waist | | | | | | |
| Hips (women) | | | | | | |
| Weight | | | | | | |
| Pinch tests | | | | | | |
| Belly | | | | | | |
| Upper arm | | | | | | |
| Thigh | | | | | | |
| Chest | | | | | | |
| Love-handles | | | | | | |
| Aerobic exercise | | | | | | |

*This material is repeated for you to fill out in the Tear-Out Appendix.*

TABLE
2-2

# First Mid-Term Examination:
# Risk Factor Questionnaire

1   Has a first-degree relative (parent, sibling, child) had a heart attack or developed coronary heart disease before age 55?

2   Has a first-degree relative (parent, sibling, child) had a heart attack or developed coronary heart disease before age 65?

3   Has a second-degree relative (grandparent, uncle, aunt) had a heart attack or developed coronary heart disease before age 65?

4   Has a first-degree relative had a stroke before age 55?

5   Has a first-degree relative had a stroke before age 65?

6   Is your blood cholesterol greater than 270?

7   Is your blood cholesterol greater than 240?

8   Is your blood cholesterol greater than 220?

9   Is your level of triglycerides greater than 200?

10   Do you smoke more than half a pack of cigarettes per day?

11   Do you have diabetes?

12   Does a first-degree relative have diabetes that started before adulthood and requires the use of insulin?

13   Do you get regular aerobic exercise, sustain an exercise heart rate greater than 150 for at least 10 consecutive minutes, with no more than two days between exercise periods, and totaling a minimum of 60 minutes per week?

14   Is your blood pressure greater than 140/90 without treatment? (Note: either a systolic, upper reading, of 140 or a diastolic, lower reading, of 90 is sufficient.)

15   Is your relative weight greater than 1.20? That is, are you more than 20 percent overweight? (See page 47 for method of calculating relative weight.)

16   Do you get 14 or more points on the Type A behavior scale? (See page 148.)

*This material is repeated for you to fill out in the Tear-Out Appendix.*

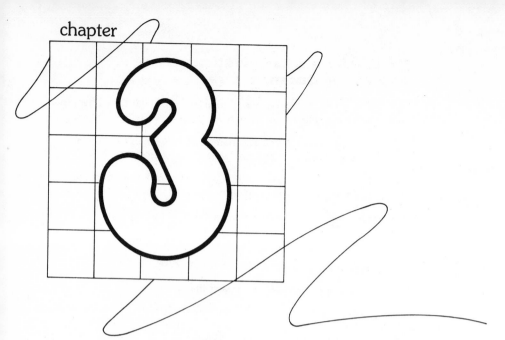

# This Week We've Got to Get Organized

A t this point you probably aren't sure whether or not you're on the 10 percent high-risk curve. By the time you've finished the book and have answered the required questions, you should be fairly confident about which curve is yours, and about how high your risk is on your own personal curve. If you're a high-risk candidate, you'll have to start thinking of your health as a top priority item. Your health program will require more intense involvement than will be demanded of your lower-risk friends. But what if your risk turns out to be relatively low? Then you'll have to be aware of and follow a sensible health maintenance program appropriate for your lower risk—and designed to keep that risk low.

Whatever your Whole Heart Program turns out to be, it will require an act of will, a commitment, and some basic knowledge of how to begin breaking bad habits and developing good habits. That's the gist of behavior modification. It starts with knowing who you are and what your habits are, and progresses a step at a time, identifying the habits that don't lead to good health, and replacing them with habits that do.

In the proverbial nutshell, that's it.

But you've been fighting the battle of the bulge all your life—and losing. And with Mark Twain, you've found smoking to be the easiest habit you've ever broken, because you've broken it so many times. Besides which, you've heard of Mickey Mouse behavior modification stuff that's not even supposed to require will power. You play this game: you reward yourself with happy activities and happy thoughts that reinforce behavior patterns you want to establish as "good habits."

But what about will power? I believe that those who claim that behavior modification does not require will power are guilty of a fundamental error. And it is this error that prevents many (or most) behavior modification programs from succeeding. It takes an act of will to start something that is not already a habit, and it takes inner controls to maintain a new habit. An act of will is where it begins. But common sense tells you that. You don't have to seek support from philosophers or psychologists for something that's just common sense. Yet there are those who might prefer some such support. So let's turn to Kierkegaard, who stated that life is a matter of Either/Or. He said that only through choice is authentic selfhood attained. There comes a time when you have to decide: Either/Or. And the decision is immediate—sudden. It occurs in an instant, and it can last a lifetime.

This is not to say that we should go around making instantaneous decisions, without thought or deliberation, when these decisions may have a profound effect on our lives. It's probably better to think of the decision in the context of the Zen idea of *satori* (or enlightenment). In one miraculous instant, the *seeker* acquires a new point of view on life. Note that I said the *seeker*. A new point of view just doesn't happen to someone passively. The seeking, at least for Buddhahood, may require many years—and then in an instant *satori* is attained.

Buddhahood is not a required goal for the reader of this brief account. Health is the goal. But the reader must be actively committed and seeking. And he or she should know that a decision, a commitment, must be made, and that commitment is best made in an instant. It is the establishment of the "new way" that may be gradual.

To move back from more exotic Eastern concepts to practical Western approaches, let's think of an experience described in the diary of William James. I have to confess to a long-standing admiration for

William James. As an undergraduate student majoring in psychology at Harvard, I took great satisfaction in knowing I was working where William James had worked, in a field in which he was a pioneer. But James, for all of his accomplishments, was not without his personal frailties and difficulties. His diary recorded that he had given some thought to suicide. This experience happened after he had obtained his M.D., and five years before he began teaching psychology at Harvard. He had reached a nadir of depression that he described: "Today I touched bottom and perceived plainly that I must face the choice with open eyes." Then he turned to Renouvier's definition of free will: "the sustaining of a thought because I choose to when I might have other thoughts." This concept served the function of a *koan* exercise in Zen. William James experienced a *satori* of sorts. He decided to accept the idea of free will and commitment. His first act of free will was to believe in free will. He was able to choose this behavior over that behavior. The new behaviors must surely have been learned gradually. But the decision to learn them came in an instant.

Another illustration from a recent giant in the history of ideas, Albert Camus. At the beginning of *The Rebel,* Camus says: *"jusque-là oui, au-delà non."* Up to this point yes, beyond it no. To play fast and loose with Camus's magnificent prose, but to be true to his concepts, he says there is just so much a human being should put up with. Then, to be a man, he must draw a line.

In many of our lives we've reached points where conditions have become intolerable. Things press in from all sides. Or, to borrow from Emerson: "Things are in the saddle and ride mankind." It's not just that being ridden by "things" is uncomfortable. It may also be a serious threat to your health. At some point you have to draw that line. Decide. Become committed. This comes in an instant.

The rest takes a little longer.

Well then, what about after the decision? Does that mean we're back to the rewards games? Let's think about it. Why do we do what we do? We don't stick our hands into fires. Why? Because it hurts, obviously. It's not a rewarding thing to do. In fact, it's a very punishing thing to do. So only a highly disturbed or intellectually deficient person would repeat such punishing behavior. But we open a refrigerator door and ladle out a dish of ice cream. Why? Because it tastes good to most of us. It's rewarding. Behavior gets established through rewards and punishments. We repeat what's rewarding and avoid what's punishing. This is going to be a major theme throughout the rest of this book.

Now the punishments don't have to be as hot as fire or the rewards as caloric as ice cream to help establish behavior. Words of praise or encouragement given first consistently, then sporadically, or just the association of previous rewarding experiences can maintain behavior. Having discussed William James and Zen and Camus, I must now acknowledge that my training in psychology was in a Harvard department more influenced by B. F. Skinner than William James. So I'm forced to take note of animal models of behavior. One with which most of us are familiar is the training of the family dog. At first to get a dog to come to you, you offer a rewarding dog biscuit, accompanied by words of praise. Then, only words of praise. And once the behavior is well established, the words are often omitted.

So let's face it, if we're talking about establishing behavior (or habits) in people, pigeons, or dogs, we're talking about rewards and punishments. And going through an emotional crisis because you're trying to use "will power" to break bad habits and establish good ones is not particularly productive. In fact, it's often counterproductive. You may end up thinking you have serious flaws in your character. That you're weak. Spineless. And altogether a disgrace to the American ideal and work ethic. That's really too bad, because that's not the problem. The problem is that you're just not understanding the simple psychological elements that underlie the establishment and modification of behavior in higher organisms.

We've already taken note that the punishment does not have to be fire, or the rewards ice cream or dog biscuits. Madison Avenue has also noted this. A pleasant memory or visual sensation or fantasy is quite effective. Stop and think of cigarette ads. Do they show a room or airplane filled with choking smoke? Do they portray the brown teeth and stained fingers? Is the smoker coughing uncontrollably with lung cancer or emphysema? Or clutching his chest while sustaining a heart attack? These images, especially the last ones, are really too much to expect of the tobacco industry. But do the tobacco ads even associate smoking with smoke? Think about it. They show a crystal mountain stream, preferably with a bubbling waterfall. Everywhere you look you find green leaves and a blue sky. And nowhere is there a suggestion of air pollution. It's a beautiful image—intended to associate the pleasant, tranquil experience (or fantasy) in the clean air with smoking. You see the ad and you want to take a deep breath of that pure, mountain air. But that's not what's being sold. Shades of 1984, doublethink, and Ignorance Is Strength! They've thrown you a curve that would be the envy of the entire pitching staff of the New York Yankees. They're selling you the visual image of clean air and giving you choking, killing smoke.

All of this is to say that if behavior modification, using only images, can work to establish destructive habits, then the rewards games (as transparent as they may be) can be employed with more than equal hope of success to establish constructive habits.

All right, we'll now assume that you've made a commitment to undertake a program of cardiovascular health, and that you have the general idea that you will have to take it a step at a time through simple behavioral techniques. Behavioral modification programs are initially quite successful for diet, smoking, and other habits. But then a curious thing happens. Having learned and established good habits, people turn around and relearn and reestablish the old habits that had offered considerable gratification in the past, which is why they became established in the first place. This is what is known in the trade as reversion. And it's disappointingly common. Where to now? Remember that in Chapter 1 it was stated that your program, to be successful, must become an integral part of your life. It must be incorporated into your frame of orientation. I suggested that your frame of orientation would be your road map and (to continue the metaphor) that the behavioral techniques would serve as signposts along the way.

I also suggested that you'll need all the help and support you can get from family and friends. A health program must be a family program to be successful. That isn't to say that you can't undertake your personal Whole Heart Program if you live alone. But if you live with others, you won't have an easy time of it if only some family members are involved and others are active or passive nonparticipants. If you're reasonably sated after supper, and an uncommitted family member offered you an eclair, it might be difficult to resist. Or if those responsible for the purchase and preparation of food for the family made all those junk-food and convenience-food delights constantly available, you'd have to have enormous, if not rigid, discipline to resist. The reason these foods sell so well is because they usually taste good. That takes us right back to habit formation: What's rewarding gets established. So, quite obviously, it's unwise to constantly confront temptation while trying to break those bad habits and establish good ones. A few saints may be successful, but you and I are not likely to qualify.

This brings us back to frame of orientation. Cardiovascular epidemiologists have been studying select populations in which a health program and life-style are very much a part of the religion itself. The Seventh-Day Adventists and Mormons are two such groups. And their morbidity and mortality statistics for cardiovascular and other major diseases are very much better than those of the American population at large.

Now I don't belong to either of these religious organizations, so I'm certainly not attempting to proselytize on their behalf. But I think they serve as a model for the success that can be achieved when a health program is incorporated into your frame of orientation—in these cases when health and life-style are part of your religion. Actually, there are threads of health programs woven throughout the history of many religions. Dietary abrogations are common, and in many cases have a valid medical basis, such as the prohibition of pork in Judaism and Islam. For decades, Fundamentalist and some mainstream Protestant churches frowned on smoking and alcohol. And most world religions have encouraged a simple, temperate, and abstemious orientation.

But such an orientation is in conflict with the demands of conspicuous consumption that fueled profligate economies for several decades. Then came the reaction of the sixties—"up to this point yes, beyond it no." People began to look inward again. All of a sudden, a segment of the population began to question the assumption that they had been put on this earth only to become bigger and better consumers. And the pendulum began to swing. Crazily at first, and banging against the sides of life-styles even more unhealthy than the one being rejected. Now, at the beginning of the eighties, the pendulum is establishing a new rhythm. An increasing number of Americans have made personal health and well-being a tenet of their life-style—a priority in their lives that has become part of their frame of orientation.

Make no mistake about this, you may make your own decision to institute changes in your life. And that decision will come in an instant—like the town drunk hitting the sawdust trail of conversion. But if the decision is to be sustained, it must have an enduring support structure—frame of orientation, belief system, religion. Call it what you will. Select the help that best meets your needs. Just be sure that the help is there.

One enduring prescription for help that I find relevant in this context is found in the Dharma. These are frequently called the Four Noble Truths of Buddha:

**1**  We must recognize that we suffer.

**2**  We must discover the cause of our suffering.

**3**  We must seek the way to overcome our suffering.

**4**  We may overcome our suffering by following a new way of life.

The first two principles correspond to case-finding and diagnosis: We must realize we suffer and find the cause. The last two principles represent treatment: We must actively seek to overcome our suffering and then follow a new way of life.

This may appear to be a curious place to start talking about meditation. A few years ago, if an M.D. had come out for meditation, it would almost have been grounds for hauling him before his county medical society for a reprimand. Be that as it may, in several of the chapters that follow we're going to rely on knowledge of the techniques of meditation. You can probably see how it would be relevant in the chapter on stress control, but it also comes up in the chapters on smoking, diet, and high blood pressure. I consider meditation to be as valuable an adjunct in general cardiovascular health as it is a technique in helping to achieve the inner control necessary for behavior modification. While meditation does not have the medical panache of an operation or injection, it does possess a long and respected tradition in the major religions of the world.

As a youngster I was told that prayer and meditation were essentials of the religious life. I knew what prayer was, but I wasn't sure about meditation. I guess I thought it had to do with thinking hard about something. I should probably note here that my own religious tradition is Christian (Protestant), because so much of our thinking about meditation is tied up with Eastern religions: Hinduism, Buddhism, and even Taoism. However, meditation also has a real place in the religions that started in the Middle East: Judaism, Christianity, and Islam. Within Christianity it was developed and nurtured by the Catholic mystics, such as St. Augustine, St. Teresa, Fray Francisco de Osuna, and Meister Eckhart. My own introduction to the technique of meditation occurred over 20 years ago from reading it all in a single sentence in Erich Fromm's *The Art of Loving.*

I know people attend courses (some fairly expensive) to learn how to meditate. You can also buy books (some of them best-sellers) devoted only to the subject of how to meditate. As far as I'm concerned, there has to be (and is) a fair amount of filler in such books, because I can't see how to improve on this one sentence in which Erich Fromm describes how to meditate: "It would be helpful to practice a few very simple exercises, as, for instance, to sit in a relaxed position (neither slouching, nor rigid), to close one's eyes, and to try to see a white screen in front of one's eyes, and to try to follow one's breathing; furthermore to try to have a sense of 'I,' I = myself, as the center of my powers, as the creator of my world."

That's it. That's the technique. I'll do a little amplifying, but the technique of meditation is all there, in one sentence.

The first bit of additional information concerns how long you should meditate. A standard recommendation is 20 minutes, but I would aim initially at 10 minutes. Next, when should you meditate? Most meditators would agree that it's good to meditate first thing in the morning on arising. There are those who meditate twice a day, while many choose to meditate only once daily. There's some difference of opinion on a second time to meditate. Some suggest bedtime, whereas others say meditation can be too stimulating at that time, and it will keep you awake. Therefore early evening is a suggested time.

I find all of that a little too formal. I think anyone who wishes to meditate can find the times that suit him or her best. I don't think that 20 minutes is either a minimum or a maximum for a single session, but I do believe that there is little to be gained by going beyond 20 minutes (and some potentially valuable work time to be lost). It is necessary from the point of view of habit formation to schedule your meditation for the same time or times each day. When subject to acute stress, you can employ a minute or so of meditative techniques at any time to help you through the episode.

The next point of technique has really already been described. As Fromm puts it, you may just sit in a relaxed position. A chair does nicely. If a lotus position were required, the majority of meditators over 30 would be out of luck. You can try modifications of cross-legged positions on the floor or in a chair, or you can just sit naturally in a chair.

Once you start trying to meditate you'll appreciate some of the requirements as well as some of the problems. One problem is having a quiet place. Most people need to be alone in a quiet room or, if outdoors, far enough away from people and noises to avoid distraction. The next problem is keeping competing thoughts out of your consciousness. The goals are to see a white screen (some see colors), to focus on the blank screen with your eyes closed, and to follow your breathing. No thoughts. Just relax and follow your breathing. If thoughts about your problems or plans for what you're going to do next enter your consciousness, you're not being very successful with your meditation. When competing thoughts enter, simply say, "No" or "Stop." Say it in your mind. Say it so forcefully that it seems that you're shouting "No" in your mind. During that moment of mind-clearing you can regain control to exclude thoughts and worries.

The *mantra* is a popular technique used in transcendental meditation, where you repeat a secret sound or word over and over again. While there may be some advantage to the secret sound, it's not clear to me how it is superior to using such words or phrases as "I = myself," or "Love," or "In" and "Out," while following your breathing. Some word or sound is useful to achieve mind control, but some people can meditate for long periods without focusing on any word or sound. The deeply vocalized sound "Ommmm" is preferred by many, but I've heard that one must be cautious in its use to avoid being abruptly transported to a remote timberline ledge in Nepal!

When you begin to practice meditation, it will be best to set aside no more than 10 minutes a session—and don't be discouraged. Your first 10 minutes may contain no more than 30 seconds of actual meditation. And if you extended your first session to an hour, you still may not have achieved more than 30 seconds of true meditation. But as you practice daily, you'll find that more and more of that 10 minutes passes in genuine meditation, not in mind-wandering and worrying. You'll be gaining progressively more control of your mind. And as you gain control of your mind, you may be able to gain greater control of every aspect of your life, your behavior, your attitudes, your reactions and responses to stress, and your ability to do what needs to be done—whether it's diet, exercise, elimination of smoking, or elimination of senseless striving and counterproductive worrying.

Now wait a minute! This appears to be getting out of hand! Sitting around for 10 to 20 minutes once or twice a day, trying to see a white screen, and trying not to think any thoughts—and like magic, you're a new person? You're controlled, confident, smarter, and a more competent human being? Don't knock it till you've tried it. But there are some people who just can't seem to get the hang of meditating. If you're one who needs some personal guidance in the technique, there are seminars and symposia offered. I can't vouch for the legitimacy or efficacy of any of them, but you should be able to inquire around until you reach an informed decision. The point I want to make is that you shouldn't conclude that meditation doesn't help if you haven't actually meditated regularly, but have only unsuccessfully tried to do it.

Because meditation is so central to the Whole Heart Program, I recommend strongly that you start as early as possible to develop this skill.

## The Game Plan

Please accept the suggestions that follow in this section as valid and valuable techniques in behavior modification methodology. You are asked to undertake your Whole Heart Program as a binding agreement. A sample contract is shown as Table 3–1 and is repeated in the Tear-Out Appendix. As is consistent with the way that habits are acquired—good ones or bad—we take it a step at a time. You're not being asked to sign a contract for the rest of your life, for a year, or even for a month. You're just being asked to sign it for a week at a time. It's preferable, even if you live alone, to have a cosigner, a helper. Why do

you think Weight Watchers and Alcoholics Anonymous have such success? Please note that if you're a smoker, your first duty has to do with
smoking cessation. It's really asking too much to expect anyone to give
up smoking and start dieting at the same time. After smoking has been
kicked, the standard Whole Heart Program contract may be activated.

A typical protocol to follow would be to renew and endorse the
contract weekly for four weeks, biweekly for another four weeks, and
then to monthly renewal. Beginning with the next New Year's Day the
endorsements could be annual. While the ultimate goal is a full lifetime
of good health, the manageable goals are distributed to be achieved a
step at a time. In the chapters that follow, you'll find schedules and
progress reports for the essential activities in your Whole Heart Program. These items are replicated in the Tear-Out Appendix. In addition,
you'll need a pocket notebook or note cards to record your activities
and dietary intake as they occur during the day.

Some people like schedules, while others find them abhorrent.
Perhaps it's already apparent that I'm one who likes them. And for this
program their use is required, as is the use of a journal. But these
things can be overdone. After graduation I looked back on my medical
school days and decided that if only I'd spent the time studying that I
spent making schedules for studying, I would have been further along.
Well, you don't have to make out the schedules, as I've done it for you.
All you have to do is fill in the blanks.

The investment is only a few minutes a day to take control of your
life and health. Eventually it will all be habit—just like swimming or
driving a car. You won't have to think about it. You'll just do it. Then
only the annual endorsements should be needed. The annual rededica-
tion and commitment.

But if you find you're slipping, go back to square one and restart
your weekly reviews. Obviously, the number of blanks I've supplied is
going to run out. When that happens, you'll have to decide whether
you feel the new habits are so entrenched that you no longer require a
record. Some will want to continue a calendar or journal of their own
design. Even a small pocket agenda can help you maintain the control
you may need.

# Three Miles, Three Sets, and a Coronary

Some people are hard to get going. And some are hard to control *once
they get going*. In a later chapter we'll review a little about a personality

type found in the coronary-prone individual. Once these people decide to do something, there's no stopping them. Everything they do, they do flat out. They work hard and play hard—and wear themselves out (and everyone around them). You know them. They haven't had a vacation in ten years, or had exercise any more strenuous than pushing an elevator button for the same period of time.

So they take that vacation. And the first day they play three sets of tennis with their teenage sons. Or if they decide to take up running, they go into it—for three miles the first time out. When I was in country practice and learning about the familial nature of heart disease, I also learned a lot about this type of person.

The small town in which I practiced was the trading center for a fine farming community, but because it was located on a beautiful Wisconsin lake not too far from Chicago, the town was a busy vacation resort as well. On only my second night in practice, I got a 2:00 A.M. call from the wife of a Chicago executive who'd played three sets of tennis on his first day of vacation.

He died on the way to the hospital.

If you think you'll have any problems dealing with the gradual, step-by-step approach to exercise advocated in the Whole Heart Program, work those problems through before starting—or don't take up the program at all. It must be the ultimate absurdity to undertake an exercise program to prolong your life and have it kill you.

TABLE
**3-1**

# Whole Heart Program

## STANDARD CONTRACT

### (Sample)

Because I'm concerned about my health, I hereby commit myself to participate in the Whole Heart Program as an act of free will.

1    My entire program is based first on the understanding that I am a mature person capable of making a decision to change my life-style to one that promotes good health. This new life-style is inner controlled and will become an integral part of my personal value system.

2    I will practice meditation for no less than 10 minutes a day, but preferably for 20 minutes once or twice daily.

3    If I have been a smoker, I have now abrogated the habit and will continue my resolve not to return to smoking.

4    If I require weight reduction, I will follow my systematic program, one step at a time, until I reach my ideal weight. I will then maintain my ideal weight.

5    As a second dietary commitment, I will follow a prudent diet or a more strict special diet, if indicated.

6    I will faithfully follow my personal exercise prescription (which in most cases will require at least 30 minutes a day, six days a week).

7    At bedtime each night I will review and record my progress and outline my program for the next day for as long a period as required (generally at least four months).

This contract is binding on the signatories for the period specified. It is the obligation of the signatories to help each other and assume responsibility for the success of the program for all participants.

The contract is considered binding and in force during the following dates:


*Dates* _____    _____    *Signatories*


*Dates* _____    _____    *Signatories*


*Dates* _____    _____    *Signatories*

*This material is repeated for you to fill out in the Tear-Out Appendix.*

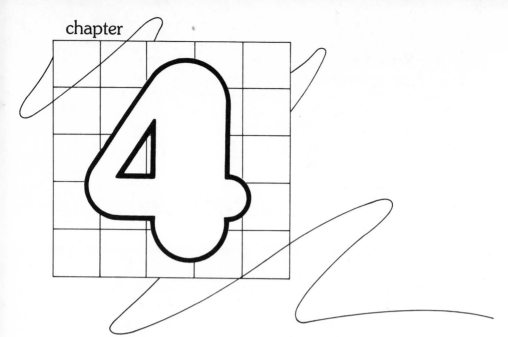

# Digging Your Grave with Your Teeth

The title is pretty strong language. And it's meant to be. This is a difficult problem and a difficult subject to write about. There are probably as many books on how to diet and lose weight as there are cookbooks. The market for both types of writing seems almost limitless. And there are also many books on low cholesterol, low fat cooking. If the answer to our dietary problems lay in writing and reading books on the subject, America would be populated only by slim, beautiful people with blood cholesterol levels of 150 or less.

But, of course, that's not the reality. The reality is that more than one in four Americans may, by a common definition, be classified as obese; and in one large epidemiologic study the *average* weight of men was found to be above the level where obesity was defined to begin.

Add to this the knowledge that the average weight of *all* Americans, men and women, comes out in about the middle of the range between overweight and obese, and you can see we have a long way to go. We'll give some frequently used definitions of obese and overweight a little later.

Being overweight is not the whole story on the American diet. The content of our diet is by the standards of good nutrition so unsound that a select committee of the U.S. Senate prepared a report voicing the opinion that our diet represented a critical public health concern. They published these findings under the title *Dietary Goals for the United States*, in 1977, and suggested significant changes in our eating habits.

This chapter and the one that follows are going to undertake the Herculean assignment of summarizing two topics, either of which could command a full book. The topics are weight reduction and maintenance diet for those at low risk and high risk of coronary heart disease.

# On Being Overweight

As you know without my emphasizing it, the market is glutted with books on how to lose weight. Many weight-conscious families (including my own) possess several such books, with hundreds of thousands to millions of words on the subject. Yet one well-known nutritionist believes that a weight reduction program can be summarized in nine words: "Eat half as much and exercise twice as much." I have no doubt that there are some people who need no more guidance than those nine words added to their strong personal commitment to lose weight.

This book will seek a middle ground and provide more than nine and less than hundreds of thousands of words on the subject of weight reduction. Before anyone undertakes a program to change his diet— which, after all, will change the way he lives—he should demand to know exactly how being at a desirable weight is better than being overweight. It would also be useful to know just what the definitions of "overweight" and "obese" are.

Second question first. One definition utilizes the information in Tables 4–1 and 4–2. You've probably seen this sort of table many times. Our tables are slightly modified from the Metropolitan Life Insurance presentation. These are called "desirable" weights for different heights and frame sizes in men and women. You will note that the weights are not "average" weights, because as we've already observed, our "average" may not be "desirable." Anyone who weighs 20 percent more than the desirable weight in this table is obese by one definition. And anyone who weights 10 to 20 percent more than desirable weight is termed overweight by this same standard.

Epidemiologic studies use these weight tables in calculating the risk of heart attack, and of course, insurance companies have found that an increase over desirable weight is associated with increased risk of death and disability from many causes. The greater the increase, the greater the risk. Now look up your weight for your height and frame size. Don't cheat on frame size. You know pretty well whether you're small, medium, or large. Please don't call yourself "large" if you can get your fingers around your wrist.

Say you're a man, 5 feet 10 inches, weighing 192 pounds, and can get your fingers around your wrist. This means you have a medium to small frame. We'd take your desirable weight *in indoor* clothing (*including shoes*) as 160 pounds. But you weigh 192. Divide 192 by 160 and you get 1.20—that is, you are .20 or 20 percent overweight. The figure 1.20 is called your relative weight. This qualifies you for obese. Let's do another problem. Say you're a woman, 5 feet 4 inches, small to medium frame, and weigh 138 pounds. A desirable weight for you would be about 125 pounds. Divide 138 by 125 and you get 1.10 (relative weight). You're 10 percent above your desirable weight, categorizing you as overweight, but not obese.

Now, wait a minute. Back in Chapter 2, we talked about a 5-foot 10-inch fullback who could weigh 210 pounds and not have a bit of fat on him by the "inch of pinch" test or by carefully measuring his skinfold thickness with calipers. Is the fullback obese? Well, not in the sense of having excess body fat. Giving him credit for a large frame and taking the top reading in that column we divide 210 by 179 and get a relative weight of 1.12. Our fullback is 12 percent over desirable weight. He falls in the 10–20 percent category called overweight, but not obese. If you use the stricter standard of a large risk factor study (The Pooling Project Research Group), the desirable weight for *any* man 5 feet 10 inches tall (height measured without shoes), but weighing in with about 5 pounds of indoor clothing (including shoes), is 157.5 pounds. Divide 210 by 157.5 and the relative weight is 1.33. Our fullback is obese by this standard to the level of being 33 percent overweight. By any standard our fullback seems to weigh too much.

What does all this mean? Does it mean you can actually be overweight, possibly dangerously overweight, without being fat? Yes, I guess it does. You see, the life insurance statistics and most epidemiologic studies just correlate desirable weight with height. Skinfold thickness doesn't usually enter the data. And being overweight from big muscles is perhaps not that much safer than being overweight from fat when it comes to risk from cardiovascular disease. In fact, a cardiovascular risk that has been well recognized by cardiologists for several decades is "body habitus" (what the layman might call "type of build")—the muscular male or mesomorph has been well appreciated to be at increased risk when compared with his slender, ectomorphic counterpart. There are, of course, many complex interactions in this whole problem, but what comes through is that "overweightness" (for whatever reason) is not as compatible with health and longevity as slimness is. As Paul Dudley White, the famed cardiologist at Harvard, was fond of saying: "A slim horse for a long race."

As I've been defining "overweight" I've been slipping in some arguments against being overweight. I'll add a few more here. Obesity and high blood pressure are associated, as are obesity and high triglycerides and high cholesterol. As for heart attacks, being overweight is a risk factor specifically for the younger patients, those in their forties, the ones with early-onset coronary heart disease. An estimate from the Framingham Study projected that for men 35 to 55 years old, a 10 percent reduction in weight could bring about a 20 percent reduction in the incidence of coronary disease.

Now I'm just going to throw out a few other observations about obesity in the United States that you may find interesting. As opposed to countries such as India, where the poor are too poor to have adequate caloric intake and are thus very thin, in the United States the poor usually get enough calories, but of the wrong kind. Often in order to obtain adequate protein they take in excess carbohydrate. While starchy foods contain protein, foods like milk and meats are richer (and more expensive) sources. Part of the problem is also simply a matter of education. Generally speaking, in America fatness correlates better with poverty, and slimness with affluence and higher education—especially among women. Lean women tend to "marry up" and fat women tend to "marry down."

Fatness is a family affair; the fatter the parents, the fatter the kids. Two fat parents make it even more likely that the kids will be fat than one fat parent does. Even biologically unrelated adopted children tend to take on the fatness of a fat family. It appears that living together and sharing undesirable dietary habits are much more likely to produce fatness than any hypothetical predisposition to being fat is. The bottom line on gaining or losing weight *for anybody* is the number of calories taken in compared with the number of calories used. It's that simple. *If you eat more calories than you burn up, you gain weight. If you burn up more calories than you eat, you lose weight.*

The conclusions are clear. If most familial fatness is related to living together and eating too much, familial slimness may be achieved by having the entire family committed to weight reduction and/or maintenance of desirable weight. It's a formidable chore for one member of a family to reduce without the commitment of all members of a family. However, even if you don't have the cooperation of the family, you yourself are ultimately responsible for what you do. When it gets to the crunch, there's no one to blame but you. And blaming someone else is just a cop-out.

As we'll point out again in the chapter for children, fatness begins early. Fat mothers have a tendency to produce fat newborn babies, and the babies tend to stay fat or get fatter during infancy. Fat babies become fat children, and fat children become fat adults. In fact, how fat you are between 10 years of age and 16 is most likely to persist until 60. About 9 to 10 percent of children under 6 years old are obese. These children are also more likely to come from lower socioeconomic levels. Mothers' attitudes toward obesity are central in this. Lean moms want lean kids, and fat moms readily accept their kids being fat. Lean mothers encourage exercise and fat mothers encourage food. Lean kids have a tendency to eat more frequently, leave food on the plate, and prefer skim or low fat milk. Fat children have high blood pressure more often than slim children, but through the simple expedient of slimming down, almost half of the kids who have high blood pressure and are at the same time fat can return to normal blood pressure levels.

# Food Facts You Need to Know

You should know that calories do count and that you've got to know how to count them. If you consume more calories than you burn up, you gain weight. Now, some of you may be able to eat half as much (cut your usual food portions in half) and exercise twice as much, and that's all you'll need to do to diet. But most of you will need to know basics of nutrition and be able to do some simple arithmetic. Nutrition tables generally give the contents of foods per 100 grams. Table A–1 in the Appendix will follow this convention. But you'll also be given the various constituents per ounce and per standard portion (since most of us aren't used to thinking in the metric system). The following conversions may also be helpful:

1 ounce = 30 grams (dry) or ml (wet)

1 cup = 8 ounces = 240 ml

1 teaspoon = 5 ml

1 tablespoon = 3 teaspoons or 15 ml

A gram of fat contains nine calories while there are only four calories in a gram of protein or a gram of carbohydrate. Table A–1 on pages 242 to 277 will give you the calories, protein, carbohydrate, fat (saturated and unsaturated), cholesterol, and sodium in common foods. This will be your more definitive nutrition guide to what's in the food you're most likely to eat. There will also be tables scattered throughout Chapters 4, 5, and 7 to call your attention to the calories, fat, cholesterol, or salt in specific foods. Table 4–3 gives a few of the most frequently eaten foods, and gives the calories and protein per usual portion—and the size of the usual portion is specified, a more handy length than Table A–1.

You would also benefit from having a dietetic scale. You'll be asked to measure and weigh things carefully, and some items don't measure easily in cups or tablespoons (dry spaghetti, for instance). But without a scale you can still make reasonable estimates. Dietetic scales cost from $2.00 up. (My family's cost $1.49 a couple of years ago.)

Since I've mentioned more than once the idea of "eating half as much," I feel I'd better qualify that before proceeding. Although most people need a more sophisticated program, the idea of simply eating half as much is sound in that the dieter stays with regular foods and avoids fad diets. If you've been reading your newspapers you've probably read about deaths attributed to various fad diets. Fad diets work for losing weight. There's no question about that. If you greatly restrict your food selection, the lack of variety will lead to a significant reduction in calories. Except you're not going to spend the rest of your life living on just goober peas and cabbage leaves. Or just hard-boiled eggs. Or just protein. Eventually you'll want to return to the land of the living and partake of palate-stimulating, balanced nutrition.

Table 4–4 gives nutritional requirements for adults and children. Where fad diets or overly zealous diets generally lead you astray is in the area of protein content, vitamins, and minerals. If you take to the idea of eating half as much, but you have only been used to getting the basic adult minimum of about 50 grams of protein per day and then you cut every food item in half, you'll begin to use up your own muscle in the weight loss. (Most Americans get much more protein than that— closer to 100 grams per day.) You'll have to be sure that in cutting your diet back, you don't allow your protein to fall below your minimum daily requirement.

But here's where some fad diets enter the picture. If protein has a minimum requirement, how about a diet that is exclusively protein? Or amino acids (the components of protein)? Or protein and fat alone? We can't adequately develop this topic in a short space, except to say that some of these approaches can be dangerous—and one, even fatal. Stay with balanced nutrition.

How about vitamin and mineral supplements while dieting? If your diet is very well balanced, a supplement will probably not be needed. However, if you're going to have to diet for a long period of time, a vitamin and mineral supplement would be reasonable to consider. I personally would use it. See Table 4–4 for vitamin and mineral requirements. You don't want to buy a supplement that contains excessive quantities of these nutrients—just get something with the minimum daily requirements, if you use a supplement at all.

Finally, you should know that the people who process and distribute food exert enormous influence over what you eat for the purpose of their greater profit. They put unwholesome products together and, through their advertising agencies, tell you how great they are. Resist this in the marketplace. Don't be manipulated. Read the labels. Be appalled! Perhaps you'll even want to become a food activist and pressure the distributors, the processors, and your legislators.

## Losing Weight

If you don't need to lose weight, feel free to skip ahead to the next chapter. The groundwork for the techniques of weight loss have been laid in the previous chapters. Let me repeat the elements:

**1**  A strong commitment.

**2**  Knowing your present dietary habits and dietary intake.

**3**  Acquiring the skills to change your dietary *habits and content* to produce weight loss.

**4**  Maintaining desirable weight through your newly acquired skills and habits.

**1 Commitment**  ○  We've already devoted considerable space to commitment. You make your decision, and make it an important part of your frame of orientation. You get all the help you can. You get a helper (the whole family can be the "helper"). Make a big deal of it, broadcast your intentions, and sign your contract. But the contract covers only short manageable periods. And within those periods you divide and conquer a day at a time. A meal at a time.

Post your weight-loss graph in a conspicuous place (see sample in Table 4–5). Draw your line for a loss of one or two pounds per week. *No more.* Then every week at the same time plot your weight on the graph. Your weight may bounce around a little, but the course should be constantly downward. And your achievement should be clearly visible to yourself and the rest of the family, because the graph should be prominently displayed (say, in the kitchen). Seeing the line go down will be rewarding and encouraging. Seeing the line plateau should be a spur to more intense efforts.

Then at the end of your diet, when your goal is achieved, you make another big deal of it. You reward yourself emotionally, and your helpers should provide considerable psychological reward. Many strokes and great praise.

And finally some very consequential material reward. Not splurging on a diet-busting indiscretion. (We so often celebrate with food and drink.) But with some new clothes for your new shape. Plan and save for it all during your diet. Keep that reward and goal in front of you every day. The new clothes should include a new bathing suit. And if at all possible financially, the reward should include a little vacation to a place where your new bathing suit and shape may be displayed. Your dieting may have actually produced enough of a saving from your usual food budget to pay for part of the vacation.

**2 Knowing your present dietary habits** ○ For three days before you start to diet, you need to keep a food diary in a pocket notebook or on 3-by-5 cards. Everything of food value that you put in your mouth should be recorded—including a careful measure of the quantity. A glass of milk? How many ounces? An 8-ounce glass or a 16-ounce glass? If the caloric count is immediately available on the package, record it on the spot. Then at night, at bedtime, you add it all up. Using Table A–1 on pages 242–277 in the Appendix and from whatever other sources you have, including the package information, you record calories, cholesterol, total fat, saturated and unsaturated fat, carbohydrate, protein, and sodium.

It sounds like a lot of work, but it's only for three days. And, after all, you're learning a whole new subject while you're doing it. You're learning about the nutritional content of the foods you've been consuming all your life. And you're learning what you eat and how much. Now, if you happen to eat unusual foods or mixtures of food, you may have to break them down into their basic constituents. The U.S. Department of Agriculture has an entire book devoted to the nutritional composition of various foods. For Table A–1 in the Appendix of this book, we've had to be selective. We couldn't give you a full book in the Appendix.

So your three-day food diary may have some informational holes in it, and may require some estimates based on the components of food mixtures. But what about when you're actually dieting? Then I would recommend that you *not* eat anything if you can't find its caloric content on the package or in Table A–1. Lately, you've probably noticed that the nutritional content of most processed foods is on the label. And the nutritional contents of as many fresh fruits, vegetables, meats, and processed foods as is practical to compile are supplied in Table A–1.

**3 Acquiring the skills** ○ Because the first week is the hardest, you should divide it into days and subdivide it into meals. And then you'll need to rededicate yourself at the beginning of every week, until your new habits are firmly established.

Your first decision in plotting your diet concerns how much you want to lose. Tables 4–6 and 4–7 give an appropriate schedule of caloric intake to lose 1 or 2 pounds per week, based on your starting weight. Let's start with our 192-pound man who needs to get down to 160. Does he want to achieve his goal in 32 weeks or 16 weeks? A lot depends on his personality. I think the "pound-a-weekers" are in the minority, so let's say our man wants to lose 2 pounds a week. From Table 4–6 we see that he needs to cut down to 2,100 calories per day. Does this represent cruel and unusual punishment? Look at Table 4–7 for women. A woman of 120 pounds takes only 1,800 calories to keep her weight at 120 pounds. So our dieting 192-pound, slightly chubby man still gets to eat considerably more than a 120-pound woman who isn't even dieting.

Six weeks later our man, who has been completely faithful to his 2,100-calorie diet, hasn't quite lost 12 pounds. Perhaps 10 to 11 pounds. Why? Because he now weighs about 180 pounds, and he needs fewer calories to maintain this weight. He needs to reduce his calories to 1,950 to continue losing 2 pounds per week. Check Table 4–6.

Please don't get hung up on the exact numbers. We have different metabolisms and people of the same weight may lose a little faster or a little slower at the very same caloric intake. These are approximations, and you'll have to play around with your own caloric requirements and make slight adjustments to fit your needs.

Five weeks later our man is now a more svelte 170-pounder, because he's been reducing his calories to the requirements of his declining weight. He's now taking 1,800 calories, and his appetite center has become accustomed to this intake. At this point our man may make a decision. He might want to go all the way down in the next five weeks, or he might want to wean himself back toward a maintenance caloric intake by increasing the calories to 2,300, with the goal of losing only 1 pound per week until 160 pounds is reached.

You can also see that if our man had stayed at 2,100 calories, the velocity of his weight loss would have been decreasing and he would now be at about 175. This weight loss strategy is completely satisfactory, as long as you appreciate what's happening. Some dieters experience a good initial weight loss and then find that each subsequent pound becomes harder to lose. So they get discouraged because they don't understand that as they lose weight they have to consume fewer calories in order to maintain their new weight.

The next point to make under skills is the one we've been talking about in previous chapters. Changing habits. If you focus only on the content of your diet—as many diet books do—you're doomed to failure. The two components of dieting, *habit* and *content*, must receive equal attention.

When you start the diet, you've made your commitment. You've got your pocket notebook and calorie counters, Tables 4–3 and A–1. You've kept your three-day food diary, so you know what you've been consuming in calories, cholesterol, and other constituents. D-Day (D for diet) is here. A Sunday or Monday is a good day to start, but any day of the week is suitable. You sign your contract with your cosigner(s), and with much fanfare you begin.

For the duration of your first contract (and for as many subsequent contracts as are necessary for you to know what you're eating), you should record in your pocket notebook (or on 3-by-5 cards) a running tally of foods. Before you put a bite into your mouth, record what you plan to eat. Know the quantity and content exactly. And take no more than the amount specified. Record all calories and protein that you consume.

An orange or 4 ounces of orange juice is 50 calories and about 1 gram of protein. Bread, depending on the type and brand, may have 60 to 75 calories and 2 grams of protein in a slice. You'll want to spread a teaspoon of polyunsaturated margarine on it—30 calories, no protein. Breakfast cereals tell you on the box what a one-ounce serving contains (usually 70 to 110 calories for unsugared cereals, and 3 to 4 grams of protein). A cup of oatmeal is 150 calories and about 5 grams of protein. Let's say you select an ounce of Cheerios—that gives you 110 calories and 4 grams of protein. A cup of skim milk (8 ounces) provides 80 calories and 8 grams of protein. Let's add it up (see list on following page):

|  | Calories | Protein (g) |
|---|---|---|
| orange juice | 50 | 1.0 |
| toast | 60 | 2.0 |
| margarine | 30 | — |
| Cheerios | 110 | 4.0 |
| skim milk | 80 | 8.0 |
| coffee or tea (without sugar or milk) | 0 | 0 |
|  | 330 | 15.0 |

That actually turns out to be quite a substantial and nutritious breakfast. You'll note that you'll not be asked to record the amount of fat or cholesterol in the food you eat while you're trying to lose weight. Your weight reduction diet will be low in fat and low in cholesterol according to the guidelines of what may be called a prudent diet and the recommendations of the U.S. Senate Select Committee on Dietary Goals.

We'll discuss this prudent diet in the next chapter. If it turns out you need to be on a maintenance diet even more restrictive than a prudent diet, then you'll have to record fat and cholesterol intake. But not at this stage. Not while you're just trying to lose weight. That chore alone requires your full attention.

Now for specific skills. You've been given the approach to behavior modification.

Here we'll catalog some of the knowledge, skills, and gimmicks used in dietary behavior modification programs.

1. Recording what you eat in advance makes you aware of your eating habits and also keeps you within the caloric restrictions of your diet. The pen and notebook must be at hand at all times. Follow the form used in Table 4–8. You see a goodie? Reach for your pen before you reach for your goodie. You don't know the caloric content of the goodie? Then don't eat it! It's that simple. You can't carry an oversized book on the composition of foods with you everywhere you go. So if you don't know what's in it, forget it—or be very sure you can make a close estimate. Your running tally of calories lets you know when you're reaching the end of your allotment. And the protein tally and exercise make certain that you don't get into a muscle-wasting problem. If you reach the end of the day with calories to spare, but not enough protein, make up for it with skim milk, plain yogurt, or uncreamed low fat cottage cheese.

2. How you eat turns out to be quite important. Apparently it takes about 20 minutes for the message that you've eaten something to get from your stomach to the appetite center in your brain. So a smaller amount of

food eaten slowly, taking 20 minutes to consume, will turn down your appetite almost as effectively as eating two or three times as many calories in half the time. Remember, take at least 20 minutes before you decide that what you're eating hasn't filled you up. Other gimmicks for eating slowly include sipping a full glass of water before starting on the food, putting the silverware (or sandwich or whatever) down after each bite, chewing each bite 15 times, and swallowing before raising food to your mouth again. Overweight people tend to devour their food rapidly. Slim people tend to pick at their food.

3. Don't allow yourself to get too hungry by skipping meals or having too small a lunch. You've got X number of calories, and you divide them any way you want in order to keep your appetite and nutritional needs satisfied. Many diet programs call for six small meals a day. Skinny people tend to nibble a lot and not eat much at a single sitting. *If you've had an ulcer, you should divide your food into six or more small feedings or you'll risk aggravating your condition.* It's certainly self-defeating to have to interrupt your diet to cure an ulcer that's recurred. You'd likely gain five to ten pounds on an ulcer diet regimen. My own approach to dieting for myself and my patients has been to advocate three small meals and three very low-cal snacks, including one at bedtime. I suggest taking low-cal snacks to work with you, so that when the hunger pangs start you don't follow the path of least resistance to the candy machine or doughnut tray. Skim milk, plain yogurt, and carrot sticks cool the hunger, provide good nutrition, and don't cost many calories.

4. Be a smart shopper. You'll eat what's available. So if you have lots of junk food around, you'll eat it. When you or your spouse shops, don't buy the convenience junk foods, the high sugar, high salt, high fat, high cholesterol stuff. Buy fresh fruits and vegetables, whole grains, lean meats, fish, and poultry. If what you buy comes in a package ready to mix or cook directly, beware. Prepared and processed foods have all sorts of additives, caloric and otherwise. But the nutritional values are usually printed on the package or can. They're listed in order according to the relative quantities of the ingredients. Whatever is listed first is the main ingredient. So a breakfast cereal that starts off with sugar (or sucrose) is more sugar than anything else.

If the high caloric stuff isn't in your refrigerator or cupboard when you open the doors, you won't be able to eat it. Your automatic reflex when you enter the kitchen may be to open the refrigerator. But instead of a pie or cold cuts or pop or cheese, have oranges, carrots, unsweetened iced tea, club soda, skim milk, low fat cottage cheese, and yogurt. In the cupboard replace the cookies, potato chips, and snack crackers with spoon-sized shredded wheat and other unsugared cereals. And you might try some dry-roasted, unsalted soybeans. If these specific food items don't appeal to you, find things that do—as long as what you select is nutritious, low calorie, and is clearly not high calorie, high salt, high fat, or high cholesterol.

**5.** Keep foods out of sight. First you should make it a rule that foods be kept only in the kitchen and that eating take place only in the kitchen or dining room, while sitting down and doing nothing else. No parking in front of the TV set with a bowl of empty calories. Your full attention must be devoted to eating and nothing else. Through meditation and through the practice of being fully concentrated on what you're doing, you'll become aware of when you're eating. It's amazing how many calories can be consumed while you're ostensibly doing something else. So the rule is when you eat you do nothing else.

Then what about parties, including those infamous cocktail parties, that are designed for doing two or more things at once? Hang on to a glass of club soda. Drink it slowly, nurse it, but that should be your only dietary crutch during conversation. Eat your allotment of low calorie snacks before going to the party, position yourself as far from the hors d'oeuvres as possible, and don't touch the food. Cling to that glass of club soda as a drowning man clings to a life preserver.

Back to keeping foods out of sight. Even after you've consigned food storage to the kitchen alone, you have to keep them out of sight within the kitchen. But since man does not live by carrots and club soda alone, you'll still have to store more tempting foods in the refrigerator and cupboards. Store them in the back. Keep them covered. Make it difficult to reach these foods. And keep the low-cal items at the front where they are most accessible.

**6.** Serving meals. While you're trying to lose weight, family style eating has to go. The exact portions you're entitled to should be carefully measured, put on the plate, and eaten. No serving bowls visible. No opportunity for seconds.

**7.** Your dietary allowance. Table 4–9 offers a basic dietary plan that provides balanced nutrition for any healthy person. And it does it in only about 1,200 calories, while providing even more protein than needed. Its only deficiency is in calories. The point is that anything you add to this basic diet will provide more food energy (calories) or, if excessive, deposit fat. It certainly won't fill you up if you're an adult used to 3,000 calories, and it would produce too rapid a weight loss for someone with that maintenance requirement. It's also as low a caloric intake as I generally recommend for adults. Most weight loss diets will permit more calories. The first food groups to add calories from would be the low calorie vegetables and skim milk. Table 4–8 appears in this chapter, and a copy is included in the Tear-Out Appendix. Just fill in the blanks so that it all adds up to the number of calories you need to eat in order to lose one or two pounds per week. If your diet calls for 1,800 calories, as in Table 4–10's sample plan, you can eat close to twice as much of the fruits, vegetables, breads, milk, fats, and oils as allowed by the basic plan of Table 4–9. However, there's no need to eat more from the meat group, which is high in cholesterol, saturated fats, and calories.

In addition to a weight reduction blank (Table 4–11), you'll find a maintenance diet blank (Table 4–12) in the Tear-Out Appendix. This is to allow you to make up new diets in accordance with changing needs, and you can make additional copies for yourself.

**8.** Feeding frustrations. Much overeating is in response to tension and anxiety. Some of us unconsciously reach for food when tense. But the circle is broken by having to pull out a pen and notebook. At least you have been made conscious of your behavior. If you can afford a few calories, take them—carrots, skim milk. Having pulled out your pen, you're still hungry and you can't afford to tally any more calories? Then take a glass of no-calorie beverage and leave the location of food. Curiously, many people actually confuse the sensations of hunger and thirst. They eat something when a glass of water or tea is really what they want. Still hungry? Try two minutes of meditation. A few warm-up exercises. Go for a walk and reward yourself mentally for your successful resistance to the temptation by conjuring up a happy scene (a beach, a mountain stream) or a happy memory. Better yet, visualize yourself at the end of your successful diet, slim and healthy. Keep that picture of the new, slim you always in mind. Associate your resistance with happy thought-rewards. But if these thoughts occasionally fail you, leave the thought-carrot and go for the thought-stick. Visualize yourself in the morgue—the victim of a sudden heart attack. Make it gory. See the family there identifying your remains. Think of the bind you've left them in. I don't advocate the thought-stick as often as the thought-carrot. But sometimes it's just what's needed.

**9.** Miscellaneous problems. Restaurants represent a major problem for those trying to lose weight and for those trying to watch cholesterol. If you're traveling away from home, eat early (to avoid getting too hungry) and select a restaurant where you can get something light. Order broiled fish, vegetables, and a salad without the usual high calorie salad dressing. You may even want to pack your own low calorie salad dressing or see if they have a diet dressing. Ask them to allow you to add the teaspoon of margarine to your baked potato. Fruit for dessert. If you can't eat early, have a low calorie snack before you go to the restaurant, and be sure the basket of rolls is kept on the other side of the table. Let your dining companions know you're dieting, but don't be aggressive about it. (Some dieters seem to get positively hostile.)

If going to a dinner party, have your concealed diet list with you, and select items on your dinner allotment. Perhaps phoning ahead to your hostess to explain your dietary resolve and to enlist her help will ease the discomfort. Don't arrive hungry. A low calorie snack before leaving will be helpful.

For those who prepare the meals and clean up afterwards, there are special problems. These problems are best handled by having helpers with you during these periods. It's entirely reasonable that the tasks of cooking and cleaning be shared. You don't have to announce that you want someone to keep you from snacking, but it should be mutually understood that only a designated caloric snack is permitted during meal preparation. A glass of tomato juice or skim milk may be nursed throughout this period or taken before the cooking begins. No-calorie beverages may be the focus of your follow-up oral gratification. A cup of tea, a club soda with plenty of ice cubes. Keep your mouth and hands busy with these items and away from sampling what you're cooking.

The cleanup may require even more control. If you have a real problem in this area, don't mess around with saving leftovers until you gain control. Dump the table scraps immediately into the food that hasn't been served, and dump that promptly into the garbage.

**10.** Putting it together. Your plan is to space your allotted calories over six feedings: three meals and three snacks. Designate the times for all six feedings in advance. Don't miss a meal and don't be late with a meal if at all possible. Don't miss the mid-morning or mid-afternoon snack either. Set the times for them, and try to stay on schedule. Say 10:00 A.M. and 3:00 P.M. Always take a bedtime snack so you don't wake up hungry in the middle of the night. Refer to the diet sheet that you filled out to meet your personal needs. If 1,800 calories is what you need, I've supplied you with Table 4–10, which is one way to divide your calories. But you know what suits you best. Divide your food in such a way that your own needs are optimally met.

Reread this section, "Losing Weight," a couple of times, including the morning you start your diet. Read it at bedtime every night for the first week. Be sure your weight loss graph and diet are prominently posted. Be sure your clothing and vacation rewards are planned. Talk about them often—especially at suppertime.

As you resist your old dietary habits and replace them with new ones, as you turn down the high-cal goodie, reward yourself in your mind. Keep seeing yourself at the end of your diet, slim and healthy, running along a beach.

When you have lost the amount of weight you proposed to lose, do your inch-of-pinch test. While you've been dieting, you've also been exercising according to recommendations in the chapters that follow. You should have good tone, good muscle mass, and no excess fat. If you don't pass the inch of pinch, you'd better reevaluate your exercise program and work at it more faithfully. And while doing that, you'd better lose until you can't find a pinch of excess fat.

When that goal is achieved, reward yourself with your new clothes. If you can't take the little vacation at that particular time, give yourself a rain check and keep looking forward to it. If you have been planning a vacation anyway, make your taking the vacation contingent on reaching your goal of weight loss. Let the whole family get on your back for holding up vacation plans.

**4 Maintaining desirable weight** ○ Finally, carefully go on what will be your maintenance diet. A blank is supplied in the Tear-Out Appendix (Table 4–12).

If you can get your spouse and family reoriented to a prudent diet that becomes incorporated into the family life-style, you've leaped the major hurdle. If you can't get your spouse to cooperate, it may not necessarily mean that he or she is out to do you harm, but it should indicate a need for serious negotiation.

Parties may be a trap. You can't expect your host and hostess to prepare a special meal or special drinks for you alone. So you'll have to develop a new habit pattern for these situations. Hard as it is, you've got to resist. Some do it unobtrusively, which is the really hard way. Others announce on entry that they're on a diet and must decline certain items. That's easier, although a trifle boorish. Follow whatever approach you find works for you.

Eating out may be a significant problem. Even low fat, low cholesterol items are often greased and sauced to an undesirable state. (Have you had fish and chips at a franchise lately?) Stick with broiled fish if you're at high risk. If you're at low risk, are no longer overweight, and are not required to eat out many times a week, then enjoy the delicious indiscretions that go with dining in restaurants.

There's good news and bad news as regards alcohol. Moderate drinking appears to be associated with slightly increased life expectancy over total abstinence, probably because it increases the "good" HDL cholesterol. Heavy drinking, of course, is associated with a greatly *decreased* life expectancy. I would say if you're at low risk, a cocktail, a beer, or a glass of wine in the evening is not a bad idea for those who don't find alcohol objectionable on some other grounds and don't have a familial problem with alcoholism. For those at high risk with high cholesterol, a similar alcohol intake may be recommended by your physician. The idea of a *little* alcohol "for medicinal purposes" is coming back.

Let's take an example of a maintenance diet. Our 160-pound man (former 192-pound chub) will feel almost stuffed on 2,700 calories. He may be a high-risk patient who will always need to be very strict about cholesterol, fats, and salt. He may be low-risk and just need to be on the prudent diet that is described in the next chapter. Whatever his next step is, he *must always be aware of what he consumes.* For the rest of his life, he must maintain awareness. He may think of himself as a recovered foodaholic, just as members of Alcoholics Anonymous introduce themselves as recovered alcoholics.

So for the first three days on the new 2,700-calorie maintenance diet, our new slim 160-pounder should record his dietary intake faithfully, just as he did before starting his diet. He should become familiar with the calories, cholesterol, fat (saturated and unsaturated), protein, and sodium of his new diet. He should weigh himself at least weekly—and do a one-day food diary and reread this chapter the first of every month for the next three months.

If there is any weight gain, he should immediately switch to his pound-a-week weight loss diet (2,200 calories for a man of 160 pounds). After several months to a year or two, the new behavior is established. It may have to be defended occasionally or frequently. You may have to read this material, do a one-day food diary, and switch to your pound-a-week diet a couple of times a year—or every few years. But you have the tools. There are diet dropouts (not as many as smoking-cessation dropouts), but you're not going to be one of them. Because your diet and health have become incorporated into your lifestyle—your frame of orientation.

Look at that slim, healthy, and incredibly attractive person running along the beach. That's you!

TABLE
**4-1**

## Desirable Weights for MEN
## Age 25 and Over

*Weight in pounds according to frame (in indoor clothing).*

| Height (in bare feet) | Small Frame (pounds) | Medium Frame (pounds) | Large Frame (pounds) |
|---|---|---|---|
| 5'1" | 112–120 | 118–129 | 126–141 |
| 5'2" | 115–123 | 121–133 | 129–144 |
| 5'3" | 118–126 | 124–136 | 132–148 |
| 5'4" | 121–129 | 127–139 | 135–152 |
| 5'5" | 124–133 | 130–143 | 138–156 |
| 5'6" | 128–137 | 134–147 | 142–161 |
| 5'7" | 132–141 | 138–152 | 147–166 |
| 5'8" | 136–145 | 142–156 | 151–170 |
| 5'9" | 140–150 | 146–160 | 155–174 |
| 5'10" | 144–154 | 150–165 | 159–179 |
| 5'11" | 148–158 | 154–170 | 164–184 |
| 6'0" | 152–162 | 158–175 | 168–189 |
| 6'1" | 156–167 | 162–180 | 173–194 |
| 6'2" | 160–171 | 167–185 | 178–199 |
| 6'3" | 164–175 | 172–190 | 183–204 |
| 6'4" | 168–179 | 177–195 | 188–209 |
| 6'5" | 172–183 | 182–200 | 193–214 |
| 6'6" | 176–187 | 187–205 | 198–219 |

TABLE
**4-2**

# Desirable Weights for WOMEN
# Age 25 and Over

*Weight in pounds according to frame (in indoor clothing).*
*For girls between 18 and 25, subtract 1 pound for each*
*year under 25.*

| Height (in bare feet) | Small Frame (pounds) | Medium Frame (pounds) | Large Frame (pounds) |
|:---:|:---:|:---:|:---:|
| 4'8" | 92–98 | 96–107 | 104–119 |
| 4'9" | 94–101 | 98–110 | 106–122 |
| 4'10" | 96–104 | 101–113 | 109–125 |
| 4'11" | 99–107 | 104–116 | 112–128 |
| 5'0" | 102–110 | 107–119 | 115–131 |
| 5'1" | 105–113 | 110–122 | 118–134 |
| 5'2" | 108–116 | 113–126 | 121–138 |
| 5'3" | 111–119 | 116–130 | 125–142 |
| 5'4" | 114–123 | 120–135 | 129–146 |
| 5'5" | 118–127 | 124–139 | 133–150 |
| 5'6" | 122–132 | 128–143 | 137–154 |
| 5'7" | 126–135 | 132–147 | 141–158 |
| 5'8" | 130–140 | 136–151 | 145–163 |
| 5'9" | 134–144 | 140–155 | 149–168 |
| 5'10" | 138–148 | 144–159 | 153–173 |
| 5'11" | 142–152 | 148–163 | 157–178 |
| 6'0" | 144–156 | 152–167 | 161–183 |
| 6'1" | 148–160 | 156–171 | 165–188 |
| 6'2" | 152–164 | 160–175 | 169–193 |

TABLE
**4-3**

# Quick Reference Calorie Counter

| | Quantity | | Calories* | Protein* (grams) |
|---|---|---|---|---|

## Beverages

| | Quantity | | Calories* | Protein* (grams) |
|---|---|---|---|---|
| Alcoholic | | | | |
| Beer, 4.5% alcohol | 12 | oz. | 150 | 1.2 |
| Beer, low carbohydrate | 12 | oz. | 70–100 | — |
| Gin, rum, vodka, whiskey | $1\frac{1}{2}$ | oz. | 100 | — |
| Mixed drinks | | | | |
| Daiquiri | $3\frac{1}{2}$ | oz. | 200 | — |
| Gin gimlet | $3\frac{1}{2}$ | oz. | 150 | — |
| Martini, dry | $3\frac{1}{2}$ | oz. | 150 | — |
| Screwdriver | 8 | oz. | 288 | — |
| Wine, sweet, 18% alcohol | $3\frac{1}{2}$ | oz. | 140 | .1 |
| Wine, dry, 12% alcohol | $3\frac{1}{2}$ | oz. | 85 | .1 |
| Nonalcoholic | | | | |
| Cola type soda | 12 | oz. | 144 | — |
| Fruit type soda | 12 | oz. | 184 | — |
| Ginger ale | 12 | oz. | 108 | — |
| Root beer | 12 | oz. | 156 | — |
| Diet soda | 12 | oz. | 1 | — |
| Noncarbonated | | | | |
| Coffee, black | 1 | cup | 0 | — |
| Coffee, milk & sugar | 1 | cup | 35 | — |
| Kool-Aid with sugar | 9 | oz. | 91 | — |
| Tea, plain | 1 | cup | 0 | — |
| Tea, sugar 1 tsp. | 1 | cup | 20 | — |

## Breads, Cereal, Grains, Pasta

| | Quantity | | Calories* | Protein* (grams) |
|---|---|---|---|---|
| Breads | | | | |
| Biscuit, baking powder | 1 | 2 in. | 104 | 2.1 |
| Cracked wheat bread | 1 | slice | 66 | 2.2 |
| French roll (hoagie) | $11\frac{1}{2} \times 3$ in. | | 392 | 12.3 |
| Hamburger bun | 1 | med. | 125 | 3.3 |
| Hard roll (Kaiser) | 1 | roll | 156 | 4.9 |
| Italian bread | 1 | slice | 80 | 2.7 |
| Muffins, blueberry | 1 | muffin | 112 | 2.9 |
| Pancakes | 1 | 4 in. | 64 | 2.0 |
| Rye, white, whole wheat | 1 | slice | 60 | 2.2 |
| Cereal, grains, pasta | | | | |
| Bran flakes (40%) | 1 | cup | 100 | 2.9 |
| Corn grits (cooked) | 1 | cup | 120 | 2.5 |

| | Quantity | | Calories* | Protein* (grams) |
|---|---|---|---|---|
| Corn flakes | 1 | cup | 110 | 2.2 |
| Farina (cooked) | 1 | cup | 100 | 2.5 |
| Macaroni, spaghetti, cooked | 1 | cup | 192 | 6.4 |
| Noodles, egg, cooked | 1 | cup | 200 | 6.1 |
| Noodles, chow mein | 1 | cup | 224 | 6.1 |
| Oatmeal, cooked | 1 | cup | 132 | 4.3 |
| Rice, white, cooked | 1 | cup | 223 | 4.1 |
| Rice cereal, puffed | 1 | cup | 60 | .9 |
| Shredded wheat, crumbled | 1 | cup | 124 | 3.5 |

## Cakes, Candy, Cookies, Desserts, Pies

| | Quantity | | Calories* | Protein* (grams) |
|---|---|---|---|---|
| Cakes from home recipes | | | | |
| Angel food, plain | $\frac{1}{12}$ | of 10 in. | 160 | 4.3 |
| Boston cream pie | $\frac{1}{8}$ | of 8 in. | 311 | 5.2 |
| Chocolate, chocolate icing | $\frac{1}{12}$ | of 8 in. | 288 | 3.5 |
| | 1 | cupcake | 160 | 2.0 |
| Sponge cake | $\frac{1}{12}$ | of 10 in. | 196 | 5.0 |
| White with coconut icing | $\frac{1}{12}$ | of 8 in. | 300 | 3.0 |
| Cakes from bought mixes | | | | |
| Coffee cake | $\frac{1}{6}$ | of 8 in. | 230 | 4.5 |
| Chocolate, chocolate icing | $\frac{1}{12}$ | of 8 in. | 312 | 4.0 |
| Honey spice, caramel icing | $\frac{1}{12}$ | of 8 in. | 360 | 4.2 |
| Yellow with chocolate icing | 1 | cupcake | 155 | 1.9 |
| Candy | | | | |
| Caramels, plain | 1 | oz. | 113 | 1.1 |
| Chocolate, milk | 1 | oz. | 150 | 2.2 |
| Chocolate coated almonds | 6–8 | | 160 | 3.4 |
| Chocolate coated raisins | 50 | | 120 | 1.5 |
| Chocolate coated mints | 1 | $(2\frac{1}{2}$ in.) | 144 | .6 |
| Fudge, chocolate with nuts | 1 | cu. in. | 90 | .8 |
| Hard candy | 1 | oz. | 110 | 0.0 |
| Peanut brittle | 1 | oz. | 120 | 1.6 |
| Cookies | | | | |
| Brownies with nuts | $2 \times 2 \times 1$ in. | | 100 | 1.5 |
| Chocolate chip ($2\frac{1}{2}$ in.) | 4 | cookies | 200 | 2.2 |
| Macaroons ($2\frac{3}{4}$ in.) | 2 | cookies | 180 | 2.0 |
| Oatmeal with raisins ($2\frac{1}{2}$ in.) | 4 | cookies | 235 | 3.2 |
| Sandwich type, chocolate | 4 | cookies | 200 | 2.0 |
| Sugar cookies ($2\frac{1}{4}$ in.) | 10 | cookies | 355 | 4.8 |
| Desserts | | | | |
| Bread pudding, raisins | $\frac{1}{2}$ | cup | 250 | 7.4 |
| Cream puffs with custard | 1 | puff | 300 | 8.5 |
| Custard, baked | $\frac{1}{2}$ | cup | 150 | 7.2 |

| | Quantity | | Calories* | Protein* (grams) |
|---|---|---|---|---|
| Doughnuts, cake | 1 | | 227 | 2.7 |
| Doughnuts, raised | 1 | | 176 | 2.7 |
| Gelatin dessert, plain | 1 | cup | 142 | 3.6 |
| Ice cream, plain | 1 | cup | 257 | 6.0 |
| Ice milk, plain | 1 | cup | 200 | 6.3 |
| Pudding, chocolate | $\frac{1}{2}$ | cup | 160 | 4.4 |
| Sherbet | 1 | cup | 250 | 1.7 |
| Tapioca pudding | 1 | cup | 221 | 8.3 |
| Pies—9-in. single crust | | | | |
|   Apple | $\frac{1}{8}$ | of 9 in. | 300 | 2.6 |
|   Chocolate & lemon meringue | $\frac{1}{8}$ | of 9 in. | 275 | 3.9 |
|   Custard | $\frac{1}{8}$ | of 9 in. | 250 | 7.0 |
|   Pecan | $\frac{1}{8}$ | of 9 in. | 430 | 5.3 |
|   Pumpkin | $\frac{1}{8}$ | of 9 in. | 240 | 4.6 |
|   Strawberry | $\frac{1}{8}$ | of 9 in. | 185 | 1.8 |

## Dairy Products

| | Quantity | | Calories* | Protein* (grams) |
|---|---|---|---|---|
| Butter | 1 | pat | 36 | — |
| | $\frac{1}{2}$ | cup | 812 | .7 |
| Buttermilk from skim milk | 1 | cup | 88 | 8.8 |
| Cheese | | | | |
|   Blue, brick, Colby | 1 | oz. | 100 | 6.2 |
|   Cheddar | 1 | oz. | 113 | 7.1 |
|   Cottage, uncreamed | $\frac{1}{2}$ | cup | 100 | 18.0 |
|   Cream cheese | 1 | oz. | 106 | 2.3 |
|   Swiss | 1 | oz. | 105 | 7.8 |
| Cream | | | | |
|   Half and half | 1 | oz. (2 T.) | 40 | 1.0 |
|   Heavy whipping | 1 | oz. (2 T.) | 106 | .6 |
|   Sour cream | 1 | oz. (2 T.) | 50 | — |
|   Substitute dry cream | 1 | t. | 10 | .3 |
| Milk, whole | 1 | cup | 160 | 8.5 |
| Milk, 2% | 1 | cup | 145 | 10.3 |
| Milk, skim | 1 | cup | 88 | 8.8 |
| Milk, chocolate | 1 | cup | 213 | 8.5 |
| Yogurt, low fat, plain | 8 | oz. | 113 | 7.7 |

## Eggs

| | Quantity | | Calories* | Protein* (grams) |
|---|---|---|---|---|
| Hard-boiled, poached | 1 | lg. egg | 82 | 6.5 |

| | Quantity | | Calories* | Protein* (grams) |
|---|---|---|---|---|
| Fried, in butter | 1 | lg. egg | 99 | 6.5 |
| Omelet, scrambled with milk and cooked in fat | 1 | lg. egg | 111 | 7.2 |

## Fish and Seafood

| | Quantity | | Calories* | Protein* (grams) |
|---|---|---|---|---|
| Clams, canned, drained | ½ | cup | 75 | 13.0 |
| Crab, cooked | 1 | oz. | 27 | 4.9 |
| Flounder, baked | 1 | oz. | 57 | 8.5 |
| Halibut, broiled | 1 | oz. | 48 | 7.1 |
| Lobster, cooked | 1 | oz. | 27 | 5.3 |
| Ocean perch, fried | 1 | oz. | 64 | 5.4 |
| Oysters, fried | 1 | oz. | 68 | 2.4 |
| Salmon, broiled | 1 | oz. | 52 | 7.7 |
| Shrimp, boiled | 10 | med. | 37 | 7.7 |
| Tuna, canned in oil | 1 | oz. | 56 | 8.2 |
| Tuna, canned in water | 1 | oz. | 36 | 8.0 |

## Fruit and Fruit Juices

| | Quantity | | Calories* | Protein* (grams) |
|---|---|---|---|---|
| Apple | 1 | med. | 80 | .3 |
| Applesauce, sweetened | ½ | cup | 116 | .3 |
| Apricots, fresh | 3 | whole | 55 | 1.1 |
| Avocado, fresh | ½ | avocado | 188 | 2.4 |
| Banana | 1 | med. | 100 | 1.3 |
| Cantaloupe, honeydew | ½ | melon | 100 | 3.7 |
| Fruit cocktail, canned | ½ | cup | 100 | .5 |
| Grapefruit | ½ | med. | 50 | .5 |
| Grapes, fresh | 20 | grapes | 54 | 1.0 |
| Grape juice | ½ | cup | 83 | .3 |
| Orange | 1 | med. | 65 | 1.3 |
| Orange juice, diluted frozen | 8 | oz. | 100 | 1.5 |
| Peach, fresh | 1 | med. | 38 | .6 |

| | Quantity | Calories* | Protein* (grams) |
|---|---|---|---|
| Peach slices, canned | ½ cup | 98 | .5 |
| Pear, fresh | 1 med. | 100 | 1.1 |
| Pineapple, canned in heavy syrup | ½ cup | 100 | .4 |
| Plums, fresh | 1 whole | 32 | .3 |
| Prune juice | ½ cup | 100 | .5 |
| Raisins, uncooked | ½ cup | 200 | 1.8 |
| Strawberries, fresh | 1 cup | 55 | 1.0 |
| Watermelon | 1 cup diced | 42 | .8 |

## Jams, Jellies, Sugar Products, Sauces

| | Quantity | Calories* | Protein* (grams) |
|---|---|---|---|
| Jam, jelly, preserves | 1 T. | 78 | .2 |
| Molasses, cane | 1 T. | 46 | — |
| Honey | 1 T. | 60 | — |
| Sugar, brown | 1 T. | 50 | — |
| Sugar, granulated | 1 T. | 46 | — |
| Syrup, maple | 1 T. | 50 | — |
| Syrup, chocolate, thin | 1 T. | 50 | — |
| Tartar sauce | 2 T. | 150 | .4 |
| Worcestershire, soy sauce | 2 T. | 15 | 1.6 |

## Meats: Beef, Lamb, Organ, Pork, Veal

| | Quantity | Calories* | Protein* (grams) |
|---|---|---|---|
| Beef | | | |
| Hamburger, lean, cooked | 1 oz. | 63 | 7.8 |
| Roasts, rump | 1 oz. | 100 | 6.7 |
| Roasts, rib | 1 oz. | 126 | 5.7 |
| Steak, round, broiled | 1 oz. | 75 | 8.2 |
| Steak, T-bone, broiled | 1 oz. | 135 | 5.6 |
| Lamb | | | |
| Lamb, roast leg | 1 oz. | 80 | 7.2 |
| Lamb chop, broiled | 1 oz. | 100 | 6.3 |
| Organ meats | | | |
| Heart, beef, braised | 1 oz. | 100 | 7.4 |
| Liver, beef, fried | 1 oz. | 65 | 7.5 |
| Tongue, beef, cooked | 1 oz. | 70 | 5.5 |

**69**

| | Quantity | | Calories* | Protein* (grams) |
|---|---|---|---|---|
| Pork, fresh | | | | |
| Loin chops, broiled | 1 | oz. | 112 | 7.1 |
| Roast, Boston butt | 1 | oz. | 100 | 6.4 |
| Spareribs, braised | 1 | oz. | 126 | 5.9 |
| Pork, cured | | | | |
| Ham, light cure, baked | 1 | oz. | 85 | 6.0 |
| Bacon, fried, drained | 2 | slices | 143 | 6.4 |
| Veal cutlet, broiled | 1 | oz. | 62 | 7.7 |

## Meats: Cold Cuts, Sausages

| | | | | |
|---|---|---|---|---|
| Bologna, all meat | 1 | slice | 73 | 3.4 |
| Brown & serve sausage | 1 | link | 72 | 2.7 |
| Country style smoked sausage | 1 | oz. | 100 | 4.3 |
| Frankfurter, all meat | 1 | frank | 134 | 5.9 |
| Salami, cooked | 1 | slice | 88 | 5.0 |

## Nuts, Nut Products, Relishes, Snacks

| | | | | |
|---|---|---|---|---|
| Cashews, roasted | 18 | nuts | 158 | 4.9 |
| Coconut, fresh | $2 \times 2 \times \frac{1}{2}$ in. | | 156 | 1.6 |
| Peanuts, roasted | $\frac{1}{2}$ | cup | 421 | 19.0 |
| Peanut butter | 1 | T. | 94 | 4.0 |
| Walnuts, English | 14 | halves | 185 | 4.2 |
| Relishes | | | | |
| Olives, green | 10 | large | 45 | .5 |
| Olives, ripe | 10 | large | 73 | .5 |
| Pickles, dill | 1 | (4 in.) | 7 | .2 |
| Pickles, sweet | 1 | (3 in.) | 50 | .2 |
| Sweet pickle relish | 1 | T. | 20 | .1 |
| Snacks | | | | |
| Crackers | | | | |
| Cheese flavored | 10 | crackers | 136 | 3.2 |
| Graham, plain | 1 | $(5 \times 2\frac{1}{2})$ | 55 | 1.1 |
| Saltines | 10 | crackers | 123 | 2.6 |
| Potato chips | 10 | chips | 114 | 1.1 |
| Pretzels, sticks | 10 | sticks | 23 | .6 |
| Popcorn, plain | 1 | oz. (4 c.) | 109 | 3.6 |
| Popcorn, buttered | 1 | oz. (3 c.) | 129 | 2.8 |

**70**

| | Quantity | Calories* | Protein* (grams) |
|---|---|---|---|

## Poultry

| | Quantity | Calories* | Protein* (grams) |
|---|---|---|---|
| Chicken, fried | 1 oz. | 70 | 8.7 |
| Goose, roasted | 1 oz. | 126 | 6.5 |
| Turkey, roasted | 1 oz. | 64 | 9.1 |

## Prepared Dishes

| | Quantity | Calories* | Protein* (grams) |
|---|---|---|---|
| Beef and vegetable stew | 1 cup | 218 | 15.7 |
| Chicken a la king | 1 cup | 468 | 27.4 |
| Chili con carne | 1 cup | 339 | 19.1 |
| Hamburger (4 oz. meat) | 1 | 416 | — |
| Lobster Newburg | 1 cup | 485 | 46.3 |
| Macaroni and cheese | 1 cup | 430 | 16.8 |
| Oyster stew | 1 cup | 233 | 12.5 |
| Pizza, sausage | $\frac{1}{8}$ of 14 in. | 157 | 5.2 |
| Soup | | | |
|   Bean with pork | 1 cup | 168 | 8.0 |
|   Chicken noodle | 1 cup | 130 | 6.9 |
|   Clam chowder | 1 cup | 80 | 2.2 |
|   Mushroom, cream | 1 cup | 216 | 6.9 |
|   Split pea | 1 cup | 145 | 8.6 |
| Spaghetti, meatballs, sauce | 1 cup | 332 | 18.6 |
| Tuna salad | 1 cup | 349 | 29.9 |

## Spreads, Margarine, Dressings, Oils

| | Quantity | Calories* | Protein* (grams) |
|---|---|---|---|
| Butter | 1 pat | 36 | — |
| Margarine ($\frac{1}{3}$ veg. fat) | 1 pat | 36 | — |
| | 1 T. | 100 | .1 |
| Margarine, diet | 1 T. | 50 | — |
| Oil, vegetable | 1 T. | 120 | — |
| Mayonnaise | 1 T. | 100 | .2 |
| Salad dressings | | | |
|   Blue cheese | 2 T. | 150 | 1.4 |
|   French | 2 T. | 132 | .2 |

| | Quantity | | Calories* | Protein* (grams) |
|---|---|---|---|---|
| Italian | 2 | T. | 166 | — |
| Russian | 2 | T. | 148 | .4 |
| Thousand Island | 2 | T. | 160 | .2 |

## Vegetables

| | Quantity | | Calories* | Protein* (grams) |
|---|---|---|---|---|
| Asparagus | 4 | spears | 12 | 1.3 |
| Beans, green or yellow | ½ | cup | 17 | 1.0 |
| Beans, baby lima | ½ | cup | 94 | 6.3 |
| Beets, canned | ½ | cup | 30 | .9 |
| Broccoli spears, chopped | 1 | cup | 48 | 5.4 |
| Brussels sprouts | 1 | cup | 50 | 5.0 |
| Carrot | 1 | med. | 30 | .8 |
| Cauliflower | 1 | cup | 28 | 2.9 |
| Corn | 1 | ear | 70 | 2.5 |
| Lettuce, chopped | 1 | cup | 10 | .7 |

|  | Quantity | Calories* | Protein* (grams) |
|---|---|---|---|
| Onion, chopped | ½ cup | 33 | 1.3 |
| Peas, green | ½ cup | 58 | 4.3 |
| **Potatoes** | | | |
|   Au gratin with cheese | ½ cup | 177 | 6.0 |
|   Baked with peel | 1 med. | 100 | 2.9 |
|   French fried | 10 2-in. pieces | 137 | 2.2 |
|   Hash browned | ½ cup | 223 | 3.4 |
|   Mashed with milk & butter | ½ cup | 100 | 4.4 |
|   Salad | 1 cup | 363 | 7.5 |
| Spinach, raw, chopped | 1 cup | 14 | 1.8 |
| Squash, summer | ½ cup | 13 | .7 |
| Squash, winter, baked | ½ squash | 160 | 2.4 |
| Sweet potato, baked | 1 med. | 176 | 2.4 |
| Tomatoes, raw | 1 med. | 40 | 2.0 |
| Tomato juice | 6 oz. | 35 | 1.5 |
| Vegetable juice cocktail | 4 oz. | 20 | 1.1 |

Note: For meats, fish, and poultry make your serving 3 ounces. You're likely to have been taking 4 to 6 ounces as your average serving, so please make this adjustment.

*The calorie and protein values are derived from different sources and brands. Check your package for more specific values of the product you are using.

TABLE
**4–4**

# Recommended Daily Dietary Allowances

*Food and Nutrition Board*
*National Academy of Sciences–National Research Council.* [1]
*(Revised 1974)*

## Vitamins

| | Age (Years) | Calories | Protein (g) | A (IU) | D (IU) | E (IU) | C (mg) | Folacin (μg) | Niacin (mg) | Riboflavin (mg) |
|---|---|---|---|---|---|---|---|---|---|---|
| **Children** | 1–3 | 1300 | 23 | 2000 | 400 | 7 | 40 | 100 | 9 | 0.8 |
| | 4–6 | 1800 | 30 | 2500 | 400 | 9 | 40 | 200 | 12 | 1.1 |
| | 7–11 | 2400 | 36 | 3300 | 400 | 10 | 40 | 300 | 16 | 1.2 |
| **Males** | 11–14 | 2800 | 44 | 5000 | 400 | 12 | 45 | 400 | 18 | 1.5 |
| | 15–18 | 3000 | 54 | 5000 | 400 | 15 | 45 | 400 | 20 | 1.8 |
| | 19–22 | 3000 | 54 | 5000 | 400 | 15 | 45 | 400 | 20 | 1.8 |
| | 23–50 | 2700 | 56 | 5000 | 400 | 15 | 45 | 400 | 18 | 1.6 |
| | 51+ | 2400 | 56 | 5000 | 400 | 15 | 45 | 400 | 16 | 1.5 |
| **Females** | 11–14 | 2400 | 44 | 4000 | 400 | 12 | 45 | 400 | 16 | 1.3 |
| | 15–18 | 2100 | 48 | 4000 | 400 | 12 | 45 | 400 | 14 | 1.4 |
| | 19–22 | 2100 | 46 | 4000 | 400 | 12 | 45 | 400 | 14 | 1.4 |
| | 23–50 | 2000 | 46 | 4000 | 400 | 12 | 45 | 400 | 13 | 1.2 |
| | 51+ | 1800 | 46 | 4000 | 400 | 12 | 45 | 400 | 12 | 1.1 |
| **Pregnant** | | +300 | +30 | 5000 | 400 | 15 | 60 | 800 | +2 | +0.3 |
| **Lactating** | | +500 | +20 | 6000 | 400 | 15 | 80 | 600 | +4 | +0.5 |

[1]The allowances are intended to provide for individual variations among most normal persons as they live in the United States under usual environmental stresses. Diets should be based on a variety of common foods in order to provide other nutrients for which human requirements have been less well defined.

| Thiamine (mg) | B$_6$ (mg) | B$_{12}$ (µg) | Biotin (mg) | Pantothenic Acid (mg) | Ca (mg) | P (mg) | I (µg) | Fe (mg) | Mg (mg) | Zn (mg) | Cu (mg) | Mn (mg) |
|---|---|---|---|---|---|---|---|---|---|---|---|---|
| 0.7 | 0.6 | 1.0 | 1.5 | 5 | 800 | 800 | 60 | 15 | 150 | 10 | 1.0 | 2.5 |
| 0.9 | 0.9 | 1.5 | 3.0 | 10 | 800 | 800 | 80 | 10 | 200 | 10 | 1.5 | 3.0 |
| 1.2 | 1.2 | 2.0 | 3.0 | 10 | 800 | 800 | 110 | 10 | 250 | 10 | 1.5 | 3.0 |
| 1.4 | 1.6 | 3.0 | 3.0 | 10 | 1200 | 1200 | 130 | 18 | 350 | 15 | 2.0 | 4.0 |
| 1.5 | 2.0 | 3.0 | 3.0 | 10 | 1200 | 1200 | 150 | 18 | 400 | 15 | 2.0 | 4.0 |
| 1.5 | 2.0 | 3.0 | 3.0 | 10 | 800 | 800 | 140 | 10 | 350 | 15 | 2.0 | 4.0 |
| 1.4 | 2.0 | 3.0 | 3.0 | 10 | 800 | 800 | 130 | 10 | 350 | 15 | 2.0 | 4.0 |
| 1.2 | 2.0 | 3.0 | 3.0 | 10 | 800 | 800 | 110 | 10 | 350 | 15 | 2.0 | 4.0 |
| 1.2 | 1.6 | 3.0 | 3.0 | 10 | 1200 | 1200 | 115 | 18 | 300 | 15 | 2.0 | 4.0 |
| 1.1 | 2.0 | 3.0 | 3.0 | 10 | 1200 | 1200 | 115 | 18 | 300 | 15 | 2.0 | 4.0 |
| 1.1 | 2.0 | 3.0 | 3.0 | 10 | 800 | 800 | 100 | 18 | 300 | 15 | 2.0 | 4.0 |
| 1.0 | 2.0 | 3.0 | 3.0 | 10 | 800 | 800 | 100 | 18 | 300 | 15 | 2.0 | 4.0 |
| 1.0 | 2.0 | 3.0 | 3.0 | 10 | 800 | 800 | 80 | 10 | 300 | 15 | 2.0 | 4.0 |
| +0.3 | 2.5 | 4.0 | 3.0 | 10 | 1200 | 1200 | 125 | 18+ | 450 | 20 | 2.0 | 4.0 |
| +0.3 | 2.5 | 4.0 | 3.0 | 10 | 1200 | 1200 | 150 | 18 | 450 | 25 | 2.0 | 4.0 |

Ca = Calcium        Mg = Magnesium
P   = Phosphorus   Zn  = Zinc
I    = Iodine          Cu  = Copper
Fe  = Iron            Mn  = Manganese

TABLE
**4–5**

# Weight Loss Chart

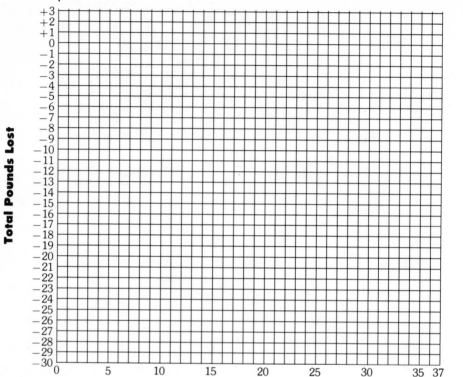

**Weeks**

---

*This material is repeated for you to fill out in the Tear-Out Appendix.*

**Beginning Weight** _____

| Date | Week | Weight | Total Lbs. Lost |
|------|------|--------|-----------------|
|      | 0    |        |                 |
|      | 1    |        |                 |
|      | 2    |        |                 |
|      | 3    |        |                 |
|      | 4    |        |                 |
|      | 5    |        |                 |
|      | 6    |        |                 |
|      | 7    |        |                 |
|      | 8    |        |                 |
|      | 9    |        |                 |
|      | 10   |        |                 |
|      | 11   |        |                 |
|      | 12   |        |                 |
|      | 13   |        |                 |
|      | 14   |        |                 |
|      | 15   |        |                 |
|      | 16   |        |                 |
|      | 17   |        |                 |
|      | 18   |        |                 |
|      | 19   |        |                 |
|      | 20   |        |                 |
|      | 21   |        |                 |
|      | 22   |        |                 |
|      | 23   |        |                 |
|      | 24   |        |                 |
|      | 25   |        |                 |
|      | 26   |        |                 |
|      | 27   |        |                 |
|      | 28   |        |                 |
|      | 29   |        |                 |
|      | 30   |        |                 |

**Goal Weight** _____

TABLE
4–6

# Calorie Intake to Lose Weight

*Calorie allowances for various weights of MEN.*

| If you weigh (pounds) | Your daily calorie intake to maintain that weight is | Your daily calorie intake to lose 1 pound per week is | Your daily calorie intake to lose 2 pounds per week is |
|---|---|---|---|
| 130 | 2300 | 1800 | 1300 |
| 135 | 2350 | 1875 | 1375 |
| 140 | 2400 | 1950 | 1450 |
| 145 | 2450 | 2025 | 1525 |
| 150 | 2500 | 2100 | 1600 |
| 155 | 2600 | 2150 | 1650 |
| 160 | 2700 | 2200 | 1700 |
| 165 | 2750 | 2250 | 1750 |
| 170 | 2800 | 2300 | 1800 |
| 175 | 2850 | 2375 | 1875 |
| 180 | 2900 | 2450 | 1950 |
| 185 | 3000 | 2525 | 2025 |
| 190 | 3100 | 2600 | 2100 |
| 195 | 3150 | 2650 | 2150 |
| 200 | 3200 | 2700 | 2200 |
| 205 | 3250 | 2750 | 2250 |
| 210 | 3300 | 2800 | 2300 |
| 215 | 3350 | 2875 | 2375 |
| 220 | 3400 | 2950 | 2450 |
| 225 | 3450 | 3025 | 2525 |
| 230 | 3500 | 3100 | 2600 |
| 235 | 3550 | 3150 | 2650 |
| 240 | 3600 | 3200 | 2700 |
| 245 | 3650 | 3250 | 2750 |
| 250 | 3700 | 3300 | 2800 |

TABLE
4–7

## Calorie Intake to Lose Weight

*Calorie allowances for various weights of WOMEN.*

| If you weigh (pounds) | Your daily calorie intake to maintain that weight is | Your daily calorie intake to lose 1 pound per week is | Your daily calorie intake to lose 2 pounds per week is |
|---|---|---|---|
| 110 | 1700 | 1200 | 700 |
| 115 | 1750 | 1250 | 750 |
| 120 | 1800 | 1300 | 800 |
| 125 | 1850 | 1350 | 850 |
| 130 | 1900 | 1400 | 900 |
| 135 | 1950 | 1475 | 975 |
| 140 | 2000 | 1550 | 1050 |
| 145 | 2050 | 1600 | 1100 |
| 150 | 2100 | 1650 | 1150 |
| 155 | 2200 | 1700 | 1200 |
| 160 | 2300 | 1750 | 1250 |
| 165 | 2350 | 1825 | 1325 |
| 170 | 2400 | 1900 | 1400 |
| 175 | 2450 | 1950 | 1450 |
| 180 | 2500 | 2000 | 1500 |
| 185 | 2550 | 2050 | 1550 |
| 190 | 2600 | 2100 | 1600 |
| 195 | 2650 | 2150 | 1650 |
| 200 | 2700 | 2200 | 1700 |
| 205 | 2750 | 2250 | 1750 |
| 210 | 2800 | 2300 | 1800 |
| 215 | 2850 | 2375 | 1875 |
| 220 | 2900 | 2450 | 1950 |
| 225 | 2950 | 2525 | 2025 |
| 230 | 3000 | 2600 | 2100 |

TABLE
**4-8** | **Daily Food Diary**

| | Calories | Protein (g) |
|---|---|---|
| **Breakfast** | | |
| **Morning Snack** | | |
| **Lunch** | | |
| **Afternoon Snack** | | |
| **Dinner** | | |
| **Bedtime Snack** | | |
| **TOTALS** | | |

*This material is repeated for you to fill out in the Tear-Out Appendix.*

TABLE
4-9

# The Basic Balanced Daily Food Plan (1,200 calories)

## Protein—Meats and Meat Substitutes

(Note the average adult requires about 50 grams of protein daily. See Table 4–4 for more exact requirements in adults and children.)

Calories 400. Protein 50 grams. Two servings of three ounces of skinned poultry, fish, or trimmed lean meat (cooked weight) provide about 40 to 60 (average 50) grams of protein. There are about 160 to 240 calories per 3-ounce serving, depending on what you select. The average would be 200 calories for each 3-ounce serving. A cup of low fat cottage cheese is equivalent or slightly higher in protein and the same in calories as a 3-ounce serving from the meat group.

## Fruits and Vegetables

Calories 200 to 300. Protein varies with vegetables. Four servings: one dark green or deep yellow vegetable (for Vitamin A) and one citrus fruit or juice for Vitamin C. A serving of most raw or cooked vegetables is about 20 to 50 calories. A serving of beans, peas, corn, or potatoes is nearer 100 calories *without* added fats.

## Breads and Cereals

Calories 200 to 300. Protein varies. Three to four servings from this group. Breads are 60 to 75 calories per slice. Cold cereals are 70 to 110 calories per one-ounce serving. Cooked cereals are 150 calories per cup. All without added milk or fat.

## Milk Products

Calories 160. Protein 16 grams. Two servings of 8 ounces of skim milk provide the above nutrition. Plain yogurt is higher in calories for the same amount of protein. Cheeses are much higher in calories, fat, and cholesterol.

## Fats and Oils

Calories 200. No protein. A total of 6 teaspoons of liquid vegetable oil, polyunsaturated margarine, or polyunsaturated salad dressing provides adequate nutritional balance.

TABLE
**4–10**

# Sample Weight Reduction Diet Plan— 1,800 Calories

## Basic Balanced Diet

_2_ Servings (3 ounces each) poultry, fish, or lean trimmed meat, or appropriate substitute. 400 calories. 50 grams of protein.

_4_ Servings fruits and vegetables. 200–300 calories.

_3–4_ Servings bread or cereal. 200–300 calories.

_2_ Servings (8 ounces each) skim milk. 160 calories. 16 grams protein.

_6_ Servings (1 teaspoon each) allowed fat (vegetable oil or polyunsaturated margarine). 200 calories.

## Additional Calories Allowed

_2–3_ Servings vegetables and fruit. 150 calories.

_3_ Servings bread. 180 calories.

_2_ Servings skim milk. 160 calories.

_3_ Servings (1 teaspoon each) vegetable oil or margarine. 100 calories.

## Sample Menu Pattern

### Breakfast:
_1_ Serving citrus fruit or juice
_2_ Servings cereal or toast
_2_ Servings allowed fat
_1_ Serving skim milk
Coffee or tea if desired

### Lunch:
_1_ Serving poultry, fish, or lean trimmed meat
_1_ Serving potato or bread
_1_ Vegetable
_2_ Servings allowed fat
_1_ Serving fruit
Coffee or tea if desired

### Dinner:
_1_ Serving poultry, fish, or lean trimmed meat
_2_ Vegetables
_2_ Servings bread
_3_ Servings allowed fat
_1_ Serving fruit
_1_ Serving skim milk

### Morning Snack:
_1_ Serving bread
_1_ Serving allowed fat
_1_ Serving skim milk

### Afternoon Snack:
_1_ Serving fruit
_1_ Serving vegetable sticks

### Bedtime Snack:
_1_ Serving bread
_1_ Serving allowed fat
_1_ Serving skim milk

TABLE
**4-11**

# Weight Reduction Plan, _____ calories

## Daily Food Plan

___ Servings (3 ounces each) poultry, fish, or lean trimmed meat, or appropriate substitute
___ Servings fruits and vegetables
___ Servings bread or cereal
___ Servings (8 ounces each) skim milk
___ Servings (1 teaspoon each) allowed fat (i.e., vegetable oil or polyunsaturated margarine)

### Morning Snack:

— _____

— _____

— _____

### Afternoon Snack:

— _____

— _____

— _____

### Bedtime Snack:

— _____

— _____

— _____

## Sample Menu Pattern

### Breakfast:
___ Serving citrus fruit or juice
___ Serving cereal or toast
___ Servings allowed fat
___ Serving skim milk

### Lunch:
___ Serving poultry, fish, or lean trimmed meat
___ Serving potato, rice, or substitute
___ Servings vegetable
___ Serving bread
___ Servings allowed fat
___ Serving fruit
___ Serving skim milk

### Dinner:
___ Serving poultry, fish, or lean trimmed meat
___ Serving potato, rice, or substitute
___ Servings vegetable
___ Servings bread
___ Servings allowed fat
___ Serving fruit
___ Serving skim milk

*This material is repeated for you to fill out in the Tear-Out Appendix.*

TABLE
**4-12** | **Maintenance Diet**

## Daily Food Plan

___ Servings (3 ounces each) poultry, fish, or lean trimmed meat, or appropriate substitute
___ Servings fruits and vegetables
___ Servings bread or cereal
___ Servings (8 ounces each) skim milk
___ Servings (1 teaspoon each) allowed fat (i.e., vegetable oil or polyunsaturated margarine)

## Morning Snack:

— _____

— _____

— _____

## Afternoon Snack:

— _____

— _____

— _____

## Bedtime Snack:

— _____

— _____

— _____

## Sample Menu Pattern

**Breakfast:**
___ Serving citrus fruit or juice
___ Serving cereal or toast
___ Servings allowed fat
___ Serving skim milk

**Lunch:**
___ Serving poultry, fish, or lean trimmed meat
___ Serving potato, rice, or substitute
___ Servings vegetable
___ Serving bread
___ Servings allowed fat
___ Serving fruit
___ Serving skim milk

**Dinner:**
___ Serving poultry, fish, or lean trimmed meat
___ Serving potato, rice, or substitute
___ Servings vegetable
___ Servings bread
___ Servings allowed fat
___ Serving fruit
___ Serving skim milk

*This material is repeated for you to fill out in the Tear-Out Appendix.*

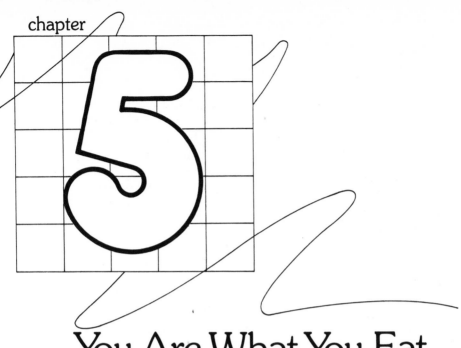

# You Are What You Eat

This chapter will give you the guidelines for a prudent diet (not a weight loss diet) that is appropriate for the 90 percent of Americans at low risk of heart attack. You'll also be given guidelines for a more strict diet for the 10 percent at high risk. Then, for about 1 percent (10 percent of those at high risk), even the strict diet won't be enough. Medication will be needed and will be described briefly in Chapter 12.

Obviously, if you require medication, you'll need to be under the care of a physician knowledgeable in this area. I would also advise the involvement of a physician if you are in the high-risk group. In Chapter 12 we'll try to put everything together to help you decide if your risk is high or low. If more than a prudent diet is needed, you should work on this with your physician and probably also with a well-informed nutritionist.

In this chapter, you will be given the general content of specific diets for high-risk problems with high cholesterol and/or high triglycerides. This information is not provided so that you will undertake your management without professional help. How can I put it delicately? Let's say some doctors are not as well trained in nutrition as others. And most doctors would resent your bringing this or any other trade book into their offices to ask them if these are the diets they will be using. In fact, you'd have to scrape some doctors off the ceiling if you presented that sort of proposal to them. You see, we doctors have very delicate egos. In a similar position, I too might even get a little testy.

So I want you to have some information to know the general dietary direction you must travel if you're at high risk. And I guess I'm giving you this material to help you be a well-informed medical consumer. I don't want you thrashing around destroying what could be a mutually rewarding patient-doctor relationship any more than I would want you to be subjected to an ill-informed, ineffectual program for managing your high risk.

Therefore, if you and your doctor conclude that you (or a member of your family) is at high risk, you might open with a very casual: "Will I be starting an NIH diet or an American Heart diet?" We'll give a few more details later.

# What's Wrong with Having High Cholesterol?

In the last chapter, you were given reasons for not being overweight. The same information should be demanded with regard to cholesterol, triglycerides, and fats connected to proteins (lipoproteins).

First there's the epidemiologic reason. Many studies, including our own, have documented that your risk of having a heart attack or stroke is increased if your blood cholesterol, triglycerides, and lipoproteins are increased. And the higher the values, the greater the risk.

But what do these fatty elements do to you? This is a very complex subject, which doesn't deter me from offering the oversimplified answer that follows. Certain lipoproteins, on which cholesterol and triglycerides are bound, interact with the inner walls of the arteries and with clotting elements of the blood to form a cholesterol and fat-rich plaque that works its way into the lining of the blood vessel. This plaque has a tendency to grow until the blood vessel is obstructed and the blood supply to whatever structure the artery serves is cut off. If the artery that is closed off serves the heart muscle, then the piece of muscle nourished by that artery dies. A heart attack results. A stroke occurs when a blood vessel to the brain is interrupted.

It is still uncertain whether the lipoprotein itself injures the inside of the blood vessel or if it is deposited in response to an injury caused by something else (such as high blood pressure or clotting elements). In fact, both mechanisms, as well as other mechanisms (mutations in the vessel lining cells or immunologic injury), may all play roles in this problem. However, what appears to be evident is that no matter how the plaque starts to form, it needs to be fed by lipids (fats) and lipoproteins. In experiments, an animal's artery may be injured by puncturing it with a tube, blowing up a small balloon on the end of the tube, and rubbing the inner surface of the vessel. If the animal has low cholesterol and lipoprotein in his blood, the vessel heals cleanly. However, if the animal has high lipoproteins, the vessel forms a plaque at the site of injury, which may build up until the blood vessel plugs up.

I should mention here that there are several types of lipoproteins. The low-density lipoproteins (LDL) are probably the most damaging. The very low density lipoproteins (VLDL) may also be involved in hardening of the arteries. But one form of lipoprotein, high-density lipoprotein (HDL), clearly protects blood vessels.

The next section will tell you in nontechnical terms how to change your diet to the diet recommended by the U.S. Senate Select Committee. These are general guidelines that don't require nearly as much dietary knowledge as you've already obtained from the last chapter. In fact, the entire program for change consists of just the seven points listed in Table 5–1.

However, I'll expect that you'll be able to apply your increasing knowledge of the composition of foods and use the tables in this book to build a very accurate and satisfying dietary program for your family.

## A Prudent Diet for Those at Low Risk

If your family history does not reveal a first-degree or second-degree relative with a heart attack or stroke before 55 years of age, the low-risk diet proposed in *Dietary Goals for the United States* (and recently revised) is appropriate for you. If you have relatives with heart attacks or strokes between ages 55 and 70, you'll want to adhere strictly to this diet. However, there is considerable room for discretion. If there is simply no heart disease or stroke in your family before relatives reach their seventies and eighties, and if you have low normal levels of cholesterol and triglycerides, I find it difficult to recommend that you must adhere strictly to the prudent diet. If I did not have high risk, I personally would be much more liberal in my diet than the Select Committee recommends. My weaknesses would be desserts, cheeses, and omelets. However, I would also keep my weight very close to the desirable weight for my height and frame.

Table 5–1 combines (and slightly modifies) elements of the original and revised U.S. Dietary Goals into a list of general recommendations for those at low risk. We'll go through these recommendations point by point.

**1.** The problem of being overweight has been discussed in the previous chapter, along with methods for losing weight to reach your desirable weight and to maintain that level.

**2.** Increase your consumption of fruits, vegetables, and grains. The time frame 1909–13 has been taken as the baseline for determining what's been happening to the American diet during this century. From 1909 to 1913 starches accounted for 68 percent of the carbohydrate in the American diet, and sugars only 32 percent. In 1976, starches were down to 47 percent and sugars up to 53 percent. The Select Committee recommendation is that fruits, vegetables, and whole grains be restored to the American diet to the level of accounting for almost half of your caloric intake. When you keep your food diary and calculate your calories, see what percentage comes from these sources. The average is only 28 percent, and you're probably somewhere near the average. That means you're going to have to figure ways to start substituting to almost double the fruits, vegetables, and whole grains in your diet and significantly reduce your caloric intake from the sources to be identified in the next paragraphs. Somehow the idea has been established in our culture that bread and other grain foods are in themselves high in calories and poor in protein. To be sure, grains are not as high in protein as meats. And if you make cakes and cookies rather than breads from grains, you end up with a lot of empty calories. But in many parts of the world, grain accounts for 80 to 90 percent of protein needs. And if I wasn't deceived by my high school history teacher, the Roman legions that conquered the world lived almost exclusively on bread. If you are trying to lose weight, you can't do it while relying almost entirely on grains and other starches for your protein. But if you're at a maintenance weight, you can be quite liberal with starches.

**3.** Decrease your refined sugar. Here's a real trap. You don't actually buy nearly as much sugar as your parents did. In 1909–13 consumers purchased 52 pounds of refined sugar per person per year. In 1971, the amount purchased was less than half—down to 24.7 pounds. But we're consuming much more sugar than we used to, not less. So where do we get it? In processed food and beverages. There's nothing like a little sugar to cover up a taste deficiency in a processed food. And so it goes. The processors doctor up our food with sugar until our palates become "hooked" on it. Until foods not sugared begin to taste unusual. Let me repeat what I say elsewhere. These corporate decisions are made for profit, not for the benefit of your health and well-being.

In 1971, we took in 70.2 pounds of refined sugar per person in processed foods, as compared with 10.3 pounds in 1909–13. In fact Americans now consume 23 pounds of sugar per person per year in beverages alone. You've got to be an aware label-reader, because the food industry sticks refined sugar into almost anything they can think of, from whole-grain cereals (some of which actually contain *more* calories from sugar than from grain) to peanut butter. So it's not just candy bars and cakes that you'll have to watch, it's a wide, wide variety of food products. So please read those labels!

**4.** Decrease the total fat in your diet from 42 percent to 30 percent. While our protein intake has stayed the same, and our total carbohydrate intake has actually decreased, it's our fat consumption that has risen dramatically in this century. Table 5–2 gives you an idea of the fat content of typical foods, and in the Appendix (Table A–1) there's a more detailed list that includes not only fat content but saturated and polyunsaturated fatty acids in each food. One gram of fat contains nine calories, while one gram of protein or carbohydrate contains only four calories. Some people, including an occasional hospital dietician, express the concern that lowering the fat content of food to 30 percent will make it unacceptably unpalatable. I agree that our palates may be accustomed to high fat content, but the Japanese live on a diet containing only 10 percent fat.

**5.** Specifically reduce saturated fats in your diet to 10 percent. This can be accomplished relatively easily by reducing your intake of animal fat. Substitute polyunsaturated margarine for butter or saturated margarine. In general, soft margarines in a tub are more likely to be higher in polyunsaturates. Read the labels and don't buy margarines that have a high content of hydrogenated vegetable oils. Hydrogenation takes unsaturated fatty acids and saturates them with hydrogen. Use cooking oils rather than solid (hydrogenated) vegetable shortenings, butter, or lard whenever possible.

Use skim milk instead of whole milk. The only exception to this is young infants, who get most of their calories from milk alone. Some essential fatty acids are needed in the diet. (It's unlikely that any baby would be taking skim milk as his only dietary source, and much more likely that he would be taking a well-balanced prepared formula.) Cut down on your quantity of red meat per serving and the number of times you serve red meat per week. Three to four times a week is plenty. Use chicken or turkey light meat and fish more abundantly. When using red meats, know how much fat they contain. You may get this information from Table A–1 in the Appendix. For example, you will find that T-bone steak contains three times as much fat as round steak, and cooked sausage contains three times as much fat as *canned* ham.

**6.** Reduce cholesterol in your diet. Cholesterol occurs only in food of animal origin. The richest common sources of cholesterol are egg yolks and liver. (Brains and kidney have even more cholesterol, but they're not consumed very often in the traditional U.S. diet.) And for that matter, liver is much less likely to be eaten than eggs are. Table 5–3 gives the cholesterol content of selected foods and Table A–1 gives a much more comprehensive list of foods with the cholesterol they contain. Let's start with eggs. (I personally love eggs.) If you're allowed 300 mg of cholesterol per day, one egg yolk pretty well shoots your entire day's allotment. But it's the egg yolk that you need to avoid—that's where the cholesterol is. On the other hand, the egg white still contains good protein. So if you want fried or boiled eggs, leave most of the egg yolk on your plate. When you scramble eggs discard two-thirds of the egg yolks. Your omelet may end up a little pale, but the flavor, to me, isn't nearly as objectionable as that of egg substitutes. But use egg substitutes in cooking where whole eggs are called for. Meats and dairy products are important sources of cholesterol. Figure about 25 milligrams of cholesterol per ounce of meat. Sadly, most kinds of fish contain 20 to 25 milligrams of cholesterol per ounce, with tuna canned in oil coming in at 30 milligrams per ounce. Whole milk is the primary source of protein for grammar school children, but it's also the major source of cholesterol, containing 50 milligrams in a 12-ounce glass. And almost half the calories of whole milk come from fat, mostly saturated. But a glass of skim milk has only 7 milligrams of cholesterol and almost no fat. Refer to Tables 5–2 and 5–3 and A–1 often until you learn what's in the foods you eat.

**7.** Decrease your consumption of salt. Since salt consumption is related to blood pressure, this will be included in the discussion of high blood pressure in Chapter 7. Those at low risk may consume five grams of salt (sodium chloride) a day, while those at higher risk must take less. Five grams of salt contain about 2,000 milligrams of sodium, which is the part of salt (the ion) that must be restricted. Five grams of salt is a level teaspoon. That doesn't mean that you should feel free to consume a level teaspoon of added salt. The five grams is all the salt recommended for your entire diet. Items such as bread and milk, for example, contain a considerable amount of salt. When you look up the salt content of a given food in Table A–1, you'll be given sodium content. Remember the prudent five-gram diet converts to 2,000 milligrams of sodium. There are, thus, 400 milligrams of sodium per gram of salt. The prudent diet for those at low risk suggests 2,000 milligrams of sodium from all sources per day.

These are to be followed after a mutual decision has been reached between you and your physician that your risk is indeed high for early-onset coronary heart disease, and that you have high levels of cholesterol and/or triglycerides that do not respond to the prudent diet alone. These diets go beyond the prudent diet in Table 5-1, and the ways in which they become more strict are specified following the same format.

There are three basic diets: one for patients with high cholesterol, one for patients with high triglycerides, and one for patients who have both high cholesterol and high triglycerides. The third diet combines elements of the first two. See Tables 5-4, 5-5, and 5-6.

There are some important points of difference between the prudent diet for the lower-risk 90 percent and the high-risk diets. For those with high cholesterol, it is recommended that your intake of cholesterol be reduced to 100 to 200 milligrams per day. You remember that cholesterol is confined to foods of animal origin and is absent in foods of plant origin. It's extremely difficult to rely on our traditional sources of animal protein, such as meat, fish, poultry, whole milk, eggs, and cheese, and control cholesterol to the level of 100 milligrams per day. However, vegetable proteins such as beans, peas, and certain grain components and "fake" meats, as developed by a number of food processors, provide excellent protein and no cholesterol.

Low cholesterol animal sources of protein include uncreamed low fat cottage cheese, part skim cheeses like mozzarella, and special low fat, low cholesterol processed cheese products (e.g., Lite-Line and Light and Lively). Skim milk provides good protein and low cholesterol, and plain yogurt has about the same amount of protein (a little more or a little less depending on how it's made). Egg whites have satisfactory protein, no cholesterol, and are very low in calories. It's the yolks you have to worry about. So figure out creative ways to use and eat egg whites. Nuts have good protein and no cholesterol but are high in calories and very high in fat.

Table A-1 in the Appendix will help you select the meats, fish, and poultry lowest in fat and cholesterol. The white meat of chicken and turkey is extremely versatile and can be used in all veal recipes as well. White fishes and tuna canned in water are low in fat and relatively low in cholesterol. (Skipjack tuna is much lower in fat than Albacore.) My advice for high-risk patients with high cholesterol is to strive to hold cholesterol to 100 milligrams per day, six days a week, but absolutely not to let it go above 200 milligrams per day. I give patients (and my own family) one day a week off from the extremely strict low cholesterol diet, but hold 400 milligrams as the absolute top limit on this day.

Doing the arithmetic, you can see that this doesn't even permit two egg yolks, let alone cholesterol from other sources.

It used to bother me (although it doesn't anymore) that some of the people who worked in my laboratory could eat two eggs for breakfast every morning and have extremely low cholesterol levels. One particular cardiology trainee, when he'd see how low his cholesterol was, would joke and say, "Maybe I ought to start eating three eggs for breakfast from now on."

Well, having read up to this point, you know enough about genetics to realize that if you're in the high-risk group, it's mainly because of your heredity. And if your cholesterol stays low despite two eggs for breakfast every day, it's also because of your heredity. We can't let our heredity concern us further. There's nothing we can do about it. We can just be grateful that we understand enough about the subject to permit us to follow the path most likely to lead to good health.

Your physician can get a stack of diets from the National Heart, Lung, and Blood Institute of the National Institutes of Health (NIH). He would also receive the physicians' handbook for prescribing specific diets. The American Heart Association provides diets for you through your physician (diets A, B, C, and D) for managing hyperlipidemias. The Appendix lists various written materials available at no cost or for nominal charges. There are many free recipe books at your heart association, and many books that you can purchase at bookstores.

Actually you'll see that there are numerous cookbooks that provide delicious low calorie, low fat, low cholesterol recipes. And just the way you handle the preparation of routine food items can make large differences in the calorie, fat, and cholesterol content of your diet. You can skin poultry, trim meat, use egg substitutes and oils in cooking in place of whole eggs and solid shortenings, and you can chill the cooked meat juices and skim off the fat to make low fat gravies and stews. Table 5–7 gives some selected hints on how to lower saturated fat and cholesterol consumption.

Please read it now and refer back to it whenever you need to.

Let me emphasize once more here that the strict diets we're talking about in Tables 5–4 to 5–6 and part of Table 5–7 are for those at *high risk*. The prudent diet in Table 5–1 is more than strict enough for the lower-risk 90 percent of the population. And even the strictest of the high-risk diets don't have to be punishing. Believe me, my family lives on one, and our diet varies between wholesome and gourmet. There are really a lot of possibilities for gourmet and ethnic cooking, especially Chinese and other Asian cookery. Even French cuisine is possible on a high-risk diet. A low calorie, generally low fat *haute cuisine* cookbook is referenced in the Bibliography (*Cuisine Minceur*). The only caution about this cookbook is that it is not specifically low cholesterol. So you'll have to be selective and make substitutions for eggs.

Delicious recipes abound, and you'll find a list of cookbooks in the Bibliography. I don't want you to feel that in undertaking a strict diet you're going to lose the real joy that we all obtain from eating. On the contrary, the increased effort that you'll be putting into your diet and cooking may very well add joy to this part of your life. I'm not sure that greaseburgers have contributed greatly to the well-being of anyone.

Please refer to the Appendix often. There's a lot of useful material there that doesn't lend itself to working into the narrative. You'll find blank diets to fill in for your prudent diet. You may also use these blanks to transcribe your physician- or dietician-prescribed diet, if you're at high risk. Let me emphasize again that you should not undertake a *high-risk* diet without the specific recommendation of your physician.

## Two Families

**Family C** ○   You remember Family C—the dentist, his wife, and five children introduced in Chapter 2. Everyone in the family had modest elevations of cholesterol and triglycerides, but the five people who were overweight (Dr. and Mrs. C and three children) had higher levels than the two children who were nearly normal in weight. Mrs. C was an excellent cook, and oriented to bringing the best in rich nutrition to her family. The C family consumed large quantities of what has been considered the traditional American diet for the past several decades.

Our first step was weight reduction for those who needed it and exercise for all. The weight reduction diet was relatively low in saturated fat and cholesterol as well. It took a lot of relearning for all the members of the family and almost a year to achieve the weight reduction goals for everybody. Mrs. C was the last to reach ideal weight, but she had started at 37 percent overweight. The hardest realization for her was that she simply couldn't eat nearly as many calories as her husband and sons. At 2,500 calories Dr. C could lose one pound per week, but at 2,500 calories Mrs. C would gain one pound per week.

Once everyone was at ideal weight, the family was first prescribed the prudent diet—the diet recommended for all Americans at low risk. This family was initially considered to be at high risk because of the family history and the total risk scores, but we still usually try the low-risk diet first. The prudent diet plus exercise was all that was necessary.

Dr. C and his wife each had 45 years of the typical American diet and life-style in which to damage their coronary and other arteries. But even considering the age they started their Whole Heart Program, we feel confident that they've significantly changed for the better their prospects for longevity, health, and quality of life. Their children should be even better served. The kids have now developed, at an early age, health habits to last a lifetime.

**Family D** ○  I'm going to introduce you to a high-risk family I've just begun to work with, to give you the other side of the coin. A simple change in diet and exercise isn't enough for some families at highest risk. Just a few days ago a 2-year-old girl was referred to us for a heart murmur. The heart murmur turned out to be an innocent (or functional) murmur. I assured the parents that every child has a heart murmur of some sort, if you listen carefully, but 99 percent of these are innocent. But I had to add something else. Although there was nothing wrong with this little girl's heart (at this time), she unfortunately had findings on her skin of a problem that meant she was at the highest possible risk for heart attack.

There were "growths" on her heels and the backs of her hands (xanthomas) that told us that she had a double dose of a gene for high cholesterol. That meant that she was subject to having a heart attack by the time she was 10 years old. It also meant that, since she had a double dose, both her parents had to have a single dose of this same gene. Her parents would be subject to heart attacks in their thirties and forties.

The cholesterol of the little girl was 1,000, her mother had 490, and her father had 300. The father smoked and was overweight. The usual Whole Heart Program of smoking cessation, diet, and exercise will be indicated. But it won't be enough. For both parents a combination of medications will be required. And for the little girl, even medications plus diet won't be sufficient. We'll have to contemplate a more aggressive approach—perhaps a surgical procedure that bypasses a large amount of blood that normally goes through the liver (portacaval shunt).

This was first performed at the University of Colorado Medical Center about four years ago on a somewhat older girl who had already had a heart attack. Since this condition is fatal early and occurs in only one child in a million, the number of these operations to date is perhaps only 50. It is obvious that one does not undertake such a procedure lightly.

Fortunately most families at high risk of coronary heart disease do not have the extremely serious situation that is present in Family D. I wanted you to have a little idea about the extreme limits of coronary disease and the modest limitations of diet, exercise, and healthful life-style. Yet it's also fortunate that with the very recent advances we've made, there is even something that can be done for the devastating genetic problem in Family D.

| TABLE 5-1 | **The Prudent Diet** |
|---|---|

*Dietary Goals and Suggested Changes for the 90 Percent of the U.S. Population at Low Risk for Cardiovascular Disease*

**1**  Avoid overweight, consume only as many calories as you expend; if overweight, decrease calories and increase expenditure (e.g., exercise more).

**2**  Increase your consumption of fruits, vegetables, and whole grains (complex carbohydrates and "naturally occurring" sugars) from the present 28 percent of calories in the average diet to about half (48 percent) of your caloric intake.

**3**  Decrease your consumption of refined and other processed sugars and foods high in such sugar by almost half (about 45 percent) to account for only about 10 percent of your total calories.

**4**  Decrease your consumption of foods high in total fat from 42 percent of calories to 30 percent.

**5**  Specifically reduce saturated* fat in your diet (from the present 16 percent to 10 percent) and partially replace this with polyunsaturated and monounsaturated fat to account for the remaining 20 percent of fat intake, by reducing intake of animal fat from meats and high fat dairy products. Eat more fish and poultry, and select lean meats low in fat (e.g., trimmed ground round in place of hamburger). Low fat and nonfat milk may be substituted for whole milk *except* in those infants whose diet is almost entirely milk.

**6**  Reduce cholesterol to about 300 milligrams per day. (The major dietary sources of cholesterol are egg yolks, meats, whole milk, and high fat dairy products.)

**7**  Decrease your consumption of salt and foods high in salt content from the present 6–18 grams per day to about 5 grams per day.

---

*Saturated and unsaturated refer to the chemical structure of the fatty acid. A saturated fat has no double bonds, a monounsaturated fat has one double bond, and a polyunsaturated fat has two or more double bonds.

TABLE
5-2

## Total Fat and Fatty Acid Composition in 100 Grams (3.5 Ounces) Edible Portions of Selected Foods*

| Food | Total Fat (g) | Total Saturated Fat (g) | Total Unsaturated Fat (g) |
|---|---|---|---|
| Avocado | 16.4 | 3.0 | 7.0 |
| **Beef products** | | | |
| T-bone steak, broiled | 43.2 | 18.0 | 22.7 |
| Rib roast, cooked | 39.4 | 19.0 | 18.0 |
| Sirloin steak, broiled | 34.7 | 15.0 | 15.0 |
| Rump roast, cooked | 27.3 | 13.0 | 13.0 |
| Hamburger, regular | 20.3 | 10.0 | 9.0 |
| Hamburger, lean | 11.3 | 6.0 | 5.0 |
| Flank steak, cooked | 7.3 | 4.0 | 3.0 |
| **Bread, cereal, grains** | | | |
| Popcorn, buttered | 21.8 | 10.0 | 10.0 |
| Biscuits, baking powder | 17.0 | 4.0 | 11.0 |
| Wheat germ | 11.5 | 2.0 | 9.0 |
| Corn bread | 8.4 | 1.0 | 2.0 |
| Pancakes, waffles | 7.4 | 3.0 | 4.0 |
| Oat flakes cereal | 5.7 | 1.0 | 4.1 |
| Hamburger bun | 5.4 | 1.0 | 4.0 |
| Bulgur (cooked) | 3.3 | .5 | 2.0 |
| White enriched bread | 3.2 | 1.0 | 2.0 |
| Whole wheat bread | 3.0 | 1.0 | 2.0 |
| Raisin bread | 2.8 | 1.0 | 2.0 |
| Shredded wheat cereal | 2.0 | .3 | 1.5 |
| Oatmeal (cooked) | 1.0 | .2 | .8 |
| Rice, brown, cooked | .6 | .2 | .4 |
| Rice, white, cooked | .2 | .1 | .1 |
| **Dairy products** | | | |
| Butter | 81.0 | 46.0 | 29.0 |
| Heavy whipping cream | 37.6 | 21.0 | 12.0 |
| Cream cheese | 37.6 | 21.0 | 13.0 |
| Cheddar cheese | 32.2 | 18.0 | 12.0 |
| Brick & blue cheese | 30.5 | 18.0 | 12.0 |
| Processed American cheese | 30.0 | 15.0 | 10.0 |
| Swiss cheese | 28.0 | 15.0 | 10.0 |
| Powdered cream substitute | 27.7 | 15.0 | 9.0 |
| Light table cream | 20.6 | 11.0 | 7.0 |
| Vanilla ice cream | 10.6 | 7.0 | 4.0 |
| Milk, sweetened condensed | 8.7 | 4.0 | 3.0 |
| Cottage cheese, creamed | 4.2 | 2.0 | 1.0 |

| Food | Total Fat (g) | Total Saturated Fat (g) | Total Unsaturated Fat (g) |
|---|---|---|---|
| Milk, whole | 3.7 | 2.0 | 1.0 |
| Milk, 2 percent | 2.0 | 1.0 | 1.0 |
| Yogurt, low fat | 1.7 | 2.0 | 1.0 |
| Cottage cheese, uncreamed | .3 | .2 | .1 |
| Milk, skim | .1 | — | — |
| **Eggs** | | | |
| Fried, in butter | 17.2 | 6.0 | 8.0 |
| Scrambled | 12.9 | 4.0 | 6.9 |
| Hard-boiled, poached | 11.5 | 4.0 | 5.9 |
| **Fish and seafood** | | | |
| Herring, Atlantic | 16.4 | 2.9 | 11.6 |
| Salmon, broiled | 13.4 | 4.0 | 4.0 |
| Ocean perch, fried | 13.3 | 1.6 | 7.0 |
| Mackerel, canned | 11.1 | 3.0 | 6.5 |
| Trout, lake | 10.0 | 2.0 | 6.0 |
| Salmon, canned | 9.3 | 3.0 | 3.0 |
| Bass, baked | 8.5 | 2.0 | 2.6 |
| Tuna, canned in oil | 8.2 | 3.0 | 2.0 |
| Halibut, broiled | 7.0 | 1.4 | 4.2 |
| Haddock, fried | 6.4 | 1.0 | .3 |
| Tuna, fresh | 4.1 | 1.0 | 1.0 |
| Clams, canned | 2.5 | .8 | 1.8 |
| Oysters, raw | 2.2 | 1.0 | 2.0 |
| Crab, cooked | 1.9 | .4 | 1.5 |
| Scallops, steamed | 1.4 | .4 | .1 |
| Shrimp, boiled | 1.2 | .2 | .8 |
| Red snapper | .9 | .2 | .4 |
| Cod, Atlantic | .7 | .1 | .4 |
| **Lamb and veal** | | | |
| Shoulder of lamb, roasted | 27.2 | 12.8 | 12.9 |
| Leg of lamb, roasted | 18.9 | 8.9 | 8.9 |
| Veal cutlet, broiled | 11.1 | 6.0 | 5.0 |
| **Nuts and snacks** | | | |
| Pecans | 71.2 | 5.0 | 59.0 |
| Walnuts, English | 64.0 | 4.0 | 50.0 |
| Walnuts, black | 59.3 | 4.0 | 49.0 |
| Almonds, roasted | 57.7 | 5.0 | 51.0 |
| Pistachios | 53.7 | 5.0 | 45.0 |
| Peanut butter | 50.6 | 9.0 | 39.0 |
| Peanuts, roasted | 48.7 | 11.0 | 35.0 |
| Sunflower seeds, roasted | 47.0 | 6.0 | 39.0 |
| Cashews, roasted | 45.7 | 9.2 | 33.8 |
| Potato chips | 39.8 | 10.0 | 28.0 |
| Coconut, fresh | 35.3 | 30.0 | 2.0 |

| Food | Total Fat (g) | Total Saturated Fat (g) | Total Unsaturated Fat (g) |
|---|---|---|---|
| Olives, ripe | 20.1 | 2.0 | 16.0 |
| Crackers, saltine | 12.0 | 3.0 | 8.0 |
| **Pies and cakes, candy, desserts** | | | |
| Milk chocolate candy, nuts | 38.1 | 15.7 | 20.0 |
| Brownies with nuts | 31.3 | 7.0 | 22.0 |
| Chocolate chip cookies | 30.1 | 8.0 | 20.0 |
| Pound cake | 29.5 | 7.0 | 20.0 |
| Doughnuts, raised | 26.7 | 6.0 | 19.0 |
| Macaroons | 23.2 | 16.9 | 6.0 |
| Pecan pie | 22.9 | 4.0 | 6.0 |
| Doughnuts, cake type | 18.6 | 4.0 | 13.0 |
| Fudge, chocolate with nuts | 17.4 | 6.0 | 11.0 |
| Chocolate cake with chocolate icing | 16.4 | 5.0 | 7.0 |
| Oatmeal cookies, raisins | 15.4 | 4.0 | 11.0 |
| Fruitcake, dark | 15.3 | 3.3 | 10.5 |
| Cream puffs with custard | 13.9 | 4.0 | 9.0 |
| Chocolate meringue pie | 12.0 | 3.0 | 8.0 |
| Apple pie | 11.1 | 3.0 | 8.0 |
| Gingerbread | 10.7 | 3.0 | 8.0 |
| Caramel candy | 10.2 | 5.6 | 4.2 |
| Strawberry pie | 7.9 | 3.0 | 8.0 |
| Sponge cake | 5.7 | 2.0 | 2.0 |
| **Pork products** | | | |
| Bacon, fried | 52.0 | 17.0 | 30.0 |
| Pork sausage, fresh | 44.2 | 16.0 | 23.0 |
| Spareribs | 39.9 | 14.0 | 19.0 |
| Ham, dry, long cure | 35.0 | 13.0 | 18.0 |
| Deviled ham, canned | 32.3 | 12.0 | 17.0 |
| Smoked sausage | 31.9 | 11.0 | 16.0 |

| Food | Total Fat (g) | Total Saturated Fat (g) | Total Unsaturated Fat (g) |
|---|---|---|---|
| Pork chops, broiled | 31.7 | 10.0 | 13.0 |
| Ham, fresh, baked | 30.6 | 11.0 | 12.0 |
| Pork roast | 28.5 | 10.0 | 13.0 |
| Chopped ham luncheon meat | 24.9 | 9.0 | 13.0 |
| Ham, light cure | 22.1 | 8.0 | 12.0 |
| Pork liver, fried | 11.5 | 3.0 | 5.0 |
| Poultry | | | |
| Chicken, dark meat, cooked | 9.7 | 2.7 | 5.6 |
| Turkey, dark meat, cooked | 5.3 | 1.6 | 2.9 |
| Chicken, light meat, cooked | 3.5 | 1.0 | 1.8 |
| Turkey, light meat, cooked | 2.6 | .7 | 1.3 |
| Salad and cooking oils | | | |
| Coconut | 100.0 | 86.0 | 8.0 |
| Cottonseed | 100.0 | 26.1 | 69.6 |
| Peanut | 100.0 | 17.0 | 78.0 |
| Sesame | 100.0 | 15.2 | 80.5 |
| Olive | 100.0 | 14.2 | 81.5 |
| Corn | 100.0 | 12.7 | 82.9 |
| Sunflower | 100.0 | 10.2 | 84.7 |
| Safflower | 100.0 | 9.4 | 86.3 |
| Spreads | | | |
| Butter | 81.0 | 46.0 | 29.0 |
| Margarine (⅓ vegetable, ⅔ animal) | 81.0 | 18.0 | 61.0 |
| Margarine (all vegetable fat) | 80.3 | 14.2 | 62.3 |
| Mayonnaise | 79.9 | 14.0 | 57.0 |
| Margarine, diet | 38.5 | 7.0 | 30.1 |
| Vegetable fats (household shortening) | 100.0 | 25.0 | 70.0 |

* Total fat and fatty acid values were derived from different sources and brands. Check your package for more specific values of the product you are using.

TABLE
5–3

# Cholesterol Content in One-Ounce Edible Portions of Selected Foods*

| Food | Cholesterol (mg) |
|---|---|
| Brains, raw | 572.0 |
| Egg yolks, fresh | 429.0 |
| Chicken livers, cooked | 233.0 |
| Kidneys, cooked | 229.0 |
| Egg, whole, fresh | 157.0 |
| Sweetbreads (thymus), cooked | 133.0 |
| Liver, beef and pork, cooked | 125.0 |
| Caviar or roe | 103.0 |
| Ladyfingers | 101.0 |
| Heart, beef, cooked | 78.0 |
| Butter | 72.0 |
| Sponge cake | 71.0 |
| Pie, lemon chiffon | 48.0 |
| Cheese soufflé | 48.0 |
| Shrimp, boiled | 43.0 |
| Popovers | 42.0 |
| Sardines, canned in oil | 40.0 |
| Heavy whipping cream | 38.0 |
| Cream cheese | 32.0 |
| Custard, baked | 30.0 |
| Turkey, cooked | 30.0 |
| Crab, canned | 29.0 |
| Cheese, Swiss | 29.0 |
| Lamb or veal, cooked | 28.0 |
| Cheese, cheddar | 28.0 |

| Food | Cholesterol (mg) |
| --- | --- |
| Beef, cooked | 27.0 |
| Mackerel, canned | 27.0 |
| Chicken, dark meat, cooked | 26.0 |
| Cheese, brick | 26.0 |
| Pork, cooked | 25.0 |
| Cheese, blue | 25.0 |
| Brownies, with nuts | 24.0 |
| Lobster, cooked | 24.0 |
| Chicken, white meat, cooked | 23.0 |
| Pancakes | 21.0 |
| Mayonnaise | 20.0 |
| Corn bread | 20.0 |
| Sour cream | 19.0 |
| Tuna in oil, drained | 19.0 |
| Frankfurter, raw | 19.0 |
| Clams, canned | 18.0 |
| Oysters, cod, flounder, halibut | 14.0 |
| Ice cream | 14.0 |
| Margarine ($\frac{2}{3}$ animal fat) | 14.0 |
| Chocolate cake with icing | 13.0 |
| Cream, half and half | 13.0 |
| Scallops or salmon, raw | 10.0 |
| Ice milk | 6.0 |
| Milk, whole | 4.0 |
| Milk, 2%; low fat cottage cheese | 3.0 |
| Yogurt, low fat, plain | 2.0 |
| Milk, skim | 0.6 |

*Cholesterol values were derived from different sources and brands. Check your package for more specific values of the product you are using.

TABLE
5-4

# High-Risk Diet for Those with High Cholesterol Levels That Do Not Respond Adequately to the Prudent Diet

**1**   Avoid overweight, as in the prudent diet.

**2**   Increase your consumption of complex carbohydrates (fruits, vegetables, grains) to about half (48 percent) of total caloric intake, as in the prudent diet.

**3**   Decrease refined sugar and other processed sugar to about 10 percent of total calories, as in the prudent diet.

**4**   Decrease total fat intake to 30 percent of calories, as in the prudent diet.

**5**   Reduce saturated fat and take twice as much polyunsaturated fat (P/S = 2/1), as in the prudent diet.

**6**   Reduce cholesterol to 100–200 mg; this is lower than in the prudent diet.

**7**   Reduce salt consumption to about 5 grams per day, as in the prudent diet.

TABLE
5-5

# High-Risk Diet for Those with High Triglyceride Levels That Do Not Respond Adequately to the Prudent Diet

**1**   Reduce weight to the lower limits of the desirable weight range for your frame size (e.g., 150 pounds for 5-foot 10-inch man of medium frame).

**2**   Maintain complex carbohydrate consumption (fruits, vegetables, whole grains) at a level of about 40 percent of calories (135 to 285 grams depending on your weight and caloric intake). Note that this is lower than in the prudent diet, but higher than in the average American diet today.

**3** Eliminate as much as possible refined sugars and processed foods high in sugar—certainly hold this to less than 5 percent of calories. Again this is lower than in the prudent diet.

**4** Total calories from fat need not be reduced to 30 percent as in the prudent diet. Fat is not restricted (except for weight loss) in the *usual* form of high triglycerides.

**5** Saturated fat is reduced in the same way as in the prudent diet (i.e., twice as much polyunsaturated fat should be used as saturated: P/S = 2/1).

**6** Reduce cholesterol to 300 mg—the same as in the prudent diet.

**7** Salt consumption should be decreased to about 5 grams per day, as in the prudent diet.

TABLE 5-6

## High-Risk Diet for Those Who Have Both High Cholesterol and High Triglycerides That Do Not Respond Adequately to the Prudent Diet

**1** Reduce weight to the lower limits of the desirable weight range for your frame size (e.g., 150 pounds for 5-foot 10-inch man of medium frame).

**2** Maintain complex carbohydrate consumption (fruits, vegetables, grains) at about half (48 percent) of total calories, as in the prudent diet.

**3** Eliminate as much as possible refined sugars and processed foods high in sugar—certainly hold this to less than 5 percent of calories. This is lower than in the prudent diet.

**4** Decrease total fat intake to 30 percent of calories, as in the prudent diet.

**5** Reduce saturated fat, as done in the other diets, to the point that twice as much polyunsaturated fat is consumed as saturated (P/S = 2/1).

**6** Reduce cholesterol to 100–200 miligrams per day, much lower than in the prudent diet.

**7** Reduce salt intake to 5 grams a day, as in the prudent diet.

TABLE
5-7

# Hints on Lowering Intake of Cholesterol and Saturated Fats

**1**  Foods of *plant origin* do not contain cholesterol and, except for coconut and palm oils, saturated fats are not high in plants. (However, vegetable oils may be artificially saturated or "hardened" by hydrogenation.) Use natural unprocessed foods of plant origin liberally.

**2**  Foods of *animal origin,* eggs, meats, and dairy products, are generally high in cholesterol and saturated fats. Eggs and organ meats are the highest in cholesterol. Shrimp is high in cholesterol, but low in fat. Use animal products sparingly, and for those you use, discard the high fat, high cholesterol portions, such as with eggs.

  **a**  Discard egg yolks.

  **b**  Do not eat organ meats (liver, kidney, brain, heart).

  **c**  Buy only the leanest meats (round steak instead of hamburger) and trim all visible fat away. Three ounces of lean red meat (cooked weight—or 4 ounces uncooked) three times per week is your allotment if you are at high risk.

  **d**  Protein-rich foods are usually taken at least twice per day. For your remaining 11 servings instead of meat use the following substitutes: use skinned poultry (the skin is high in cholesterol and fat), preferably chicken or turkey white meat. (Avoid duck and goose—too fatty.) Use white fish. (But avoid lobster and shrimp and go easy on other shellfish.) Use low fat, uncreamed cottage cheese and, more cautiously, processed low fat, low cholesterol cheeses, such as Lite-Line. Even those at high risk may use Parmesan, mozzarella (part skim), and ricotta (part skim) in moderation. Cheddar or Swiss, and other similar cheeses, use no more than 2 ounces per week. Use vegetable proteins such as beans, peas, and "fake meats."

**3**  Totally exclude butter and lard. Avoid palm and coconut oil products (e.g., whipped toppings, some nondairy creamers). Use liquid oils and margarines high in polyunsaturates (especially those that come in tubs). When a recipe requires a hardened oil, use the least saturated forms (e.g., corn oil stick margarine). Stay away from hydrogenated margarines and shortening. Avoid prepared deep-fried foods and fried snack foods.

**4**  Use skim milk, not whole milk, not 2 percent milk. No cream.

**5**  Avoid ice cream, cream pies, commercial cakes, and other sweets made with eggs and fat.

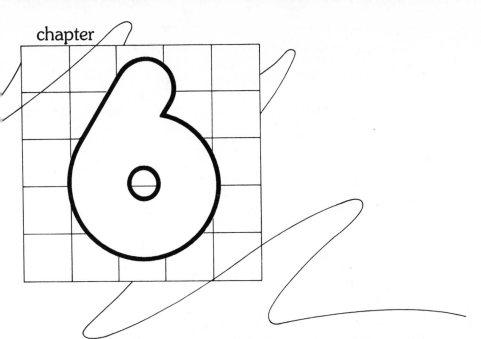

# Warning: The Surgeon General Has Determined...

he chapter title, as I'm sure you recognize, is taken from the routine warning that has been printed on cigarette packs and has appeared in cigarette advertisements for years.

But with the publication of the new report of the Surgeon General on *Smoking and Health* (January 11, 1979), an even stronger and more provocative statement has been made. The report tells us that "smoking is the largest preventable cause of death in America." In fact, *346,000 deaths per year* in the United States are attributed to smoking. The majority of these excess deaths, 225,000, are from cardiovascular diseases; 80,000 deaths are from lung cancer; 22,000 deaths from other cancers; and 19,000 deaths from chronic lung disease. The cause of death of more than one out of every six Americans is smoking. The massive review of thousands of studies presented as the most recent report of the Surgeon General is an impressive indictment.

Let me just fire off some of the findings.

**1** There are about 54 million smokers in the United States.

**2** While smoking in men has declined from 53 percent in 1964 to 38 percent in 1978, it has not declined comparably in women, but has remained at about 30 percent.

**3** "Women who smoke like men die like men who smoke." Lung cancer has increased fivefold among women since 1955.

**4** The percentage of girls aged 12 to 14 who smoke has increased eightfold since 1968. We are now experiencing what could be termed a smoking epidemic among teenage girls. Among youngsters of both sexes, 18 years and younger, there are currently over 6 million regular smokers (100,000 regular smokers are 12 years and younger). One out of three youngsters is a regular smoker by age 18.

**5** Evidence is accumulating that smoking during pregnancy has an adverse effect on the developing fetus, the newborn infant, and the growing child.

**6** Children who do not smoke but are subjected to the smoke of parents and others have more respiratory illnesses than those children not so exposed.

**7** Children who do smoke are more likely to smoke if their parents and older siblings do. And they are more likely to get hooked for life if they start as youngsters. Mortality rates from all causes are significantly higher among those who start smoking early in life. Hardening of the arteries (atherosclerosis) in the coronary arteries and aorta is positively associated with cigarette smoking, and premature atherosclerosis is associated with early initiation of smoking.

**8** The risk of heart attack is ten times greater in women who both smoke and use oral contraceptives.

**9** Blue-collar workers are susceptible to increased risk from the combined effects of smoking and toxic industrial agents (e.g., asbestos, rubber, various dusts).

**10** Minority groups smoke more and have higher death rates.

**11** The bill for the health damage caused by smoking costs this country approximately $27 billion a year.

The foregoing was just some of the bad news. Selected items will be amplified in this chapter. Some of the good news is:

**1**    Thirty million Americans have stopped smoking since the first Surgeon General's report on the health hazards of smoking, published in 1964. Even mulish doctors have gotten the message—64 percent of smoking doctors have stopped smoking (one of the highest quit rates I know).

**2**    If you stop smoking and live for 15 years after stopping, your death rate becomes the same as that of someone who has never smoked.

## Smoking Hazards to Health Other Than Cardiovascular Disease _____

Although this book is concerned with diseases of the heart and blood vessels, I'd be derelict in my responsibility to you if I didn't point out some of the very serious consequences of smoking as it affects health in general. First, death rates, *no matter what the cause of death,* are higher in smokers than in nonsmokers. For example, middle-aged smokers (ages 35 to 54 years) have a death rate from all causes that is 2.6 times greater than that found in nonsmokers. (The death rate from coronary heart disease in this age group is 4.7 times higher in smokers than in nonsmokers.)

Cancer is the second largest disease category in which smoking plays a major role. If it were not for smoking, certain common cancers, such as cancer of the lung, would be quite rare. Between 90 and 95 percent of the approximately 90,000 annual deaths from lung cancer in America are directly attributable to cigarette smoking. You should also know that only 10 percent of lung cancer victims live for five years after the diagnosis is first made. In fact, 70 percent of lung cancer patients die within a year of their diagnosis. Cancer of the throat is another smoking-related disease—about 3,500 deaths were estimated for 1978. Almost all cancer of the throat is in smokers. Cancer of the mouth was estimated to cause 8,400 deaths in 1978—and again the great majority of deaths were in smokers. We can go on down the line with the cancers of the esophagus, kidney, bladder, and pancreas. Smoking has been implicated in all of these.

Peptic ulcer is found almost twice as often among smokers as nonsmokers. Chronic lung disease (e.g., bronchitis, emphysema), highly associated with cigarette smoking, is second only to coronary heart disease as a cause of Social Security–compensated disability. The lung disease may be long-term and severely disabling, characterized by a constant, exhausting struggle just to breathe. Cigarette smoking is calculated to be responsible for 19,000 deaths each year in this group.

As I reread the previous few paragraphs, there's a tone that could be interpreted by some as scare tactics. I know scare tactics are largely ineffective, so I'm trying to avoid that approach. A simple statement of the evidence is what I'm striving to achieve, while resisting, as far as I'm able, too much editorializing.

## Pregnancy and Infant Health

For over a century there has been concern voiced about the potential hazards of tobacco to the pregnant woman and her developing fetus. However, it has been during the past decade that evidence has accumulated most rapidly. In fairness it should be noted that there has also been a certain amount of controversy regarding the effects of smoking during pregnancy. The weight of evidence is overwhelming that maternal smoking during pregnancy decreases fetal growth, yielding babies who weigh less, have smaller heads, and are shorter. Recent studies have also shown that the death rates in infancy and early childhood are increased among offspring of smoking mothers. A very recent study also suggests that malformations so severe that they cause fetal death more often than infant death are found in the miscarriages and premature infants born to smoking mothers. An enzyme called aryl hydrocarbon hydroxylase appears to be stimulated by smoking and may play a role in both the development of cancer and malformations. Illnesses in infancy and childhood are increased, and physical and mental development appear to be impaired in the children of smokers.

## Smoking and Cardiovascular Disease

I've used the terms *hardening of the arteries, atherosclerosis and arteriosclerosis* almost interchangeably. This is a good place to tell you that both atherosclerosis and arteriosclerosis produce hardening of the arteries, but arteriosclerosis is a more general term encompassing several processes. Atherosclerosis is the more specific term for the type of lesion that is most often associated with heart attacks, involves the lining of the artery, and is usually associated with fat deposits. A number of studies show cigarette smoking to be associated with increased prevalence and extent of atherosclerosis in coronary arteries in humans. Cigarette smoking is also strongly associated as an independent risk factor in heart attacks. The more you smoke, the greater the risk. This is what is called "dose related" or "dose response."

All of the precise mechanisms through which smoking produces heart attacks are not yet elucidated. Smoking appears to lower the protective HDL and to raise the damaging LDL cholesterol. *But smoking also contributes to heart attacks in people whose coronary arteries do not show advanced hardening.* Four of the possible mechanisms may be pointed out. Smoking is thrombogenic, that is, it is capable of stimulating the formation of blood clots that could participate in plugging up arteries. Next, smoking, with its production of carbon monoxide, deprives the heart muscle of the oxygen it needs to work (and to survive). Smoking may produce immunologic injury (as in hypersensitivity or very severe allergic reaction) to the blood vessels and conducting system of the heart. Finally and potentially the most important mechanism of smoking injury is spasm. Smoking may cause coronary arteries to clamp shut in spasm, even though the arteries themselves may appear to be relatively healthy.

Cigarette smoking is a risk factor for problems involving blood vessels other than the coronary arteries. Atherosclerosis of the major artery of the body—the aorta and the blood vessels of the brain and limbs—is also accelerated by smoking. Smokers also have a higher cholesterol level than nonsmokers. Women taking oral contraceptives have a 6 times greater risk of having a stroke and twice the risk for heart attack as compared with those not on the Pill. But when you add smoking to the equation, the risk of stroke is 20 times greater and the risk of heart attacks is 10 times greater.

In the 15 years that have elapsed between the first and second reports of the Surgeon General on the dangers of smoking, it has become incontrovertibly evident that smoking is not only a major contributing factor in cardiovascular disease, but is the most striking, preventable, environmental hazard causing death and disability in America. The Surgeon General's second report confirms this.

# Young Children and Other Innocent Bystanders

Unfortunately, it's not just the smoker whose health is endangered by his habit, but the people around him (or her). For the bystanders, this is termed "involuntary smoking." Some more of the jargon of smoking are the categories of "mainstream" smoke (that smoke sucked through the tobacco by the smoker) and "sidestream" smoke (the smoke given off into the air by the burning tobacco). Certain constituents of tobacco smoke are much higher in mainstream than in sidestream. And one particularly noxious constituent, carbon monoxide, is best absorbed by directly inhaling mainstream smoke. Cyanide is another poison that comes through mainstream in greater concentration than in sidestream.

However, there's a paradox here: Most of the pollutants from tobacco are in higher concentration in sidestream smoke. Thus, while the innocent bystander gets a relatively lower concentration of smoke (unless he's in a room that is literally smoke-filled), the smoke he does breathe has a higher concentration of nicotine, tar, aniline, dimethyl nitrosamine, and all those other destructive agents. Even carbon monoxide, which is best absorbed by inhaling, is still present in higher concentration in sidestream than in mainstream smoke. From the point of view of the health of your heart, if you have to breathe in an enclosed space filled with cigarette smoke, you'll find that you're inhaling a substantial dose of carbon monoxide and nicotine, both of which have been implicated in the development of atherosclerosis. Measurements have been made of significant increases in the blood carbon monoxide and in the urinary excretion of nicotine from nonsmokers cooped up with smokers.

Obviously the smoker gets much more sidestream as well as mainstream smoke, by the very act of having a cigarette around his face. But if you're a nonsmoker, you must beware of closed spaces. Commercial airplanes used to represent a real health disaster when the food trays included giveaway cigarettes, so that even some nonsmokers lit up in self defense. Now with no more giveaways and separate seating for nonsmokers, there's a little better opportunity to breathe.

The immediate effects on the nonsmoker of involuntary exposure to cigarette smoke run the gamut from eye irritation (69 percent), headache (32 percent), nasal irritation (29 percent), and cough (25 percent). These symptoms may be classified anywhere from annoying to distressing. But there's another possible immediate effect noted in the Surgeon General's report that is quite serious. Some individuals with coronary heart disease experience angina (the chest pain that may precede heart attack) when exposed to the cigarette smoking of others. So if you have coronary heart disease, don't get yourself trapped in smoke-filled spaces.

Children may be more susceptible to air pollutants than adults due to their greater breathing capacity for their body weight. Kids who are trapped in houses, apartments, and family cars with smoking parents have more respiratory illness than those whose parents don't smoke. This is a short-term effect, and one can only project what the long-term effect may be of this constant low dose of tobacco smoke exposure as it relates to cancer and heart disease.

## Older Children

As was pointed out earlier, 30 million Americans have kicked the cigarette habit. But this is not causing the tobacco industry to weep briny tears. There's always a new hooked generation to replace the old. Teenage boys smoke as much now as they did when the first Surgeon General's report was published in 1964. But more frightening is that teenage girls are smoking much more than they did before the public health warning was issued.

Children under 10 to 12 years of age often have an evangelical zeal against smoking. They delight in lecturing their parents, and act for all the world like they'd never fall into the same trap. Then they become teenagers, and they take up the habit. Why? The first influence in order of importance appears to be parental smoking. After years of exposure to smoking and hearing excuses for smoking, even kids who were once strongly against smoking succumb. (Smoking can't be all that bad—Mom and Dad are still alive.) The next most important influence is older siblings, and then peer pressure.

Mass media appear to exert considerable influence. Although television and radio advertising by the tobacco industry has been banned, the money has been transferred to magazines, newspapers, billboards, and so on. Then there is the image of smoking in movies and television. Exciting and interesting people doing exciting and interesting things are portrayed as smokers.

Although some surveys show that teenagers deny the importance of the "forbidden fruit" motivation, adults should easily be able to remember back to the teenage years and appreciate this contributing factor. If maturity and smoking are seen as being related, kids can feel that they're more mature if they smoke. But if the image can be conveyed that mature, competent, and confident people don't smoke and don't need to smoke—that true maturity and *not smoking* are what are related—then the unfortunate association may be undercut. But there's always the value of smoking as an act of rebellion. The teenager seeking his own identity needs to defy authority to some extent. Regrettably, the hypocrisy that surrounds smoking in the adult world makes this an ideal forum for defiance.

What we really need to recognize about smoking in relationship to children is the system of rewards that goes into establishing a habit that on the surface is both unpleasant and self-destructive. We'll get into that in the section on why anybody (including a kid) smokes.

There are a few more problems that are pertinent to children. The age of onset of smoking continues to decrease. And the earlier you start to smoke, the more likely you are to become addicted. In 1968, about 6 percent of kids between 12 and 14 years old smoked. In 1974, the rate had doubled to 12 percent of children at this early age who were *regular* smokers. As strange as it may seem, over three-quarters of teenagers who smoke feel that it is bad for them and wish they had never started. Most teenagers believe that smoking is habit-forming but—here's the hooker—the majority do not feel that they themselves are becoming addicted. Or that if addiction occurred, it would not represent an imminent threat to their health. Children and young adults can look around them and see that their parents and friends who smoke are not immediately dropping over on the spot with heart attacks or lung cancer. What may happen to you when you are "old" has no relevance to those who live in the present day of instant-on.

## Smoking Behavior

**Why Anyone Starts to Smoke and Why Anyone Has Difficulty Stopping** ○ In Chapter 3 we spent some time on how habits are established through rewards and punishments. We've discussed dietary habits and will talk about habits of exercise in subsequent chapters. But with smoking we get into the big leagues of habits. Here we have to start talking about addiction (or dependence, if that word sounds better).

First, there's something about the chemistry of tobacco itself that reinforces its use. Many studies of why people continue to smoke come under a behavioral model, the *nicotine addiction model.* Like Shakespeare's Cleopatra, tobacco creates an appetite that only it can satisfy. The something in tobacco that does this is probably nicotine, and possibly some other ingredients. Certainly, nicotine-free tobacco substitutes, like lettuce leaves, don't seem to have the same effect. Evidence has been piling up during the past decade that tobacco is a bona fide "dependence-producing substance" complete with a withdrawal syndrome. Those who are dependent on nicotine have a certain tolerance of tension and anxiety, but it's probable that nicotine doesn't actually reduce anxiety or "calm the nerves." It appears that the calming effect of smoking is mainly due to relieving the withdrawal symptoms of *not smoking.*

Various symptoms have been attributed to the tobacco withdrawal syndrome, and these include headache, nausea, irritability, drowsiness, fatigue, insomnia, diarrhea, constipation, and increased appetite. Inability to concentrate is frequently reported. While these symptoms are not as dramatic as those found in heroin withdrawal, ex-smokers report that they are unpleasant enough to add a significant burden to their efforts to break the habit. My belief is that if a smoker is forewarned and prepared for what to expect from withdrawal, he will be much better able to cope with his problem.

The *social learning model* of smoking has received major attention in studies of why people start smoking and in intervention programs to terminate smoking. Back to Pavlov's dogs and Skinner's pigeons. Habits may become established through rewards and punishments, but how can a punishing habit become established? We all know that the first cigarettes smoked are usually unpleasant. However, if smoked in the environment of greater rewards (social approval, esteem income, role modeling, presumed self-realization, peer pressure, and so on), the unpleasantness of smoking is an easily surmountable obstacle. Think of exercise. At the very beginning there may be a few aches and pains, but if we keep in mind that soon we'll be feeling better for having become involved in exercise, the aches become quite bearable. So smoking itself can become the positive reinforcement for smoking, just as exercise can become its own reinforcement.

The behavioral theory may now get a little more difficult to follow. But what happens is that cigarette smoking becomes associated with many activities and emotions. When you are having a cup of coffee and a pleasant chat with friends, the cigarette becomes part of the ritual of friendship. And there's the old Army motto: "Take ten and smoke 'em if you've got 'em." After a couple of hours of painful physical activity, here comes a much-needed rest. And with the welcome rest comes a cigarette. As I've noted before, advertising agencies understand the behavioral principles involved. So they try to associate smoking with green meadows, sparkling brooks, and liberation. In order to change smoking behavior, there must be an understanding of how the behavior became established.

Smoking, while initially unpleasant and ultimately destructive, can take place as a pleasurable experience for many years without immediately noticeable adverse consequences. Steady-state behavior is said to exist, a dynamic equilibrium between positive reinforcement and negative withdrawal symptoms. Anything that happens in the environment that has previously been associated with smoking becomes a cue for lighting up. The cup of coffee, the glass of beer, the welcome break in tedious routine, tension, anger, anxiety, socialization. Out come the cigarettes—the reward, the relief. And the ultimate punishment is too far away to worry about.

# Strategies Against Smoking

There are two categories of people and two strategies to consider in reducing the enormous impact of smoking on the health of the nation. The first category includes individuals who have not yet started smoking or are just beginning to smoke. The strategy for such people is education. It is assumed that an intelligent, reasonably well-adjusted individual is able to respond positively to a clear presentation of the problem that smoking represents. Education includes the example and influence of others. If someone doesn't start smoking by the time he hits his mid-twenties, the battle is won. The second category of smokers encompasses the so-called dependent smokers—the addicted, the hooked. The strategy here is psychosocial intervention.

In the second category of concern, there are certain characteristics common to those who are successful in stopping smoking. The successful ex-smokers are:

1   Low on neuroticism and nervous oral habits

2   Low on extraversion, sociability, and need for arousal

3   Low on anxiety and worries

4   High on need for achievement

5   High on internal (rather than external) orientation—inner-directed rather than other-directed

6   High on personal adjustment and life satisfaction.

The personalities of those who are likely to fail to stop smoking would of course be the opposite of those who succeed. They would be high on neuroticism, low on need for achievement, other-directed, and so on. In addition they are more likely to be: female, younger, lower in education, and heavy smokers who started smoking early in life. They are more likely to list the cost of smoking as a more important reason for stopping than health.

Many other features have been observed in those who are successful in stopping smoking:

1   Having higher education

2   Coming from a higher socioeconomic level

3   Having many friends who are nonsmokers and fewer friends who are smokers

| **4** | Church-going |
|---|---|
| **5** | Knowing someone whose health was adversely affected by smoking |
| **6** | Having children in the household |
| **7** | Being married (men only) |
| **8** | Starting smoking late |
| **9** | Light smoking |
| **10** | Having personal adverse health effects from smoking (e.g., cough) |
| **11** | *But the strongest of all influences in causing individuals to stop smoking is having a heart attack.* This event is a frightening experience, which relates clearly to smoking. And there's no smoking allowed in a coronary care unit. So by the time a patient is discharged he or she has gone through the withdrawal syndrome, with a lot more to occupy thoughts and concerns than the next cigarette. |

We've had tests in many of the other chapters, so we'll go through one here (Table 6–1) on the assumption that if a smoker understands some of the reasons why he smokes he may be able to attack specific aspects of his personal problem. Obviously, if you're not a smoker, skip the test. This particular test is slightly modified from one designed by Daniel Horn, Ph.D., director of the National Clearing House for Smoking and Health, Public Health Service, and is based on a model developed by Silvan Tomkins, Ph.D.

Those of you who have now taken the test are alerted to some of the reasons underlying your smoking habit. It's consistent with what we know about behavior modification to find a substitute desirable behavior to replace an undesirable behavior (i.e., smoking). The trick then is when the usual cue for smoking presents itself, to be prepared to give a substitute response. For example, if handling the cigarette is an important part of your habit, put something else where you usually carry your cigarettes. When you reach for your cigarettes, you should always find the cigarette substitute—a pen and small pad of paper for doodling is often effective.

Let's take the six items on the score card in Table 6–1, one at a time. You may have scored high on all the items or only on one or two. The more items you have high scores on, the more your work is cut out for you.

**1) Stimulation** If you need a cigarette to get you going in the morning or to pick you up during the day, the best substitute-stimulator is exercise. This gives you an additional important health benefit while replacing a health hazard. Every time you reach for a cigarette do one or more of your 10–20–30 exercises (see Chapter 9, page 161). Start making the association. Desire for a cigarette becomes the cue to exercise. Head rolls, shoulder shrugs, arm wraps, toe stands. These are nontiring and stimulating—and can be done almost anywhere. If the urge is particularly strong, do more exercises, including pushups or running. These are tiring and can't be done just anywhere, but have even greater conditioning benefits. A cup of tea or a small glass of juice can replace the wake-up cigarette, or be judiciously taken during the day. This drink can be a substitute stimulator, although the person with a two-pack habit can't have 40 cups of tea or 40 glasses of juice.

**2) Handling**   We've already used this as an example. I offered the pen and pad suggestion, but women (and some men) who start feeling anxious when their hands aren't busy may find knitting or crocheting helpful. These items, of course, can't be kept in cigarette pockets. A silver dollar is favored by some, or a medallion, a piece of jewelry. If you're a "handler" find something that's specifically suitable for you and use this substitute for as long as necessary until the handling behavior is extinguished. A file card with reasons not to smoke can do double duty for "handlers."

**3) Relaxation**   Here's a behavioral twist that would appeal to Big Brother's Ministry of Truth. We've already pointed out that cigarettes have been deliberately put into association with relaxing situations, such as "take ten," the coffee break, the end of a satisfying meal, pleasant socialization, green meadows—the whole bit. This is what helped to establish the feeling that an essentially unpleasant activity was a pleasant experience. Thus, when the end of an enjoyable meal comes along, and good conversation continues, cigarettes are lit. I think that for this association what is necessary is to understand the basis for the behavior. It's not the cigarette that makes the meal and the conversation satisfying—it's the meal and the conversation themselves. The cigarette, by irritating your eyes and throat, can actually spoil the pleasant ambience, although some may feel they enjoy the taste of cigarettes. When tempted to light up to "complete" whatever the picture of relaxation may be, say to yourself forcefully: "Don't spoil it." Allow the pleasurable event to stand on its own without adding an artificial association. Use your stimulation substitutes (like a cup of gourmet tea) and your handling substitutes if these are among your needs, but let the pleasurable event stand on its own without spoiling it.

**4) Crutch: tension reduction**   This need is in many ways the opposite of the previous one. Here you smoke not when you're feeling relaxed but when you're feeling tense. How did this association come about? We all feel tense and anxious at one time or another. So how does smoking get into the picture? There are plenty of possible explanations. The stimulation and handling and the conditioned association with pleasur-

**116**

able events can all contribute. Then there's the association with the syndrome of withdrawal—which includes anxiety and tension. If cigarette smoking relieves the tension of withdrawal, why shouldn't it be worth trying for any kind of tension? Well, except for the tension of withdrawal, a cigarette has no value beyond minor and transient distraction. You must keep that fact in mind. You should also try to minimize the struggle with the conditioned association between tension reduction and smoking. So you can see that it might not be productive to decide to stop smoking when you're filling out your income tax. If your life appears to be constantly tense, you'll just have to pick the time that's slightly less tense, and get on with it.

**5) Craving: addiction**   This is the tough one. Many smokers do not have a strong addiction, but for those who do, you're going to suffer when you stop. You'd better be as emotionally and physiologically prepared for it as possible. The craving appears to be as bad and to last longer when you stop after tapering gradually than when you stop cold turkey. If you taper gradually you go through withdrawal for as long as you're tapering. Those who have looked into this problem contend that the symptoms of withdrawal can be severe for as long as the tapering lasts. Many programs advocate the cold-turkey method of stopping for those strongly addicted. The craving will be most intense the first two days and will diminish over the remainder of the week. For the other five categories of reasons why people smoke, the recommendation would be to stop smoking in your usual work and living environment. For those strongly addicted you may need to take a week off, a family vacation with all the members of the family supporting you while you fight your personal battle. A lot of exercise and diversion during this period will be essential. Further recommendations regarding the cold-turkey method will follow in a few paragraphs.

**6) Habit**   Smoking cigarettes is like driving a car or riding a bicycle or opening a refrigerator door when you enter the kitchen. The behavior follows a pattern that becomes so automatic that a thought process does not appear to intervene. Why shouldn't it be automatic? If you're just a pack-a-day smoker, you light up 7,300 times a year. There are very few behaviors you can think of that are repeated that many times. And all of this lighting up is cued from routine activities and emotions with which smoking has become associated. This means you've got to deliberately set out to break the patterns. Think of it in terms of a golf or tennis stroke that you've been doing wrong for years. You've got to get your brain and nerves and muscles to follow a new path—to unlearn the old stroke and replace it with a new stroke. So for a while don't take your coffee break in the same place, don't sit in your usual chair to watch TV, do get up immediately after eating—substitute a new environment of cues. Whenever you reach for a cigarette, look around you and see what set off the Pavlovian dog-salivation behavior. (That's the level you're functioning at, you know, when you reach for a cigarette.) If the environmental cues are such that they can be avoided, do it. Avoid places and situations that call for a cigarette response. If the environment can't be avoided, have a substitute ready—something different to associate with that particular environment. For example, maybe you've always wanted to learn another language. Have a pocket book ready and pull it out in the cigarette response environment. Learn a few words and put the book away. Make that your Pavlovian substitute for as long as it is necessary. (You may actually even learn a new language. Who knows?)

## Getting Psyched Up to Quit

If you smoke, the little test you've taken has given you some ideas as to why you smoke and some specific points of attack. There are a few more questions that need addressing. We mentioned dose response earlier in the chapter. Most studies are quite clear on the point that the more cigarettes you smoke, the greater your risk. Inhalers appear to have a greater risk than those who don't inhale. Filter tips and low tar cigarettes may be less dangerous. And cigarette smokers seem to be at greater risk for most problems than pipe and cigar smokers, except for cancers of the mouth.

You've also probably been bombarded with TV ads about profit-making and nonprofit programs to help you quit smoking. You can get the idea from the ads that these programs are based on behavior modification. Most are positive modifications of the type I've been discussing. But some are negative modifications—that is, they are based on developing a painful or highly unpleasant association with smoking behavior. "Aversive" is the term for these less desirable negative techniques.

There are also pamphlets and booklets you can obtain from your Heart Association, Lung Association, Cancer Society, and the federal government—all containing step-by-step programs for kicking the habit. You can also attend group programs sponsored by the American Cancer Society. And if you have an Adventist hospital in your area, they have a good group program (which has also been adopted by the Lung Association).

You'd probably like to know how successful these various programs can be. I'll have to be honest with you. Almost all formal programs, with few exceptions, have a quit rate of about 40 percent at the end of the program—and 18 months later, the quit rate is down to only

20 percent. Behavioral psychologists have not taken kindly to this affront to the methods of behavior modification, so they've gone back to the drawing board and have returned with a concept that I discussed with you earlier: *working on habits is not enough.* Internal controls must be present and functioning to make behavior modification succeed. Back to belief systems. You've got to incorporate your new lifestyle into your system of values—your religion.

We rely heavily on behavior modification, through standard psychological techniques, as it relates to cardiovascular health. But if you were asked to choose one method for smoking cessation—behavior modification or an informed and responsible decision (act of will?)— which would you prefer? The data suggest that those who stop on their own, spontaneously, do better and have a lower reversion than those who participate in some formal treatment programs.

There is an ongoing research project in heart disease prevention called the Multiple Risk Factor Intervention Trial (abbreviated MRFIT and usually called Mister Fit) that has run into a totally unexpected snag. Patients judged to be at risk of coronary heart disease have been divided into two groups. In one group, all the stops have been pulled and a truly aggressive, state-of-the-art approach to attacking the risk factors has been followed. Then there's the control group. Obviously, conscience and ethics do not permit allowing the people in the control group to be deceived that a rich diet, no exercise, and smoking are appropriate options of medical management. This control group is called the "usual treatment" group. The people are merely told that they should follow the usual nonaggressive standards of care that are currently being used in many medical practices. They are told that smoking is a significant health hazard, but they are not enrolled in a group program for smoking cessation. They're just given the facts on smoking and allowed to reach their own decision.

So what happened? The control group, on the basis of a presentation of the facts and no other help achieved a long-term quit rate of about 35 percent; this is higher than any of the previous group cessation training programs. The controls were concerned, motivated, and did it all on their own. That's the good news on stopping smoking.

And there's even better news. The high motivation in the MRFIT program *plus* aggressive behavior modification techniques led to an even higher long-term quit rate—about 43 percent. So there's the problem. The control group is stopping smoking almost as well as the aggressive treatment group. Therefore it will be hard to test the effects of smoking when there is so little difference between the two groups. From the point of view of the patient and physician interested in preventive programs, this scientific snag is of less concern. What's enlightening is that through high motivation great changes in behavior can be made. And with internally controlled behavior modification even more can be accomplished.

One other influence on quitting smoking that has been studied should be mentioned: meditation and relaxation training. A group of 2,000 meditators were studied in Boston. Before meditation training 48 percent were smokers; after 21 months of meditation only 16 percent smoked. That puts this group's quit rate even ahead of that of doctors.

## Kicking the Habit

As you can tell, I've been leaning toward the cold-turkey method of quitting, but for those who are not strongly addicted, there is a five-week program that has been as successful as any and is distributed as a brochure from the American Heart Association and your local heart association office. Whatever works for you is what you should follow, including enrolling in a group program. I can only repeat that the best results *seem to be* associated with stopping spontaneously, cold-turkey.

**1.** The first step, as if I hadn't mentioned it many times, is developing the motivation, the inner control. Sit down and go over the reasons not to smoke. Then write down the main reasons that apply to you, your life, and your family. Look at the reasons. Keep them on a card in the place where you would carry your cigarettes. Pull the card out when your habit calls for you to reach for your cigarettes. (If handling is part of your problem, you can use the card for this purpose too, but you'll wear out a few cards before you're through.) The reason for not smoking should always be in front of you and become more and more an important part of your value system.

**2.** Announce your decision to stop smoking to all family members and friends. Ask them to help you with your resolve. Make up a one-sentence contract that you will sign as a binding agreement to stop smoking. Find one or two people who will agree to be partners with you in your efforts, cosigners of your contract. If they are smokers trying to stop at the same time or ex-smokers, all the better. This is an underlying principle in the success of Alcoholics Anonymous. But a loving spouse who has never been a smoker can often be your supportive partner.

**3.** Select your day to quit, based on what you know about your habit. Try not to pick a time when you're under a lot of pressure. And if your score card and your own knowledge of your habit suggest that you have a strong addiction, don't start on a workday. If you can't take a week's vacation, at least start on a weekend. Remember, if you quit smoking away from your usual environment in order to fight addiction better, you'll still have to fight the battle back at work and at home, because the habit-cues will be around you and will need to be extinguished where they are.

**4.** Get your replacement habits all lined up and ready to activate based on what you already know about your smoking behavior and what you determined on your smoker's test. Reread the specific behavior modification techniques suggested in the previous sections. Think of some of your own that might meet your needs even better. Then write the best techniques on another card to have with you at all times. Another card to pull out and read when your habit calls for you to reach for cigarettes.

**5.** Meditate. It would be to your advantage to have already started meditating regularly 20 minutes per day *before* you try to kick the habit. You'll have gained in mind control, and you'll also be able to call on the techniques of meditation when needed to resist the craving. Close your eyes. See the plain white screen in front of you. Breathe deeply, evenly. Exclude all thoughts from your mind. Just follow your breathing. In. Out. Repeat whatever word or sound you've selected for your mantra. Breathe in and out. A minute or two of this exercise will usually suffice and should be available to help you through the most difficult first few days and whenever needed later.

## TABLE 6-1 | Why Do You Smoke?

Here are some statements made by people to describe what they get out of smoking cigarettes. HOW OFTEN do you feel this way when smoking them? Circle one number for each statement. It's necessary that you answer every question.

| | | Always | Frequently | Occasionally | Seldom | Never |
|---|---|---|---|---|---|---|
| A | I smoke cigarettes in order to keep myself from slowing down. | 4 | 3 | 2 | 1 | 0 |
| B | Handling a cigarette is part of the enjoyment of smoking it. | 4 | 3 | 2 | 1 | 0 |
| C | Smoking cigarettes is pleasant and relaxing. | 4 | 3 | 2 | 1 | 0 |
| D | I light up a cigarette when I feel angry about something. | 4 | 3 | 2 | 1 | 0 |
| E | When I have run out of cigarettes I find it almost unbearable until I can get them. | 4 | 3 | 2 | 1 | 0 |
| F | I smoke cigarettes automatically without even being aware of it. | 4 | 3 | 2 | 1 | 0 |
| G | I smoke cigarettes to stimulate me, to perk myself up. | 4 | 3 | 2 | 1 | 0 |
| H | Part of the enjoyment of smoking a cigarette comes from the steps to take to light up. | 4 | 3 | 2 | 1 | 0 |
| I | I find cigarettes pleasurable. | 4 | 3 | 2 | 1 | 0 |
| J | When I feel uncomfortable or upset about something, I light up a cigarette. | 4 | 3 | 2 | 1 | 0 |
| K | I am very much aware of the fact when I am smoking a cigarette. | 4 | 3 | 2 | 1 | 0 |
| L | I light up a cigarette without realizing I still have one burning in the ashtray. | 4 | 3 | 2 | 1 | 0 |
| M | I smoke cigarettes to give me a "lift." | 4 | 3 | 2 | 1 | 0 |
| N | When I smoke a cigarette, part of the enjoyment is watching the smoke as I exhale it. | 4 | 3 | 2 | 1 | 0 |
| O | I want a cigarette most when I am comfortable and relaxed. | 4 | 3 | 2 | 1 | 0 |

**P**  When I feel "blue" or want to take my mind off cares and worries, I smoke cigarettes.

4  3  2  1  0

**Q**  I get a real gnawing hunger for a cigarette when I haven't smoked for a while.

4  3  2  1  0

**R**  I've found a cigarette in my mouth and didn't remember putting it there.

4  3  2  1  0

## Score Card

When you have completed the test, score yourself:

**1**  Take the numbers on the first line and add across; that is, add the numbers for A, G, and M and put the total in the last column.

**2**  Follow the same procedure for each line.

Scores can vary from 0 to 12. Any score 8 and above is high; any score 4 and below is low.

____ + ____ + ____ = _____
A       G       M                    Stimulation

____ + ____ + ____ = _____
B       H       N                    Handling

____ + ____ + ____ = _____
C       I       O                    Pleasurable Relaxation

____ + ____ + ____ = _____
D       J       P                    Crutch: Tension Reduction

____ + ____ + ____ = _____
E       K       Q                    Craving: Addiction

____ + ____ + ____ = _____
F       L       R                    Habit

*This material is repeated for you to fill out in the Tear-Out Appendix.*

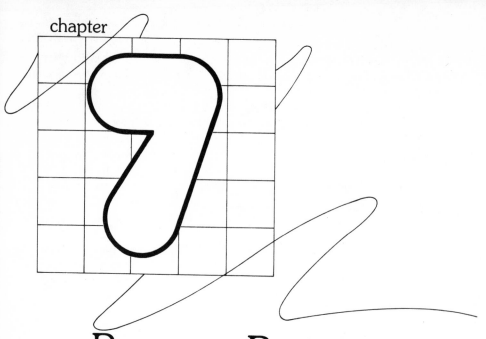

chapter

# Pressure, Pressure, Pressure

High blood pressure (hypertension) is a treacherous and potentially devastating condition. Although approximately 24 million Americans suffer from this condition, many are not aware of it. That's the treacherous part. You can appear to be the picture of health, but under this glossy surface the canvas is beginning to fray.

So what if you've got high blood pressure; what can it do to you? It can damage the inside of your blood vessels to allow cholesterol and other fats to leak into the wall (and in fact be pushed through the damaged areas under excessive pressure). Through a series of interactions between constituents of the blood and blood vessels, the arteries begin to narrow and may eventually plug up, depriving critical organs of their blood supply. As mentioned earlier, if the organ is the heart, you get a heart attack; if it is the brain, you get a stroke. Or if the organ is the kidney, you get kidney failure. The high pressure by itself can burst weakened or defective blood vessels (again, if it's in the brain, a stroke results).

There are many causes of high blood pressure. A category of conditions, called secondary hypertension, includes such problems as discrete narrowing of a segment of the major blood vessel of the body (coarctation of the aorta), kidney disease, and certain tumors. The various causes of secondary hypertension can be readily identified by your physician. But this category is only a small part of high blood pressure. The great majority of cases come under the heading of primary or essential hypertension. That really sounds impressive. If you name something, people get the idea that you know a lot about it. But *essential hypertension* means high blood pressure of unknown cause. At least until recently. Now we don't have to fake it so much with a term that means: we don't know. We're really beginning to understand a lot about the cause of "essential hypertension." (From now on when we use the term *high blood pressure,* we are almost always referring to essential hypertension.)

But back to cause. To begin with, high blood pressure runs in families. Surprised? It seems that everything we write about in this book "runs in families," and high blood pressure is no exception. Then, within the category of essential hypertension, there are complex interactions between salt (sodium), the kidney, blood volume, stress, blood chemicals, and hormones. Indeed, it will probably be possible in the near future to divide the category of essential hypertension into several etiologic subgroups. And that's about as deep as we will go for the purposes of this book.

Now we've got to say what blood pressure is, and what high blood pressure is—that is, how high is high. For blood to move through blood vessels or for water to move through a pipe, there has to be some pressure behind it, such as a gravity column or a pump. The fluid, whatever it is, exerts its pressure in all directions, including against the wall that confines it. Blood in humans is propelled by a pump (the heart). Blood pressure may be most accurately measured by putting a needle or tube inside the artery and connecting it to a manometer. But it may also be measured, with only a slight sacrifice in accuracy (and with much less pain), by compressing the artery with a blood pressure cuff.

Most physicians accept 140/90 as the beginning of high blood pressure. Anything below this is generally accepted as "normal." The 140 part is the systolic pressure, the force of the heart when it contracts and pushes blood out. The 90 part is the diastolic pressure, the resistance of the blood vessels to the flow of blood. The numbers 140 and

90 are measured in millimeters of mercury (mmHg). But when a conservative estimate of 24 million Americans with high blood pressure is made, this is based on adult blood pressures greater than 160/95. So that's one of several levels selected to be the beginning of high blood pressure. Let me say here that the top number and bottom number are of equal importance, so if either the systolic or diastolic pressure is elevated, high blood pressure is said to be present. I should also note that there are some data to support the idea that when adult blood pressures exceed a level as low as 120/80, risk of cardiovascular disease begins to increase. Our data indicate significant risk beginning at 140/90, so our policy is to treat pressures above 140/90.

The higher the pressure the greater the risk: 180/120 represents more risk than 160/100, which in turn is a more serious risk factor than 140/90. Blood pressure has a tendency to increase with age. Certainly this is evident throughout childhood and is associated with growth. Whether or not the magnitude of increase in childhood is inevitable may be debated. However, the progressive increase in blood pressure in adult life among Americans, Europeans, and Japanese is not the universal experience in many other cultures.

Figures 7–1 and 7–2 show how blood pressure increases during childhood in American boys and girls. You'll see that the pressure stays about the same for the first five to six years of life. Then it begins to climb and plateaus at a higher level in the teens. Selected percentile curves are plotted in the grids to give an idea as to what low, average, and high blood pressures are for various ages. Let me say right here that someone with low blood pressure is generally to be congratulated, not treated. The fiftieth percentile is, of course, the midpoint of blood pressure levels, and those in the ninety-fifth percentile have blood pressure readings higher than 95 percent of the American children from whom these data were taken. The ninety-fifth percentile is usually agreed to represent high blood pressure, and the ninetieth percentile is considered "borderline or suspicious." Therefore, an 8-year-old child with a blood pressure of 125/85 would be considered to have high blood pressure on two counts, both systolic and diastolic. A blood pressure of 125/80 would still be high on the basis of the systolic pressure. A blood pressure of 120/80 would be in the ninetieth percentile range—"suspicious," but not clearly elevated by our definition. What's important here is really not what any one blood pressure reading shows, because there are many variables and potentials for error. The important consideration is the *persistence of the range of blood pressure.* If the systolic pressures in our hypothetical 8-year-old child are *frequently* found to be in the range of 120 to 130, then there is reason for concern.

It is difficult to determine at an early age if a child will have high

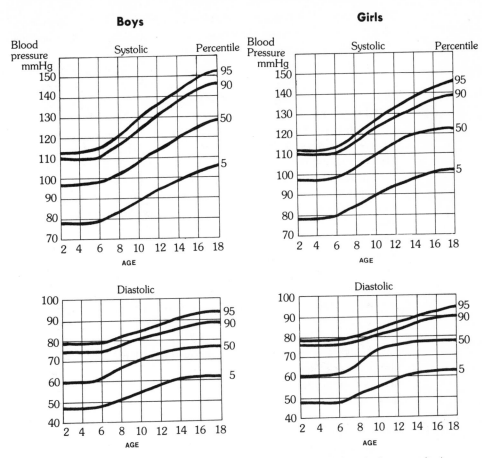

*Figure* **7-1,** On the left are the systolic (upper reading) and diastolic (lower reading)
*Figure* **7-2:** pressures in boys. Figure 7-2 on the right shows similar pressures in
girls. The fiftieth percentile on the graphs represents the average
pressure for the various ages displayed along the horizontal line.
Pressures at the ninety-fifth percentile should be considered as high
enough to require follow-up examinations and possible attention.

blood pressure at a later age. The blood pressure has a tendency to
bounce around during childhood so that a child could have a normal
pressure one year, an abnormal pressure the next, and be back to normal the following year. This is what is called a failure of "tracking" of
blood pressure. It appears that many kids who have a single or even occasional abnormal reading will not necessarily have high blood pressure as adults. However, there is also a tendency for those younger
people who will eventually have permanently fixed high blood pressure
in their thirties or forties to have blood pressure readings that are sometimes high and sometimes normal. This is called *labile blood pressure,*

and one can almost visualize that the influences leading to high blood pressure are being resisted by the body's homeostatic wisdom, an inclination toward maintaining a normal pressure.

In fact, there are data to suggest that the battle against high blood pressure may be lost fairly early. Irreversible changes involving the blood vessels interacting with the complex factors that produce high blood pressure may become fixed even in childhood. This is why early intervention may prove to be a necessary preventive strategy.

Well then, how do you decide if a high blood pressure reading, whether in adult or children, is a cause for concern? First, there's a chance for error in just taking the blood pressure, so it's routine for many physicians to take two or three readings and then to record the lowest of these. Some advocate recording the first pressure obtained (perhaps to identify the most labile individuals). Others take a pressure early in the examination and repeat it later, recording the second pressure, whether it happens to be higher or lower. If the recorded blood pressure is high, two subsequent visits, one to four weeks apart, are recommended—at which time the routine of the first visit is repeated.

If the blood pressure is found to be elevated during three visits, a search for possible causes is indicated. If the patient is a child, and the blood pressure is demonstrated to be elevated on consecutive annual examinations, it may be suspected that high blood pressure is beginning to "track." It then becomes an important consideration whether or not high blood pressure is present in other family members. If high blood pressure is running in the family and a given patient shows occasional high readings, the safest course is that the patient should be considered at risk and a low salt diet instituted. We'll get into that in the next section.

## Heredity, Salt, and Stress

I don't want you to believe that all the answers are in with regard to essential hypertension any more than I want you to think, on the other hand, that there's nothing known about the cause and treatment of this disorder. When I was younger, I used to be impressed with the "objectivity" and "sophistication" of physicians and other assorted professors who would respond to a question with: "We simply don't know the answer to that yet." I've since come to learn that this statement frequently means that it's only the speaker who doesn't know the answer to the question and, furthermore, that he doesn't even know the current state of knowledge of the subject. So we can talk for a long time about how complex a problem hypertension is and how little we know about it, or we can concentrate on some of the things that we do know that have practical consequences in prevention and treatment.

Often physicians and other biomedical scientists, especially geneticists, search for lower animals to use as models for what happens in humans. These models are called animal homologies. Now it's not invariable that what happens in one particular animal (say, a mouse) will also happen in the same way in another animal such as a rabbit or baboon or human. But these animal homologies are extremely useful aids in understanding *possible* disease mechanisms in humans. There are some interesting strains of rats (ALR and SHR) that give us ideas on what may go into producing high blood pressure in humans. First there's hereditary predisposition. Some rats don't get hypertension, but ALR and SHR strains do. So if you start off with unfavorable heredity and add salt and stress, you end up with a rat with high blood pressure. And in the SHR strain, the high blood pressure leads to stroke. In the ALR strain, the high blood pressure produces plaques in the blood vessels, similar to those found in humans, that plug up the blood vessels and can lead to heart attacks.

So one strain gets strokes and the other gets more generalized hardening of the arteries. And other strains of rats can be subjected to stress and salt and not get high blood pressure or any other apparent adverse changes. Until it's demonstrated that this sort of model doesn't apply to humans, I submit that this is a reasonable way to look at high blood pressure and its consequences in many human families. So, my idea of the first line of defense against high blood pressure is to control both salt and stress.

**Salt**  ○  The U.S. Senate Select Committee published dietary goals for the United States, some aspects of which we discussed in Chapter 5. One of the six goals was to reduce salt consumption to approximately three grams per day from the present intake, which may be two to six times that high in American diets, and eight to ten times that high in Japanese diets. This original recommendation has been revised to reduce salt to five grams per day. Yet in some tropical cultures, which you would think would require considerable added salt because of heat and sweating, the intake is about one-half gram of salt per day. And these people do not suffer the effects of heat or high blood pressure. In fact, a committee of the National Academy of Sciences suggested the human need for salt is indeed about one-half gram per day. Clearly, salt added to food is an acquired taste, and the body's need for salt is much less than we have been led to believe.

**Prudent salt diet** ○ Without any sacrifice in legitimate dietary needs the goal of five grams of salt per day (2,000 mg of sodium) can be met by anyone who does not have a rare disease involving salt requirements (such as an adrenal disorder). I should point out that table salt is roughly 40 percent sodium and 60 percent chloride, and one gram of salt contains 400 mg of sodium. But a salt intake of about four grams per day is the level found by some investigators to be associated with increasing blood pressure among *susceptibles,* so there are differences of opinion about reasonable salt consumption. Most Americans consume between six and eighteen grams of salt each day.

To achieve a prudent salt diet really doesn't take much. All you need to do is:

**1** Add little or no salt to table food and use little or no salt in cooking.

**2** Don't eat foods with visible salt on them such as potato chips, pretzels, and other salted snack foods.

**3** Become familiar with foods high in sodium and avoid them or use them sparingly.

I'll amplify the third item in a moment, but here I must make the point that if you personally don't have high blood pressure, and you don't have high blood pressure, stroke, or heart attacks in your family, you don't have to be as strict about low salt ingestion as those who have these individual or familial problems.

The following guidelines would be appropriate. The most careful salt restriction would be for those high-risk people who actually have high blood pressure. These people should be under a doctor's care and should be consuming three grams of salt or less per day, depending on severity. The next category, those who have normal blood pressure, but a positive family history of cardiovascular disease, could use salt more liberally, but should stay at an intake level between three and five grams. The final category, those who have neither high blood pressure nor a positive family history, could use salt much more liberally. Although five grams is the maximum currently recommended by the Select Committee, I feel that these people should be permitted considerable latitude and opportunity for salt indiscretion.

Please start to familiarize yourself with Table 7–1, High Sodium Foods to Avoid or Use Sparingly. This table is adapted from the report of the U.S. Senate Select Committee. You know from the experience of your own taste buds that a lot of these foods are salty. But food substances like catsup, pickles, and sardines may not have occurred to you as being high in salt. For example, a typical McDonald's lunch—a hamburger (with pickle, catsup, and mustard), french fries, and a shake—contains almost four grams of salt. Thus in one meal you can consume more than is prudent for a high-risk individual to take in 24 hours—and almost as much as is recommended for *anyone* to take in an entire day.

Table 7–2 is also taken from the committee report on dietary goals and gives you a few things to keep in mind. Review Tables 7–1 and 7–2 periodically while establishing your personal Whole Heart Program until the information in them is pretty well second nature to you.

**Stress Control** ○ The need for stress control and the use of meditation and relaxation techniques in hypertensive patients has been popularized by Dr. Herbert Benson in his widely read book *The Relaxation Response*. Up to now I've been emphasizing preventing high blood pressure from ever occurring, even in individuals at risk. You should know that low salt diets and meditation are used also in the treatment of patients who already have high blood pressure. The techniques of meditation have been described in Chapter 3, and they are to be regarded as an essential part of your program for preventing high blood pressure as well as heart attacks. At this point please refer back to pages 40–42 to refresh your memory about meditation if you are not already incorporating it into your life-style.

**Potassium** ○ When we have been talking about salt we really have been talking about sodium—sodium chloride is the salt and sodium is the positively charged ion (or cation) in the molecule. There is some preliminary evidence that another cation, potassium, may be useful in preventing high blood pressure. Certain societies in which hypertension rarely occurs not only have a low sodium diet but also have a high potassium diet. This idea will require considerable investigation, but common foods that are rich in potassium include orange and other citrus juices, tomato juice, and bananas.

**Obesity** ○ High blood pressure and obesity are strongly associated. The overweight person is borrowing trouble from many directions, and high blood pressure is as important a complication as any.

# The Pill and Related Female Hormones

With the population explosion posing such a threat to our future, the world obviously needs a safe, effective contraceptive. And oral contraceptives have proved to be among the most effective and convenient agents to meet this need. The problem is safety, but so far there isn't a safer *convenient* alternative. The IUD certainly carries risks, and its track record of effectiveness leaves a bit to be desired. The diaphragm with spermicidal jelly is less convenient, but is effective and safe, and is easily a possible choice for women who are concerned about their health.

The Pill is a hormonal preparation made up of progestogen and estrogen or less commonly progestogen alone. The term *the Pill* may be generalized to include various female hormone pharmaceutical preparations that may be taken by mouth or by injection. It acts on blood clotting factors, the lining of blood vessels, blood fats (triglycerides), and blood sugar. It interacts with hormones that influence blood pressure and with smoking to produce a risk greater than the additive effects of the two factors (synergy).

Specifically what can the Pill do to you? First, it can cause blood clots in the deep veins in your legs (thrombosis). This is bad enough, but the devastating complication of this is that a piece of blood clot can break off and travel to your lungs (embolism). Embolism in the lungs can lead to death—and indeed deaths have been ascribed to this problem in women taking female hormones. The risk of having a clot in a deep vein is five times greater in young women taking oral contraceptives than in those not taking the Pill.

High blood pressure is another problem for about 5 percent of users of oral contraceptives (OC). It may take six months before the blood pressure begins to climb, so those who begin OC therapy should have frequent blood pressure readings during this critical period, and at longer but regular intervals thereafter. Patients with a family history of high blood pressure or with kidney disease or toxemia of pregnancy should avoid oral contraceptives. High blood pressure, in addition to putting a strain on the heart, damages blood vessels and is associated with stroke. Another cause of stroke is the plugging up or thrombosis of blood vessels in the brain. Women taking oral contraceptives have an approximately sixfold increase in stroke.

Then there is the problem with heart attack. If you already have traditional risk factors, such as high cholesterol and smoking, oral contraceptives add synergistically to the risk. The chance is 2.8 times greater that you'll have a heart attack if you're on the Pill in the age group from 30 to 39 years than if you are not. And if you're taking oral contraceptives and are 40 to 44 years of age, the risk is 4.7 times greater for heart attack as compared with women not taking hormones. Then, if you're a smoker as well, the risk is increased much more, as was pointed out in Chapter 6.

You should also know that if you are exposed to these hormones while pregnant, the chance that your baby will be born with a congenital malformation, most often a heart defect (such as a hole in the heart or a "blue baby" problem), is increased two to three times. How would you be exposed to these hormones during pregnancy? In the past they've been given as pregnancy tests, and some physicians today think that they can help maintain a pregnancy if there is a threatened spontaneous abortion or a history of this problem. But no woman should allow herself to be given a hormonal pregnancy test or hormones to maintain a pregnancy. The FDA has taken a strong position in this matter. And no woman should start taking the Pill without being certain that she is not pregnant.

# Treatment

Throughout this book prevention is our theme, but in order to prevent a serious consequence resulting from a risk factor, the preventive strategy may be to treat the risk factor.

In our drug-oriented society, it's natural to assume that there must be a pill for high blood pressure. And this is, in fact, the case. But let me emphasize that the techniques that prevent high blood pressure from ever getting started, which don't involve drugs, are the first line of defense in treatment as well.

**1) Salt restriction**   For the patient with high blood pressure a low salt diet of three grams per day (1,200 milligrams of sodium) may be surprisingly effective. A more strict salt reduction, down to one-half gram per day, may be tried by your doctor if the more liberal salt diet is ineffective.

**2) Stress control**   Patients with high blood pressure who meditate have been found to experience unequivocal decreases in levels of pressure.

**3) Exercise**   A considerable body of experience confirms that regular exercise reduces blood pressure in many patients.

**4) Weight reduction**   The overweight patient with high blood pressure may find his pressure return to normal or drop considerably as his weight returns to normal.

**5) The Pill**   Oral contraceptive hormones can drive blood pressure up to surprisingly high levels in women sensitive to this hormonal effect. Such women do not need an additional pill to lower their pressures; they need to relinquish a pill, the Pill, for another form of contraception.

**6) Secondary hypertension**   There are literally dozens of causes of high blood pressure other than the type we've been talking about, primary or

**133**

essential hypertension. Your doctor is in a position to search for these specific causes and eliminate them. However, I'll remind you again that most cases of high blood pressure are due to primary hypertension, not secondary hypertension.

**7) Drug therapy**  If blood pressure can't be lowered without drugs, be grateful that there are now available many excellent medications to treat the problem. Don't be reluctant to use them. Your physician can prescribe a program for you that should be highly effective in most cases.

TABLE
7-1

# High Sodium Foods to Avoid or Use Sparingly

Meats: Salted or smoked meats, bacon, bologna, corned beef, ham, luncheon meats, sausage, and salt pork.

Fish: Salted or smoked fish, anchovies, sardines, dried cod, and herring.

Peanut butter, unless low-sodium dietetic.

Flavorings: Commercial bouillon; catsup; chili sauce; celery, onion, or garlic salts; meat extracts, sauces, or tenderizers, unless low-sodium dietetic; prepared mustard; relishes; salt substitutes; cooking wine.

Cheeses: Processed cheese, cheese spreads, Roquefort, Camembert, and other strong cheeses.

Vegetables: Pickles, sauerkraut, and any other vegetables salted or packed in brine.

Miscellaneous: Breads or crackers with salt topping, potato chips, popcorn, pretzels, salted nuts, other salted snacks, and olives.

TABLE
7-2

# Sodium: Some Points to Remember

1 Milk, meats, fish, cheese, and eggs are quite high in sodium.

2 Vegetables, breads, and cereals have moderate amounts of sodium. There is considerable variation among the different vegetables.

3 Fruits and fats are low in sodium or have only trace amounts.

4 Highly salted snack foods should be avoided.

5 Halve the amount of salt, soy sauce, and monosodium glutamate used in cooking and at the table.

6 Do not add salt to foods already salted in freezing and canning.

7 Try different flavorings instead of salt, except those listed in Table 7-1.

8 Do not use a salt substitute unless a physician has recommended it.

9 When eating out or buying prepared canned or frozen foods, try to avoid those with an unlisted salt content.

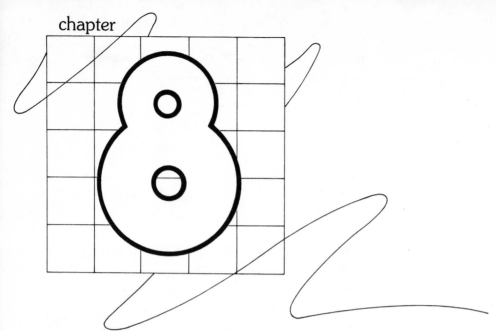

# Relax-You'll Live Longer

The role of emotional stress and behavior patterns as a contributing cause of coronary heart disease is more controversial than some of the other risk factors we've discussed. Intuitively, and on the basis of many indirect studies, one would predict that stress would be damaging to the heart and blood vessels of man. However, except for a surprisingly few investigators, interest in stress and behavior has not received major attention in cardiology.

Dr. Hans Selye of Montreal has devoted at least three decades to the study of stress, emphasizing the important role of hormones in the response to stress and in the consequent production of physical damage. Meyer Friedman and Ray Rosenman have proposed and popularized the concept of Type A behavior as a factor in coronary heart disease. But for some reason, these ideas do not find their way into standard textbooks of cardiology. One reason could be that the epidemiologic studies that test the role of stress in the etiology of coronary heart disease are as troublesome to design as they are to interpret. A cholesterol value of 270 is a neat quantitative measure. A "sense of time urgency" is more difficult to quantitate. Certainly, if it were only Drs. Friedman and Rosenman who could correlate Type A behavior with coronary heart disease, it would be impossible to persuade those holding an adversary position; however, other groups are coming to similar conclusions. The Western Collaborative Group Study (which included Rosenman and Friedman as investigators, but which also encompassed many other scientists—some quite skeptical) looked specifically at Type A behavior, and found a statistically significant association with clinical coronary heart disease.

Of course, Type A behavior isn't the only way to look at the influence of emotional stress on the heart. Certain components of the Type A personality have been selected for a self-administered test by one group. Other groups have used different standard personality tests and inventories in evaluating people who have had coronary events (retrospective studies) and in following people who eventually went on to have heart attacks (prospective studies). Some tests are given by a trained interviewer and others are filled out by the patient without assistance.

It would serve no useful purpose to review the criticisms of studies attempting to relate emotional stress to heart disease. It is sufficient to repeat that there is no such thing as a perfect epidemiologic study, and that an experienced epidemiologist can find even more flaws in the behavioral studies than in other risk-factor studies.

I should also point out that, although I'll concentrate on the Type A concept, I'm not suggesting that this approach to analysis of emotional stress as it relates to heart disease is superior to other methods. It happens to be the format I've used in our own epidemiologic studies—and it's far and away the most familiar approach to lay readers. If someone was to be able to clearly define "uptight" in a way that would fully capture the spectrum of the coronary-prone patient, I'd be glad to use that concept. As a matter of fact, what many of us probably understand by the label "uptight" would fit the coronary-prone personality quite well. However, since so much effort has been invested in the concept of Type A behavior, let's stick with that.

## Type A Behavior

The best way to assess Type A behavior would be to have an interviewer trained by the Friedman-Rosenman group administer a test that takes about 15 minutes. One study of coronary heart disease in American monks compared the conclusions reached by such trained interviewers with conclusions reached by co-workers (other monks) and supervisors (abbots) who had been familiarized with the concept of Type A. In our own studies, we have modified the Type A format so it could be used as a self-administered test. Our feeling has been that co-workers and family members, who have spent a considerable amount of time with a given individual, and who have been given an orientation to the concept of Type A behavior, can give a reasonably reliable assessment. We've also concluded that self-administered personality tests, while limited, can be informative.

An observation that should come as no surprise to those who've become accustomed to a major theme of this book is that Type A behavior is familial. Familial doesn't necessarily mean entirely genetic. A child growing up in a Type A environment is likely to have something rub off on him regardless of his genetic makeup. However, it's also quite clear that among children and adults living in the same environment, some may evince striking Type A patterns while others may be more Type B. Somewhere in here Type A and Type B are going to require definition. This can best be done initially by describing a Type A person—the sort of profile the monks and abbots had in mind as they rated their co-workers by knowing them and knowing how they acted.

So here goes. A Type A person never has enough hours in the day to achieve all that he or she feels must be done. He tries to do more and more in less and less time. This has been called the "sense of time urgency"—the harried feeling that you can't get it all done, and that whatever you're doing isn't enough, because you should be doing three other things (in three other places) at the very same time. On top of this is often a thick layer of hostility and anger. Very often the hostility is suppressed so that it's not all that obvious. And when hostility is expressed, the Type A person can readily rationalize how justified the hostility is.

The Type B person is the opposite of Type A, but this doesn't mean that he's incapable of accomplishing anything. He just does his work without feeling stressed and harried, and is perfectly satisfied that what he's doing at the time is the right thing to be doing. There isn't the constant feeling of being torn in different directions.

Friedman and Rosenman believe that there are slightly more Type A individuals in America than Type B. So Type A isn't confined to what most of us would identify as high stress occupations. Type A behavior is an attitude, an approach to life. You can feel uptight and stressed by almost anything that happens in your environment, or you can approach the same situations with calm confidence. I'm often astounded to observe how tense patients are in their approach to their occupations, many of which I would visualize as being very low-key. Can you imagine having a florist tell you that his is a "pressure cooker" occupation? Let me repeat: it's not what you do, *it's your attitude toward what you do.*

Part of your attitude toward what you do comes from your position. The concept that many people have of a stressed individual is the high-powered executive type, trying to balance a dozen deals on a knife-edge. To an extent this is true. But the high-powered executive pushes things downhill. He clears off his desk by piling the stuff on the desks of his underlings and dashes off to the club to play squash or racketball and sit in the sauna before going to a cocktail party. Then the underlings devote their evenings and nights to doing the executive's bidding while seething with rage they can't express if they want to keep their jobs. I'm reminded of a cartoon of an executive chomping on his cigar, confidently telling his physician: "I don't get ulcers, I give them."

The same may be said about heart attacks. Being high enough up in the pecking order, high enough on the socioeconomic ladder, has a protective influence not only on your coronary arteries but on every phase of your health and well-being. Illness correlates with lower status, lower education, and lower income. It's an unfortunate fact of life, supported by data from many epidemiologic studies.

But on an individual basis it doesn't have to be true. Whatever your status, if you approach life with confidence and satisfaction, feeling good about yourself and what you're doing, you can free yourself from a lot of the damaging stress of striving that is counterproductive. Easier said than done? Panglossian oversimplification? We'll discuss that later.

Table 8–1 shows a recent version of the questions we've used in our family studies to test for Type A behavior and stress. We've evaluated them by dividing the scores into four parts. (A study by another group divided the responses into five parts.) What we found was that we could discriminate between heart attack victims and those free of heart disease by comparing the top category (most Type A) with the bottom category (least Type A). The middle two categories appeared to be more neutral. So if you divided the groups for comparison into one composed of 4+ and 3+ and another composed of 2+ and 1+, it was not possible to discriminate for heart attack at a statistically significant level between the two groups. A 4+ Type A compared with a 1+ did, however, reveal a difference. Most of the questions in Table 8–1, including much of the wording, come directly from the work of Friedman and Rosenman, but we put in some of our own variations and additional questions. The questions about jobs and job satisfaction are not strictly relevant to Type A behavior, but come from another inventory of personality and stress. However hybrid the questionnaire is, this is representative of what we have used and tested.

The scores derived from these tests and shown at the end of Table 8–1 have been found to have a correlation with coronary heart disease in our own studies. For every yes add 1 point. The score is 0 for a no. A 4+ Type A individual in our series collects 14 or more points. A 1+ individual, who would be much like a Type B in behavior, would score 3 points or less. As I mentioned earlier, the 3+ and 2+ categories do not discriminate between those who had heart attacks and those who didn't, but they do help an individual to know about where he is on the scale. On first reading, some of the questions may seem to describe exaggerated conditions, but we've found these tests useful. The middle ground in the final evaluation balances out the extremes.

## Acute Stress

In addition to the chronic tension that a Type A individual subjects himself to as part of his orientation to living, there are acute episodes that add significantly to the burden we are all called to carry. Acute emotional outbursts and rages have been repeatedly associated with acute coronary events. These associations have been more anecdotal than the result of controlled observations. However, they are compatible with what we know of pathophysiology.

We've all heard of wives or husbands who have died within a year of the deaths of their spouses. A scale of stress of adjusting to change has been developed by two psychiatrists in Washington, Thomas Holmes and Richard Rahe. This scale has received considerable attention in the lay literature. Table 8–2 displays certain selected stresses and their impact on health from the Holmes and Rahe Social Readjustment Scale. You'll note that some of the "stresses" of adjustment come from good things happening to a person, not just bad things. It has been observed that 10 times more widows and widowers die during the first year after the death of spouse than other men and women in their age group do. It has also been found that the rate of illness is 12 times higher in divorced persons than in married persons during the year following divorce.

Efforts have been made to project the number of points on this scale that can be tolerated, in say a year, before having an adverse effect on health. You can imagine how difficult this sort of estimate would be, and how many confounding variables could interfere with the estimate. So we won't allow ourselves to get sidetracked on this issue. The point is that a person at high risk of coronary heart disease should be aware of the potential role of acute social stresses on his cardiovascular health and should try to minimize the accumulation of too many such stresses in relatively short periods of time—as much as it is within his power to do so.

It almost goes without saying that we should be at least as concerned about acute physical stresses. In the exercise chapter I point out that sudden, high-output exertion unfavorably changes the electrocardiogram even in young men in reasonably good condition. The better conditioned you are, of course, the better your cardiovascular system is able to respond to physical stress. Cold is another acute physical stress that requires mentioning. Again, we've all heard of men dying while shoveling snow or hurrying through sub-zero cold for a bus. And again, these are anecdotal reports, since no one is likely to do a study on the risks of snow shoveling in heart patients. We do know, however, that plunging a hand into cold water is such a good method of driving the blood pressure up that it can be used as a screening test.

Fatigue is another acute stress that may justifiably be avoided by those at risk. And there are environmental hazards that are becoming more common in our environment. Days of high carbon monoxide air pollution are all too familiar to those living in urban areas. Under such acute conditions the high-risk heart patient will do well to minimize exertion and demands on his compromised cardiovascular system.

## Stress Interactions

I'm not going to spend as much time as might be desired by many epidemiologists in defending the idea that acute and chronic stress and associated behavior patterns and attitudes are not good for your heart. I'll just resort to a Pascalian maneuver and say you're better off without stress no matter what it does to your heart—except as it may mobilize you for "fight or flight." We'll sneak up on that particular concept as we go along.

Most stress in modern society is considered unproductive or counterproductive. The relief of the symptoms that accompany stress has become strongly emphasized in contemporary medicine and in the pharmaceutical industry. The big bucks for the drug companies don't come from digitalis, but from tranquilizers. Many Americans feel, and rightly so, that they're trying to survive in a stress-ridden society. And to an extent this is true. The coronary arteries of the florist who views his job as a pressure cooker can suffer injury just as real as the coronary arteries of someone undergoing what almost any objective observer would classify as real stress. A Vietnamese refugee, for example.

For many thousands of years our ancestors lived like Vietnamese refugees. They were called on to mobilize their physiological resources to survive by fight or flight. (The phrase "fight or flight" comes from the American physiologist Dr. Walter B. Cannon.) Those who survived were quite likely to have had the better physiology with respect to fight or flight. Obviously "survival of the fittest" would depend on a number of other variables, but the ability to mobilize for fight or flight would have to have been a useful adaptive mechanism throughout the history and prehistory of early man. And it is still useful to man today under certain conditions.

What happens when the fight-or-flight response is evoked? Adrenalin pours into your bloodstream; you start burning body fuel stores; your heart rate, breathing rate, and blood pressure go up, bringing increased blood flow to your arms and legs. You're now prepared for fight or flight—for survival.

But what if you're constantly stimulated to a fight-or-flight response? Visualize rats in a cage with electrodes shooting electric current into their brains. When the electricity hits a certain area of the brain of rats it stimulates a fight-or-flight response. Swedish researchers demonstrated that after prolonged and repeated shocks the blood pressure of the rats becomes permanently elevated. A potentially useful reaction has led to a damaging result. While we're not rats, we are participating in the rat race. In restrained society we're constantly stimulated by the stresses of life, but not allowed to give full expression to our fight-or-flight response. We can't feel free to punch people out—and we can't run from our troubles. We've got to hang in there and do something that is not really natural in the perspective of the biology of fight or flight. We suppress and internalize a natural response that has great benefit for survival under primitive conditions, but this response would be disastrous if given free rein in polite society.

So in one sense our condition is as unnatural and confining as is the condition of the rats in the cage with the electrodes sending constant shocks into the brain. What if that same area of the brain of the rat is permanently altered? Friedman and Rosenman report that such rats not only exhibit stress behavior, but their cholesterol levels rise. Studies such as these require further evaluation and should be carried out over a long enough period of time to see if changes in the blood vessels occur that could lead to heart attack or stroke.

# Social Support Structures

Another variable that deserves comment has been as interesting to cardiovascular epidemiologists as it has to sociologists. The traditional social support structures throughout history have been the family, the community, religion—groups of people with common background, interests, and shared systems of value. In many societies these structures are still in place. But in mobile America large segments of the population find themselves without the benefit of such support. To cite just one example, the frequency rate of coronary heart disease is three times as high among those who migrate from the farm to urban white-collar jobs as in those who remain on the farm. I should point out that these differences could not be accounted for on the basis of differences in diet, exercise, smoking, or other risk factors.

A satisfactory discussion of this subject could occupy an entire book, and yet some points have to be made in a brief space. To put it succinctly: It's not good for your physical or emotional health to be without social support. Independence is great. Being free from the oppressive meddling of family, co-workers, neighbors, and church is in many ways to be desired. And yet to be alone, or to be alone in a nuclear family, without the knowledge that there are those close by who care can become intolerable. Damage to health and personality lies at one extreme of this continuum. And at the other extreme is escape from freedom, losing oneself in a cause or group or cult that is perceived as being greater than self.

Obviously, reading a few paragraphs on the subject isn't sufficient basis for making enormous changes in your life with respect to a support structure. However, it may be a stimulus for you to begin thinking about the problem. Something you might do for openers is ask yourself: Whom could you turn to in a crisis? If the bottom dropped out of your life today what would you do? Who could really be counted on to help? If there are relatives, neighbors, friends at work and at church who are close to you, and if you have a confident "religious" orientation, your social support structure is likely to be quite adequate. If not, you should know that your health and well-being are compromised by the lack of such a structure.

But what can we do about stress? It won't go away, you know.

The best thing we can do is try to manage stress and your perception of what constitutes stress.

In Chapter 2, I began to introduce you to some families who illustrate problems in coronary heart disease and management. In Family E, the index patient who came to us (because of an abnormally high cholesterol level discovered at a screening) was a 46-year-old physics professor from a university in the area. Right off the bat he made our risk assessment more difficult because he had been raised in an adoptive home and knew nothing of his biologic parents and family.

We took our risk-factor history at the first visit and checked his triglycerides when we repeated his cholesterol study. Professor E smoked about 30 cigarettes a day (down from 40) and had been trying unsuccessfully to kick the habit for several years. He had already lost 10 pounds, but was still about 10 pounds overweight. Also for the past two years he had been halfheartedly "trying to get back into shape" through a poorly designed program of sporadic and punishing exercise. He came across as a very uptight, Type A individual who had to finish half of my sentences for me. As yet he'd been experiencing no symptoms of coronary heart disease.

We asked him to return in a week with his wife and children to receive the results of his blood study and to allow us to study their blood lipids and lipoproteins. Just because this man did not have biologic parents or brothers and sisters to study didn't mean we couldn't still get some genetic information about him. We could learn something from his children, and also start the entire family on the Whole Heart Program. Studies of the professor's lipids and lipoproteins confirmed that his cholesterol was indeed high (320), as were his triglycerides (260) and lipoproteins. His wife had a normal cholesterol (185) but a slightly elevated level of triglycerides (165). She was about 25 pounds overweight, so her triglycerides would very likely respond promptly to a weight reduction diet.

The problem now was to determine if the professor had the single gene abnormality (which seems to carry a higher risk and requires more aggressive treatment than the multifactorial inheritance type). Just on the basis of the high level, one would predict that the single gene variety was present. Two ways to distinguish the types are a family study and a trial of response to diet and therapy.

The family study was the tip-off. Although there were only two children, one had high cholesterol (290) and borderline triglycerides (145), while the other had a cholesterol of 150 and triglycerides of 65. This put the professor and his 16-year-old son in a very high risk group with presumed single gene abnormalities. But here's the problem: Nobody was sick. A screening test was performed and a blood abnormality showed up, and then someone at the medical school (me) starts talking about drastically changing how they live.

Professor E and I discussed the implications of his risk score, and his response was very positive. This positive response deserves a comment. It is a well-appreciated fact in epidemiology that lower socioeconomic and educational levels are associated with increased risk for many diseases, including cardiovascular disease, while higher educational and economic levels mean lower risks. Well-educated people are more likely to respond to rational medical programs; and those with adequate financial resources are in a position to do something meaningful about their health care.

Professor E and his family responded in spades. Mrs. E completely changed the dietary program of the family and everyone accepted it with a minimum of resistance. The professor stopped smoking (cold-turkey) and learned how to exercise in a productive and nonpunishing way. But there was still a significant problem: his job. We had several talks about it. Research funds were becoming extremely difficult to attract, and after almost 20 years of substantial grants, Professor E was, for the first time in his career, without research support. Add to the problem with grants a new, heavy-handed department chairman who was causing more than a little turmoil. His job was no longer the source of satisfaction it had previously been. He had followed the advice of André Maurois to make his job the center of his life—and at mid-life, the center was crumbling.

Then the subject changed abruptly away from this painful direction and somehow the name of another member of the physics department came up. I casually asked about this man, because I had known someone of the same name who was getting his Ph.D. in physics at the time I was getting my M.D. It turned out to be the same person. The most vivid memory I had of this nuclear physicist I'd known years before was that he was addicted to science fiction. I mentioned this to Professor E and his expression changed completely. Ten years fell from his eyes and the corners of his mouth. He began to talk about science fiction, to which he also was apparently addicted—and we talked about the writing of science fiction. As a graduate student he'd published a paperback science fiction novel and over the next several years had written a number of short stories, one of which had been included in an anthology. But he hadn't written anything in 10 years. Now his age returned to his eyes and mouth.

Over the next three months Professor E lost 10 pounds, down to his desirable weight. By a combination of diet and medications his levels of cholesterol and triglycerides were reduced considerably—although not completely to normal. His commitments to not smoking and to rational exercise were being maintained. He looked happy and relaxed. But before I could take credit for the change, he told me that he'd reached a decision. He was writing stories again and he had found a new teaching job at a small college—a lower-paying job that some might consider him overqualified for. But this new job would give him more time for his family, for writing, and, of essential importance, it would provide relief from the turmoil of the university politics that had been stressing him so. Then he thanked me—I guess for listening, because I certainly didn't go as far as suggesting he find a different job. However, as I look back on it, it seems to have been an excellent decision (and one that would have been entirely appropriate for me to have been more involved in).

Professor E's story was my not-too-subtle way to get into the problem of stress at work. Your job and your home life are probably your two major sources of satisfaction and frustration. If you're happy both at work and at home, you have an optimal situation for your health and well-being. If you're dissatisfied and frustrated in both areas, your life is probably hell. While a great deal of satisfaction in one area can offset a certain amount of frustration in the other, we should strive to make both areas as congenial as possible.

How's work going? Few would answer that their jobs are incredibly rewarding. Most of us find our jobs somewhere between satisfactory and tolerable. But if you feel your job is tearing you up inside, it probably is. And for your health and well-being you may have to consider making some changes. Easier said than done. You have to make a living. You may not be able to get another job as readily as Professor E. There are bills to be paid. You have to eat. But a new job may not be the answer. Maybe the change you need to make is in your attitude toward your present job. Are you doing everything you can to make your job rewarding? Think about it. Don't dismiss this immediately as a meaningless suggestion. Think about it.

But what if, after giving this question serious consideration, you conclude you're working hard to make your job rewarding and you're still being torn up? Then talk to your spouse and a valued friend or two for a frank appraisal of your situation. Be sure you give them all the facts as objectively as possible. If they believe you're out of step, then you'll have some work to do on yourself. Again I resort to William James, who said: "The greatest discovery of my generation is that human beings by changing the inner attitudes of their minds can change the outer aspects of their lives."

All right, say you've given it your best shot, but your job situation is intolerable, and can't be improved by anything within your power. Then it's time to make a change. But do it in a way that is to *your* advantage.

Don't lash out. Don't burn bridges. Bide your time and quietly look for a better situation. Perhaps it will take only three months, as in the case of Professor E. Maybe it will take as much as a year or two. Don't rush, but don't take too long either.

This sort of advice is easy for professional types to make and to follow. Professors are frequently changing jobs, jumping from one university to another. But there are people in the world who are stuck in intolerable work situations and can't change. They simply don't have the mobility or marketable skills. They suffer grinding oppression in jobs they hate. And they pay the price. I'm sorry I got into this—because I don't have an answer.

If our environment is life-threatening, then we've got to try to get out—like the Vietnamese refugee. There are intolerable situations less drastic than war that may also require a change of environment. But almost any environment today carries with it considerable stress. So we must develop some skills in handling tension on a day-to-day basis. As was suggested in the previous section, it is certainly preferable to live and work within a highly supportive environment. But whatever our environment, we must be able to cope.

## Back to Meditation

In Chapter 3, I introduced you to meditation. If you haven't had the opportunity to try the technique and wish to review that section now, it begins on page 40. Meditation is a cornerstone of the Whole Heart Program. It is almost essential to start the day off with meditation. After you've mastered the technique, you can take short "mini-meds" when you feel you're getting uptight. One or two minutes of even breathing with the eyes closed and the mind cleared will help you recover from or prepare for a moderately stressful event. You might also consider building a midday break into your schedule in which you exercise and take ten minutes off to clear your mind through meditation. The midday break is indispensable if you're a flagrant Type A, scoring 14 or more points on the scale in Table 8–1. You really must shut down your striving mechanism for an hour in the middle of the day. No martini business lunches or brown-bag conferences. Mentally hang up a "gone fishin' " sign and leave the rat race for an hour. Both your job and your health should benefit.

As part of your rehabilitation, keep checking yourself on the questions that you answered yes to in Table 8–1. This is part of your self-awareness. It's not that you're supposed to just treat the symptoms while the disease continues to rage inside. But as you become aware of what you're doing, you should be able to exert progressively more control over the disease as well as the symptoms. Take satisfaction in doing one thing at a time, and taking as much time as it requires to do it well, and don't allow that twisting pain to invade your consciousness—that pain that says you should be doing three other things in three other places. Work at being calm while waiting in lines and following slower cars. Cool it. Be aware of your symptoms. And watch them decrease as you gain control of your attitudes and your life.

TABLE
**8-1**

## Type A Personality Questionnaire

PLEASE TAKE YOUR TIME ANSWERING THESE QUESTIONS. It is important to give as frank an answer as possible. Feel free to ask your spouse or friends how you should answer the question. Some of these items, such as the way you talk, may not be apparent to you, but would be to those who know you well.

1 Do you feel there are not enough hours in the day to do all the things you must do?

( ) yes    ( ) no

2 Do you always move, walk, and eat rapidly?

( ) yes    ( ) no

3 Do you feel an impatience with the rate at which most events take place?

( ) yes    ( ) no

4 Do you say, "Uh-huh, uh-huh," or "yes, yes, yes, yes," to someone who is talking, unconsciously urging him to "get on with it" or hasten his rate of speaking? Do you have a tendency to finish the sentences of others for them?

( ) yes    ( ) no

5 Do you become unduly irritated or even enraged when a car ahead of you in your lane runs at a pace you consider too slow? Do you find it anguishing to wait in line or to wait your turn to be seated at a restaurant?

( ) yes    ( ) no

6 Do you find it intolerable to watch others perform tasks you know you can do faster?

( ) yes    ( ) no

7 Do you become impatient with yourself as you are obliged to perform repetitive duties (making out bank deposit slips, writing checks, washing and cleaning dishes, and so on), which are necessary but take you away from doing things you really have an interest in doing?

( ) yes    ( ) no

8 Do you find yourself hurrying your own reading or always attempting to obtain condensations or summaries of truly interesting and worthwhile literature?

( ) yes    ( ) no

9 Do you strive to think of or do two or more things simultaneously? For example, while trying to listen to another person's speech, do you persist in continuing to think about an irrelevant subject?

( ) yes    ( ) no

**10** While engaged in recreation, do you continue to ponder your business, home, or professional problems?

( ) yes ( ) no

**11** Do you have (a) a habit of explosively accentuating various key words in your ordinary speech even when there is no real need for such accentuation, and (b) a tendency to utter the last few words of your sentences far more rapidly than the opening words?

( ) yes ( ) no

**12** Do you find it difficult to refrain from talking about or bringing the theme of any conversation around to those subjects that especially interest and intrigue you, and when unable to accomplish this maneuver, do you pretend to listen but really remain preoccupied with your own thoughts?

( ) yes ( ) no

**13** Do you almost always feel vaguely guilty when you relax and do absolutely nothing for several hours to several days?

( ) yes ( ) no

**14** Do you attempt to schedule more and more in less and less time, and in doing so make fewer and fewer allowances for unforeseen contingencies?

( ) yes ( ) no

**15** In conversation, do you frequently clench your fist or bang your hand upon a table or pound one fist into the palm of your hand in order to emphasize a conversational point?

( ) yes ( ) no

**16** If employed, does your job include frequent deadlines that are difficult to meet?

( ) yes ( ) no

**17** Do you frequently clench your jaw, or even grind your teeth?

( ) yes ( ) no

**18** Do you frequently bring your work or study material (related to your job, not to school) home with you at night?

( ) yes ( ) no

**19** Do you find yourself evaluating not only your own but also the activities of others in terms of numbers?

( ) yes ( ) no

**20** Are you dissatisfied with your present work?

( ) yes ( ) no

## Score Card

4+ = 14 or more points
3+ = 9–13 points
2+ = 4–8 points
1+ = 3 or fewer points

*This material is repeated for you to fill out in the Tear-Out Appendix.*

TABLE
8–2

# The Stress of Adjusting to Change

| Events | Scale of Impact |
|---|---|
| Death of spouse | 100 |
| Divorce | 73 |
| Marital separation | 65 |
| Jail term | 63 |
| Death of close family member | 63 |
| Personal injury or illness | 53 |
| Marriage | 50 |
| Fired at work | 47 |
| Marital reconciliation | 45 |
| Retirement | 45 |
| Change in health of family member | 44 |
| Pregnancy | 40 |
| Sex difficulties | 39 |
| Gain of new family member | 39 |
| Business readjustment | 39 |
| Change in financial state | 38 |
| Death of close friend | 37 |
| Change to different line of work | 36 |

| Events | Scale of Impact |
|---|---|
| Change in number of arguments with spouse | 35 |
| Mortgage over $10,000 | 31 |
| Foreclosure of mortgage or loan | 30 |
| Change in responsibilities at work | 29 |
| Son or daughter leaving home | 29 |
| Trouble with in-laws | 29 |
| Outstanding personal achievement | 28 |
| Begin or end school | 26 |
| Change in living conditions | 25 |
| Revision of personal habits | 24 |
| Trouble with boss | 23 |
| Change in work hours or conditions | 20 |
| Change in residence | 20 |
| Change in schools | 20 |
| Vacation | 13 |
| Christmas | 12 |
| Minor violations of the law | 11 |

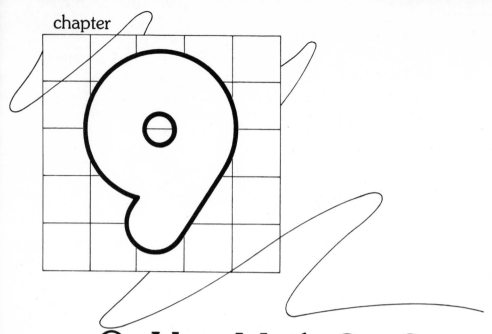

chapter

# On Your Mark, Get Set...

I think that this chapter and the one that follows are the two I've been looking forward to writing the most. In fact, I've written them many times already—in my head—as I run. As you have seen in Figure 2-1 (page 12), many risk factors interact to increase your susceptibility to heart attack and stroke. But fortunately a prescription such as exercise combats a number of these risk factors. And each component of your Whole Heart Program has a similar potential, producing a formidable defense when working together.

Well, what may you reasonably expect regular *aerobic* exercise to do for you? Among other things, it can:

**1** Improve the performance of your heart, lungs, and general circulation.

**2** Improve the coronary collateral circulation and possibly coronary blood vessel size.

**3** Improve your blood lipid and lipoprotein profile, decreasing cholesterol, triglycerides, and the undesirable low-density lipoproteins, while raising the desirable and protective high-density lipoproteins.

**4** Favorably influence blood clotting mechanisms by increasing fibrinolysins and decreasing platelet stickiness.

**5** Help you lose "fat weight" while maintaining and improving muscle mass and tone.

**6** Make the heart less vulnerable to rhythm disturbances.

**7** Lower blood pressure.

**8** Reduce stress and tension. (Some psychiatrists prescribe aerobic exercise instead of drugs in therapy.)

**9** Favorably influence hormonal and metabolic mechanisms, glucose tolerance, thyroid function, and catecholamines.

**10** Make you feel joyfully alive, give you a sense of well-being, and make you more physically attractive.

My personal conclusion is that it is the exercise and diet revolutions and the decrease in smoking among men in the past 10 to 15 years that have already produced an impact on heart disease mortality in the United States. The above list has provided what I would consider compelling reasons to get involved in a regular exercise program. But you'll also need some further practical information.

Getting into good physical condition through exercise is not as difficult as you may think. But it's also not as easy as some popular trade books and magazine articles would lead you to believe. Let's explore the idea that 30 minutes a week is all you need to invest. Under special circumstances that may indeed be *almost* true. If you start out cold and go quickly up to a training heart rate between 70 and 85 percent of your maximal rate, sustain it for 10 minutes, and then go back immediately to your normal activities, you may eventually achieve something approaching a moderate level of conditioning doing that every other day. That is, *if* you can accept such a psychologically unrewarding program, and *if* you don't cause yourself some damage by going too abruptly into such strenuous activity.

The Whole Heart Program requires an investment of a minimum of 30 minutes—not per week, but per day, six days out of each week.

Add 10 minutes for changing clothes and a shower and you're up to 40 minutes. Too much? You don't have the time? There's still more. Your Whole Heart Program also requires about 20 minutes for meditation. That's a full hour out of your busy schedule six days a week. On the seventh day you can rest (from the exercise). Or you can spend as many hours as you want in recreational exercise.

Well that's just too much, you say. Your schedule is already so full there's no way you can fit another hour a day into it. If this is really true, then it becomes even more imperative that you do just that. *Take an hour away from the hassle and invest it in saving your life.* This hour absolutely must not be looked on as just another hour to add to your other conflicting demands. You must not think of it that way or approach it that way. This hour is yours. It's for you and your life and your well-being. It's first priority. There's nothing you have to do that's more important. Your wife or husband or kids have something for you to do during that hour? No! The hour is yours! But it's ultimately for them, too. Because if you die, then you certainly can't do anything for them again. But the demands of your job, your responsibilities, that briefcase full of work? That late meeting? To hell with it! The job, the briefcase, you fit those things *around your hour.* You don't try to fit the hour into your "busy schedule."

The first item on your busy schedule is the hour for you, your life, your health, and your well-being.

If it sounds like I'm ready to leap off the page, grab you by the lapels, and punch you out until you get the idea, you're right. Because I'm talking to myself and my family, too, and we know about the demands of job and family. And we struggled trying to figure out how to fit even ten minutes of exercise into our lives, three times a week. Ten lousy minutes that could probably do us as much harm as good. But we had the wrong idea. Let me repeat it one more time. *You don't fit the hour into your schedule. You fit the schedule around your hour.*

But a full hour all at once? Well, that part isn't necessary. The hour can easily be divided into segments. Most people feel that meditation is best accomplished on arising. But some may prefer a 20-minute period at noon or in the early evening. (Others may desire two 10-minute periods.) The flexibility and strength exercises don't cause much of a sweat, so some can be done at times that suit you best—before going to work or during a lunch break. The aerobic run usually requires the time to change clothes and shower, and it also requires 3 minutes of flexibility warm-up and sometimes a couple of minutes of stretching cool-down, so that segment will take a minimum of 30 minutes.

It's obvious from what you know about yourself and human nature that you can't begin the day by saying, "Sometime today I'm going to take my top priority hour." Remember I said you fit your other work around your hour. So before you go to bed at night, when you're filling out your progress report for your heart program, you designate the time you plan to schedule your exercise for the following day. After a while it becomes automatic—a habit. But until it's established you'll have to be a compulsive schedule-maker.

# Where Do You Start?

In Chapter 2, we obtained some basic information on your physical condition. And in Chapter 4 we made further determinations concerning your weight and how much overweight you may be. It has also been pointed out repeatedly that diet and exercise are inseparable if you're going to lose weight in a way that will promote your health rather than undermine it.

But next I'm going to throw you a curve and tell you that you can't safely do vigorous exercise if you're significantly overweight, out of condition, and over 35 years old. Contradictory? No, just very cautious. In fact, I must add the disclaimer you'll see in almost all books written for lay consumption. If you're over 35 years old, you should have a stress test (usually treadmill) under the supervision of a physician before getting into vigorous exercise. The same precaution goes for you if you're in the 20 to 35 age range and have any of the risk factors shown in Table 9–1. So, if you're over 35 or have risk factors and want to get started right now while you're psyched up and ready to go, what do you do while waiting for your appointment for a stress test? That's where the stages and sequences of conditioning may offer guidance. Read Table 9–2 and find the description that fits you best. You may get a preliminary insight by noting that a 70-year-old who is aerobically trained fits into the same stage as a 20-year-old who gets no exercise (Stage III). If none of the descriptions clearly accommodates you, select the one that comes closest. And if still in doubt, assume you're in the poorer stage of conditioning. You may then begin your program by selecting the appropriate table and sequence of conditioning, and proceeding to the point where medical clearance must be obtained.

In reading the tables you will doubtless have questions about definitions, such as physical life-style, interval training, and aerobics. So we'll get one of these out of the way now, and get into interval training and aerobics in the next chapter.

Until recently, the American life-style might have been characterized by: Never run when you can walk; never walk when you can stand; never stand when you can sit; and never sit when you can lie down. For several decades we were a spectator society interested in watching others be physically active in sports, but dedicated to saving our energy. Saving it for what? It shouldn't take an exercise physiologist or cardiologist to tell you that the less physical work you do, the less physical work your body becomes capable of doing. And the converse is also true: The more physical work you do (up to defined limits), the more you become able to do. Your body accommodates to doing almost nothing or to achieving remarkable physical feats. It just depends on what you train it to do. Demand little and you get little. Demand a lot and you get a lot. That's the homeostatic wisdom of the body.

Maybe you're one of those who has developed habits of "saving your energy," waiting for elevators rather than walking a couple of flights, or backing your polluting gas guzzler out of the garage to go a few blocks. If you are, you probably also hire someone to mow your lawn to save your valuable time (so you can plop in front of the TV set, stuff your face with high calorie, high cholesterol, and high salt goodies and watch other people get some exercise). Or when you're outside and have some time, you just lie in the sun rather than exert yourself. Whatever you do, you do it with the least expenditure of your energy possible—and probably with the maximal expenditure of oil and other nonrenewable resources.

This is what I'd call a nonphysical life-style. And it's still the life-style of too many Americans—possibly even you. We can all speculate as to how we were sold on such a physiologically unsound way to live. But let's not. Let's just turn from it as quickly as we can.

Well then, what's a physical life-style? Just the opposite. Look at your activities and ask yourself how you can perform them in a way in which you can extract some good exercise.

You'll have to make entries in your journal as to what your daily activities are and try to decide how you might have achieved exercise from what you did. I've given only some simple examples such as taking stairs rather than elevators and walking or bicycling in preference to using the automobile, whenever possible. But you know what goes on in your life and the opportunities you have for exercise. A few more possibilities will come to mind as we go along.

# Stretching and Flexibility Exercises

These exercises may be started with safety at any age or stage. And since walking and stretching and flexibility exercises are the only physical activities suggested for those in Stage V, while waiting for medical clearance, it's reasonable to discuss these early in the chapter. Stretching and flexibility exercises are also the warm-up part of the 10-20-30 exercises as well as the warm-up for running.

On the way to the Eighth World Congress of Cardiology, which was held in Tokyo in September 1978, I stopped over in Hong Kong for a few days, and had the opportunity to observe some interesting exercise rituals. Knowing how polluted the air would be from auto exhaust when I arrived in the evening, and realizing how hot and humid the weather was, I knew I'd have to run very early in the morning, before the pollution became unpleasant. (I should note here that wherever I travel I take my running shoes and running clothes.) So my first morning in Hong Kong, before six and before sunrise, I was out running and trying to find a congenial area for this activity. I made a turn up a steep road toward St. John's Cathedral and the central government offices. Here there were trees and grass. A small park in the middle of a very crowded city. And here, before dawn, were countless residents of the city—exercising. I kept running uphill along Battery Path and saw signs pointing to the botanical and zoological gardens. All along the route were the early-morning exercisers, and when my run finally led me into the gardens, the paths were so choked with people exercising that I had to slow down to a jog to avoid a collision.

Running slowly I was able to study what they were doing—these were mostly older men and women. No stiff hup-two-three-four, Germanic-Swedish routines. Nothing that an American gym teacher or army drill sergeant would recognize as exercise. Just gentle stretching movements. Almost like a ballet. The men would sometimes go through a series of movements that would end with striking a pose reminiscent of the martial arts. But everything was basically stretching and flexibility. And each person was performing his individual routine. As I returned, running along Garden Road, I encountered my first fellow runners—Caucasians and younger Chinese.

I must admit that I was intrigued by this approach to exercise. And when I arrived in Tokyo I witnessed a slightly more vigorous variant of Asian exercise in the very small park near my hotel. The early-morning activities here were more directed, coordinated, and less individualized.

But the emphasis again was on stretching and flexibility rather than strength. The runners in Tokyo were out a little earlier, perhaps because the pollution becomes even more formidable as the day progresses than in Hong Kong.

As I'm writing now I can still see vividly the gentle exercisers along Battery Path, and I conclude that it's a very pleasant way to begin the day. But since I don't know the exact routines, I can only offer American versions of stretching and flexibility exercises, which are presented in the sections that follow. Of course, you can devise your own routines. The principles underlying all of these are to develop a full range of motion around joints and articulations *without* straining against resistance (head and neck, shoulders, trunk, hips, and knees), and to stretch muscles rhythmically in a natural flow that involves every part of the body.

These exercises have intrinsic value in producing good muscle tone, in maintaining mobile joints and suppleness, and in producing a sense of well-being. They are also necessary preludes to the more vigorous (or ballistic) of the 10-20-30 exercises—and to running. If you have been on your duff ever since you got your high school gym teacher off your back, you should ease back into exercise as painlessly and pleasantly as possible. This is especially true if you're over 35. You can't just barrel into an activity like a teenager. Your muscles and joints will rebel and you'll end up with a punishing experience (sprains, strains, and pains). And as we've already discussed, desired behavior gets established through rewards, and undesired behavior gets discouraged through punishment. Don't get these two reinforcement mechanisms turned around.

## Gym Teachers and Exercise = Punishment

Yet isn't that what happens? Hasn't that been the experience of most of you? Exercise is equated with punishment. And who's responsible for that? I submit that the responsibility rests on the muscular shoulders of the nation's third greatest collective health hazard: gym teachers and coaches. Not only do they make exercise an unpleasant experience, with their damned hup-two-three-four routines, but they have traditionally used exercise as a deliberate punishment. "You left your locker open, give me twenty-five push-ups." "You're clowning around, give me two fast laps. And if it's not fast enough, you'll have to give me two more." So when kids finally get out from under the thumbs of the frustrated jocks who teach physical education, what do they do? If they're not genetic jocks themselves, they avoid exercise like the plague it was shown them to be.

But what if a kid has an enduring love for athletics that will not be quenched by a gym teacher? He gets to play football for as long as his joints, bones, and nerves can handle it. But a lot of these kids may wash out with injuries that not only prohibit future participation in that particular blood sport but impair their ability and their pleasure in many healthful exercises.

Not long before he died, I had the pleasure of having dinner with the dean of American cardiologists, Dr. Paul Dudley White. Dr. White had maintained a lasting interest in the state of health of Harvard graduates, particularly ex-athletes, so I took this opportunity to ask him about the current findings of his studies. He pointed out that an entire eight-oar Olympic gold-medal-winning crew had returned to Harvard for their fiftieth class reunion. Most of them were still rowing—but single-sculling, rather than pulling in an eight-oared boat.

The ex–football players presented another situation. Their involvement in exercise had rapidly diminished in many cases. With heavy muscles and heavy appetites to support, they'd deposited a lot of fat that could not be burned off by getting 22 guys together in a board room for a scrimmage. Their morbidity and mortality data were disastrous when compared with classmates who had prepared for and had continued to participate in exercise throughout their entire adult lives. But so many gym teachers and coaches have great difficulty in conveying this message to their charges—in preparing people for a lifetime of exercise. We'll discuss this problem in more detail in the chapter for kids.

## Exercises for Strength

In this category are a variety of exercises, including the vigorous ballistic exercises (typical calisthenics). A little of this goes a long way unless you have some conditioning goal in mind in which physical strength is essential. These exercises are valuable for kids, generally useful for men, and less appealing for women. However, these exercises cannot be avoided entirely.

After a patient has had a heart attack and has been in bed for a required period of time, he or she must very gradually work into a rehabilitation exercise program. Joints and muscles must be babied while there is a gradual achievement of function to a level that permits the patient to exercise on his own at home.

I'm sure you have no problem visualizing the rationale and wisdom of such a course of action. What you may not realize is that many Americans, even relatively young ones, are in such deplorable physical condition that they must be approached in almost the same way that the recovering heart attack patient is. A young woman, a medical student on a summer fellowship assisting in my program, was helping me with our tables for age- and stage-specific conditioning. She asked: "Where do you put people who are not a bit overweight, who are young, and who are in terrible physical condition?"

I was quite surprised by the question, so I countered with: "I wasn't aware that there are many such people."

Her answer: "The majority of my classmates are in that category. And most women my age fit the description. They may look slim and trim and tanned and healthy, but the most exercise they get is rubbing on suntan lotion."

Well, I haven't personally done a well-designed study to validate this medical student's contention, but I have made some subsequent observations through her perspective, and I'm inclined to believe that she may be right. Please do not try aerobic running or vigorous ballistic exercises *until your muscles and joints are ready.* You get your joints ready by performing gentle stretching and flexibility exercises for a couple of weeks. Then follows muscle building. Only after flexibility and strength are achieved through gradually increasing function in an incremental exercise program should you consider aerobic running and vigorous exercise.

# Walking

This is a suitable starting point for any age. Together with the stretching and flexibility exercises. This is where your beginner's program starts if you're over 35 and don't qualify for Stage II. Even those younger than 35, particularly sedentary young women in Stage III, may have to begin with walking in order to achieve some nonpunishing exercise.

First you have to lay out a measured course for yourself. The odometer on your car or bicycle, or a pedometer, will help you determine the distance for 1 mile, 1.5 miles, and so on. Then you begin walking. The first day you walk a mile at a completely comfortable pace and see how long it takes you and how fast your heart rate is at the beginning and end of the walk, and ten minutes later. Be sure your recovery heart rate returns to below 100 within ten minutes after completing the walk. If it does not return to below 100 at ten minutes, even this minimal exertion is too much for you, and you should decrease your walking distance and rate until you have a medical examination.

After one to eight weeks of daily comfortable walks of 1 mile (depending on your progress, your age, and your stage of conditioning), you may increase the distance to 1.5 miles—again checking your heart rate before, immediately after, and ten minutes later. If your recovery rate is satisfactory, just maintain a comfortable pace without trying to improve your time until you have medical clearance. After you have medical clearance (or if you don't require it), you may begin walking more briskly and even intersperse slow jogging for short distances according to the schedule in Table 9–3. As you'll note in the table, Level 1 is the lowest. You start walking 1 mile, increase to 1.5 miles, still walking, and then increase to walk/run for 1.5 miles. The final stage is to have a longer period of walk/run, of unspecified distance but presumably greater than 1.5 miles. The schedule is just a general guide to you. This is the beginning of interval training.

We'll return to Table 9–3 later. You'll note that I've been extremely cautious in my walk/run prescription for those over 60. This isn't because 60- and 70-year-olds can't do aerobic training even if they haven't exercised in decades. It's just that there is a wide variation in physical capacities in this age group, and I feel more comfortable with the idea of an individualized exercise prescription for those just starting to exercise at ages beyond 60. For some people over 60 a walking program and stretching and flexibility will be as far as they should ever go with exercise. For others interval training and full aerobic conditioning are possible, and the programs in this book are entirely suitable. This is where personal medical input will be desirable for an individual prescription.

## 10-20-30 Exercises

### Stretching, Flexibility, and Strength ○ Running and other aerobic exercises are the keys to the health of your heart. However, a balanced health program requires that you have adequate strength and tone in your muscles, and a good range of motion in your joints. Most people can't just go out and run. It would be punishing and self-defeating. Stiffness and injuries will occur that will prevent you from running.

In this section we'll go through exercises suitable for men, women, and children. These are for warm-up, strength, and flexibility. The 10-20-30 merely refers to the number of times each exercise is performed in the series. The first principle of exercise is: Make it nonpunishing. Easy victories, small victories, a step at a time is the way to proceed. For the younger person who is currently exercising vigorously, the warm-up activities will seem close to ludicrous. The point is that they're designed to be such easy victories that anyone can start exercising at any time of the day—dragging out of bed in the morning, dragging home from work at night, during lunch hour. Warm-up exercises should be performed daily.

## Warm-up

**1) Ten head rolls**  Stand comfortably, feet apart, belly sucked in, and begin by simply rolling your head around ten times. Put your chin on your chest, let your head lean to the right side, then let it fall to the back, to the left, and return to the front. Five times starting to the right, followed by five times starting to the left. Anybody (unless there is a spinal defect) can roll his head around. This is clearly an easy victory to start your exercise program.

**2) Ten arm circles**  Consider your straight arm as a propeller. Do a full circle with your right arm, reaching forward, above, and behind, as if you were doing a backstroke in swimming—five times with your right arm. Then reverse the direction for five forward strokes (in the direction of the crawl in swimming). Repeat the same routine with your left arm (Figure 9–1).

**3) Ten arm wraps with arm flings**  This works on the range of motion of your shoulders in another plane. Extend your arms straight out to the side, shoulder level, parallel to the floor, bring them in, wrapping them around your body, then snap them out to the sides again—all at shoulder height (Figure 9–2).

**4) Ten Chinese trunk twisters**  Feet apart, raise your arms straight up over your head and rotate your body at the waist, reaching to the right, stretching back, coming forward to the left and bending over reaching toward the floor (see Figure 9–3). The secret of this exercise is gentle rotation. No stiff-kneed ballistic, touching the toes, "hup-two-three-four." Just gentle rolling. As you warm up, your hands may begin to touch your toes and the floor as your body circles around. But the object is easy stretching, not toe-touching. To avoid getting dizzy do only five in one direction before doing five in the other direction.

**5) Ten knee hugs**  Standing on your left foot, lift your right knee up and pull it to your body with both hands (Figure 9–4). Do the same with your left knee. Alternate right with left until ten knee hugs have been completed.

**6) Ten toe stands**  Simply stand up on your toes (as high as you can) ten times. In this exercise and the next one you may want to support yourself by holding on to something.

**162**

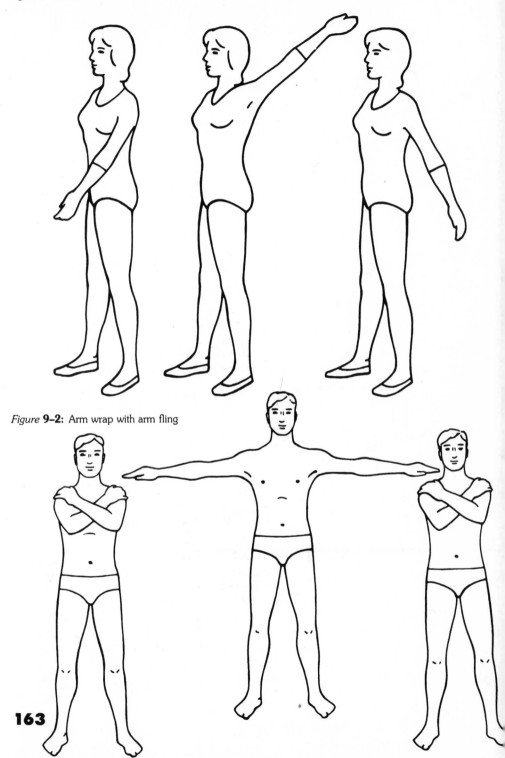

*Figure* **9–1:** Arm circle

*Figure* **9–2:** Arm wrap with arm fling

**163**

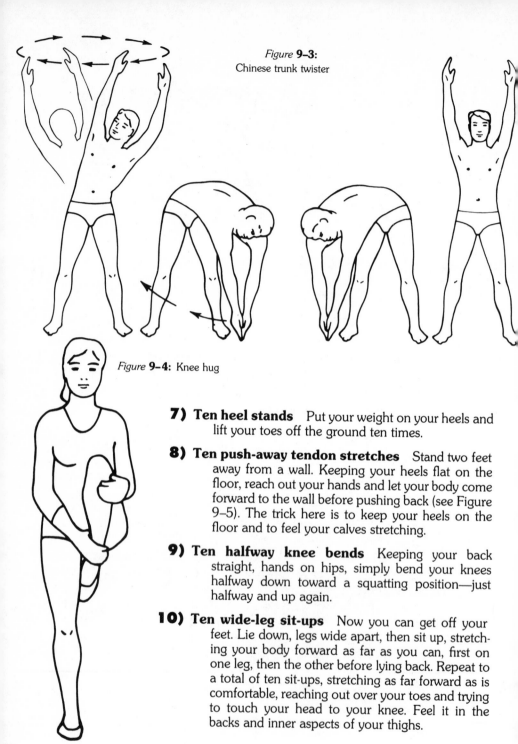

*Figure* **9–3:**
Chinese trunk twister

*Figure* **9–4:** Knee hug

**7) Ten heel stands**   Put your weight on your heels and lift your toes off the ground ten times.

**8) Ten push-away tendon stretches**   Stand two feet away from a wall. Keeping your heels flat on the floor, reach out your hands and let your body come forward to the wall before pushing back (see Figure 9–5). The trick here is to keep your heels on the floor and to feel your calves stretching.

**9) Ten halfway knee bends**   Keeping your back straight, hands on hips, simply bend your knees halfway down toward a squatting position—just halfway and up again.

**10) Ten wide-leg sit-ups**   Now you can get off your feet. Lie down, legs wide apart, then sit up, stretching your body forward as far as you can, first on one leg, then the other before lying back. Repeat to a total of ten sit-ups, stretching as far forward as is comfortable, reaching out over your toes and trying to touch your head to your knee. Feel it in the backs and inner aspects of your thighs.

**164**

*Figure* **9–5:** Push-away tendon stretch

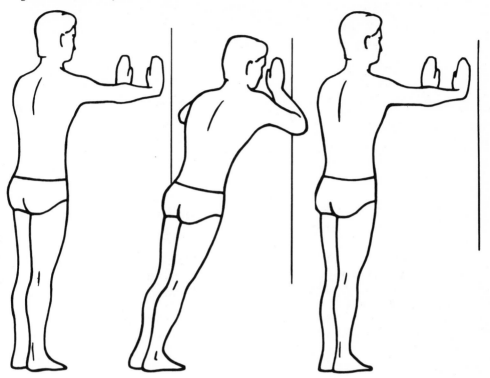

This is the basic warm-up routine that may be followed by men, women, and children before running or other aerobic exercise, and before a more intensive strength and flexibility workout. When you're just starting out learning a warm-up routine, take as long as you may need to perform the series. After the routine is established, it should require around three minutes. A good competitive Type A individual can probably do the series in 38.4 seconds. But by now you surely realize that's not the object of the exercise. In fact there are those who would advocate that rather than do a series of ten stretching exercises, such as the push-away tendon stretch and the wide-leg sit-up, it would be advisable to simply hold the maximally stretched position of each exercise for three minutes. I guess this is what ballet dancers do at the bar. Some of you may wish to substitute three-minute "holds" for a series of ten "stretches."

**Cool down** ○ If you have a long aerobic workout, a 30-minute run or greater, you will probably find it useful to cool down by performing a few each of your warm-up exercises. For shorter workouts the cool-down is optional, and most people don't find a need for it. This is something you'll have to determine for yourself.

## Strength and Flexibility

There are many good routines for strength and flexibility: the Royal Canadian Air Force and the West Point exercises have loyal followings. The goal of programs of this type is to exercise major muscle groups. A secondary gain is a small amount of cardiopulmonary and lactic-acid, anaerobic conditioning (see pages 175–77). I refer readers to the paperback editions of these two exercise programs (see Bibliography) for more details and variations on the four basic muscle-group exercises. This part of the 10-20-30 exercises should be performed at least every other day and should be preceded by the warm-up exercises.

**1) Chinese trunk twister**   You've already been introduced to this one in the Warm-up section. An adequate workout with this exercise is accomplished by doing it 30 times. You've done 10 in your warm-up, so you just repeat 20 more in your workout. Few people will have trouble doing a full 30 twisters a day. But if you do, take your time and ease into it, increasing your performance by 2 or 3 with each workout until you

*Figure* **9–6:**
Bent-leg sit-up

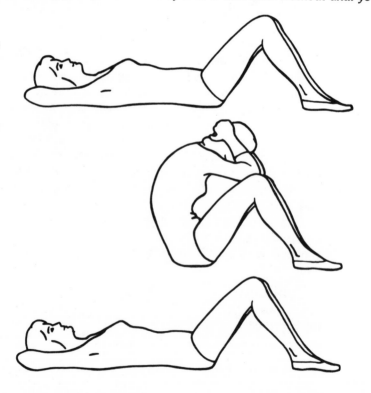

reach 30. Some days you'll do warm-up, strength and flexibility exercises, and running. Other days you may limit yourself to just warm-up and running, and still other days only warm-up with strength and flexibility exercises. The trunk twister is something you'll do every day.

**2) Sit-ups**  There are several possible ways to do sit-ups. Youngsters who start right off with the bent-leg sit-up may find it easy to do (see Figure 9–6). But most older individuals will find the straight-leg sit-up easier (see Figure 9–7). Some of you may feel pretty tough and want a little variety. You can try the chair sit-up in Figure 9–8. Again, many of you will be able to do a full 30 sit-ups without going through a progression. If you're at a suitable teenage maintenance level, you'll want to stay with your 50 or 60 sit-ups. There's no point in regressing to a lower maintenance level. There are those who will have all they can do to accomplish 10 of the sit-ups shown in Figure 9–7. The routine for individuals in this group would be to progress to 30 straight-leg sit-ups before trying to progress to bent-leg sit-ups. Try to increase your number with each workout, even if it's only 1 more each time. And then maintain your level at 30 straight- or bent-leg sit-ups.

**3) Butterflies**  There are a number of alternative exercises for the back muscles, which you can find in various sources, such as the West Point and Royal Canadian Air Force books. For this exercise you merely lie on your belly with your arms extended out from the shoulders and raise your legs, arms, head, and chest as far off the floor as you can (Figure

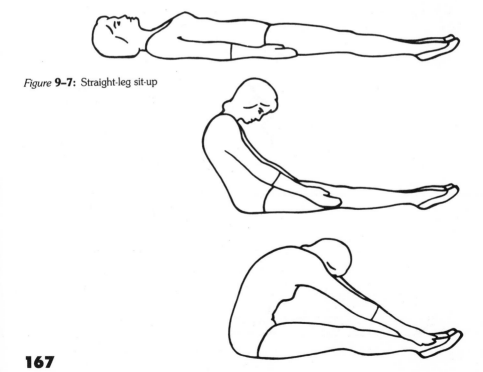

*Figure* **9–7:** Straight-leg sit-up

9–9). The maintenance level of 30 can be done by most people at the very beginning, but if you don't find this comfortable, start at 10 or 20 and work your way up at a rate of 2 or 3 more at each workout.

**4) Push-ups**   This is the exercise that will progress most slowly for those who are out of condition. Your ultimate goal can be 20 or 30 depending on your age and disposition. If you're able to do 30 immediately, that's a good level to maintain. If you have to struggle to do 10 or 15, then just take it easy, work your way up slowly, and increase by 1 or 2 a week. The classical push-up is performed as illustrated in Figure 9–10. In the prone position put your legs together, place your hands on the floor, three or four inches outside each shoulder, and distribute your weight between your hands and your toes. Push up until your elbows are

*Figure* **9–8:** Chair sit-up

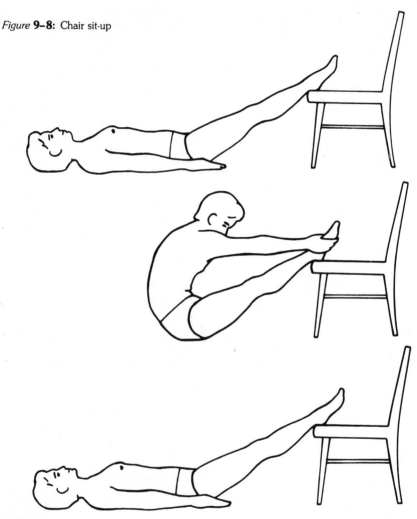

straight, and let yourself down until your nose or forehead just barely touches the floor. Keep your back straight. When you let yourself down, your belly and chest *should not touch*—only your nose. Figure 9–11 shows the push-up often advocated for women. My youngest daughter wrinkles her nose disdainfully at this "female push-up." The difference between this and the classic push-up is that the weight is distributed between the hands and knees rather than between the hands and toes. It's certainly easier, but not very challenging for girls and young women in reasonably good condition. As with other exercises there are variations you might prefer as you work into them, such as the eight-count push-up, the hand-clap push-up, and others that are illustrated in the supplemental reading. The supplemental reading and exercises are for variety only. What is covered in this book is quite adequate for a basic routine.

*Figure* **9–9**: Butterflies

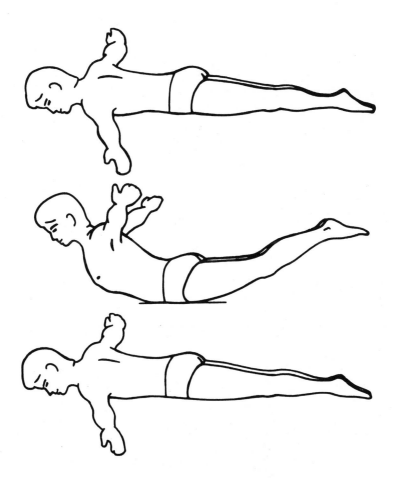

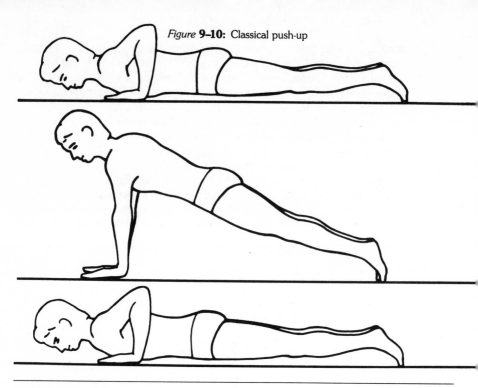

*Figure* **9–10:** Classical push-up

*Figure* **9–11:** Bent-knee
     push-up

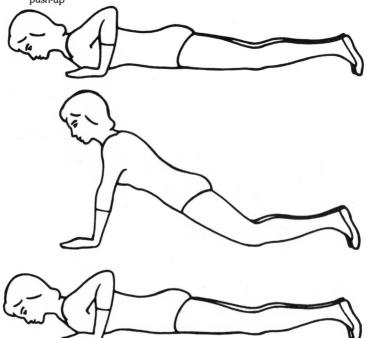

TABLE
9-1

## Risk Factors Requiring Medical Clearance for Patients Over 20 Years of Age Who Wish to Enter Aerobic Training

**1** Known heart disease

**2** Risk factors

    **a** Early-onset coronary heart disease ($<55$ years) in first-degree relatives

    **b** Blood pressure $>140/90$ at rest

    **c** Cholesterol $>250$

    **d** Obesity $>20$ percent overweight (relative weight $>1.20$)

    **e** Cigarette smoking

TABLE
9-2

## Stages of Entry into Conditioning

| | Ages | Condition |
|---|---|---|
| **Stage V** | Over 60 | Not currently participating in regular aerobic exercise |
| | 50–60 | 10 percent overweight, nonphysical life-style, no exercise or irregular exercise (e.g., weekend golf) |
| **Stage IV** | 50–60 | Desirable weight, physical life-style, weekend and some weekday exercise |
| | 25–50 | $>20$ percent overweight, nonphysical life-style, no exercise |
| | 35–50 | 10–20 percent overweight, nonphysical life-style, irregular exercise |
| | 45–50 | 5–10 percent overweight, physical life-style, irregular exercise |

| **Stage III** | Over 50 | Desirable weight, physical life-style, regular aerobic exercise |
| | 35–50 | 5–10 percent overweight, physical life-style, weekend and some weekday exercise |
| | 40–50 | Desirable weight, physical life-style, weekend and some weekday exercise |
| | 30–40 | 10–20 percent overweight, physical life-style, irregular exercise |
| | 20–35 | Desirable weight, nonphysical life-style, no exercise or irregular exercise. *Risk factors.* |
| **Stage II** | 35–50 | Desirable weight, physical life-style, regular aerobic exercise |
| | 25–35 | Desirable weight, physical life-style, weekend and some weekday exercise |
| | 6–25 | > 20 percent overweight, nonphysical life-style, irregular exercise |
| **Stage I** | Under 35 | Desirable weight, physical life-style, regular exercise, no risk factors |

*Note: If you do not find the description of a stage that completely meets your particular circumstances, select the one that is closest. When in doubt, assume that you fall into the poorer stage of conditioning.*

TABLE
**9-3**

# From Walking to Running

*Start at Level 1 and work to Level 4. Increase from lower heart rates, shorter distances, and shorter exercise periods to higher heart rates, longer distances, and longer exercise periods.*

|  |  | Level 1<br>Walk | Level 2<br>Walk | Level 3<br>Walk/Run | Level 4<br>Walk/Run |
|---|---|---|---|---|---|
| **Ages 6–49** | Distance |  |  |  |  |
|  | (miles) | 1 | 1.5 | 1.5 | — |
|  | Minutes | 17–12 | 25–18 | — | 40–20 |
|  | Weeks in Level | 1–4 | 2–4 | 2–4 | 2–4 |
|  | Heart Rate |  |  |  |  |
|  | (percent) | 60–70 | 60–70 | 70–85 | 70–85 |
| **Ages 50–59** | Distance |  |  |  |  |
|  | (miles) | 1 | 1.5 | 1.5 | — |
|  | Minutes | 17–12 | 28–20 | — | 40–20 |
|  | Weeks in Level | 4–6 | 4–6 | 4–6 | 4–6 |
|  | Heart Rate |  |  |  |  |
|  | (percent) | 60–70 | 60–70 | 70–85 | 70–85 |
| **Ages 60+** | Distance |  |  |  |  |
|  | (miles) | 1 | 1.5 | medical |  |
|  | Minutes | 25–20 | 35–30 | supervision |  |
|  | Weeks in Level | 6–8 | 6–8 | and individual |  |
|  | Heart Rate |  |  | prescription |  |
|  | (percent) | 60–70 | 60–70 |  |  |

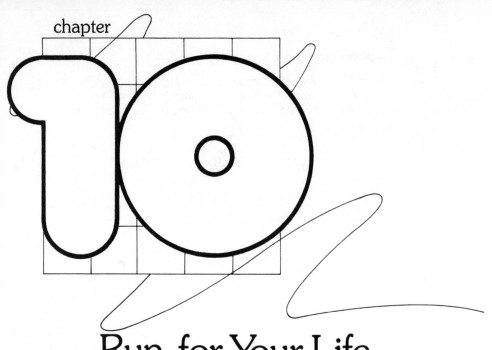

# Run for Your Life

The title of this chapter captures much of the spirit of the exercise revolution. And I think it may well be able to deliver what it promises. But when we speak of running, we really mean any good aerobic exercise. Running is just the most common and most convenient. So far we've got you stretching and walking and strengthening your muscles, all of which are good for you—and all of which are necessary preludes to aerobic exercise. We've also had you thinking about what stage you're in, so you can follow an exercise prescription appropriate for you. But now let me tell you that in one series, over half of the adults who started an aerobic exercise program had to quit because of severe joint and muscle problems. It is absolutely essential that you are prepared for running through a strength and flexibility program. If you need more help than this book is able to provide, you may require the assistance of a professional in orthopedics or physical medicine. *Do not allow imprudent exercise or injury to disrupt your program.*

Now we'd better stop and give you a few more definitions.

# Interval Training
# and Aerobics

First, the idea of interval training is really very simple and it's entirely compatible with your personal experience. If you work for half an hour at a pace near the limits of your physical capacity, you collapse. If you work for five minutes at a similar pace, then rest, work another five minutes, then rest, and so on, you get the same amount of work done without collapsing. The only other difference is that it takes longer if you alternate rest periods with periods of vigorous exercise.

Now, I'm required to introduce you to some very simple principles of energy and exercise—the three energy systems, ATP-PC, lactic acid, and oxygen. The first two systems, ATP-PC and lactic acid, rely mostly on stored energy and do not depend extensively on oxygen. Therefore these are called *anaerobic*—meaning without oxygen. The third system requires oxygen and is therefore called *aerobic*. And that's a term you're probably familiar with from the work of Dr. Kenneth Cooper, who has done so much to popularize aerobic exercise.

ATP (adenosine triphosphate) is the actual source of energy for muscles. If you need to use your muscles for a burst of exercise lasting only a few seconds, you use the ATP-PC system. PC stands for phosphocreatine, which like ATP is stored in muscle and can be instantaneously converted to ATP. But only so much ATP and PC can be stored. An event such as the 100-yard dash totally depletes this system.

So how can you exercise for more than ten seconds? Well, sugar is also stored in muscle and can be used for energy without requiring an immediate supply of oxygen. But when exercise demands exceed the capacity of the body to utilize oxygen, the sugar breaks down into a product called lactic acid. This lactic acid system is relied on extensively for vigorous exercise lasting from one-half to three minutes, such as the 440- and 880-yard dashes. It allows you to run 440 yards faster in one burst than you could run 440 yards over and over again as part of a two-mile run. However, you pay a price for this. You accumulate what has sometimes been called an oxygen debt to signify that you have not reduced the products of exercise to a relatively nontoxic state. You have withdrawn more energy from your account than can be immediately replenished by oxygen.

Lactic acid is toxic. It's what gives you that painful feeling of fatigue. When I was competing in track in high school and college, my events were the 440 and 880. For many of those years I didn't know that it was possible to run without being in agony. But when I discovered cross-country, I found that I could run four miles at a somewhat slower pace than the 440 and feel reasonably good at the end. At the time I didn't understand why. Now, of course, it's clear. For about the first three minutes of intensive exercise the predominating energy system is lactic acid. After three minutes you switch into the aerobic oxygen-using system. The 440 and the 880 are events that rely on the lactic acid system. And lactic acid hurts. So my advice to those of you entering the Whole Heart Program is to stay out of the lactic acid system—because, as you've been reading over and over, punishment discourages the establishment of a behavior. Only the perception of a greater reward permits a person to tolerate pain and punishment. For those who may become dedicated runners there are great rewards to offset pain. But don't start off with pain if you want to give yourself a fair chance to get your program established.

There are two ways to avoid excessive fatigue and pain from lactic acid. One is to intersperse rest periods to cancel your oxygen debt. And the other is to increase your pace very slowly. If you're at a stage where running for even a short distance at a slow pace is painful, then you should give yourself frequent periods of relief by slowing to a walk or stopping. What's happening is that your conditioning is so poor that your blood level of lactic acid rises as much from a little exercise as it does from vigorous and intense exercise in a person who is well conditioned.

Once you're in good physical condition, you can still profitably use interval training to permit more intense exercise than you could sustain for long periods. Instead of running 2.5 miles nonstop at eight minutes per mile you may wish to break the distance up into four runs of 220 yards, two of 440 yards, and a run of 1.5 miles, with a rest period between each run. Under these circumstances each of the short runs could be at a slightly faster rate than the continuous run and would thus offer a higher intensity of training. Another advantage to this type of training is that you actually benefit from rest periods in that the oxygen-pulse, as it reflects the amount of blood pumped by each beat of the heart, is higher during the recovery period immediately following exercise than it is during the exercise itself. Some people prefer interval runs to continuous runs, even after they're well conditioned, as an aid to improving their conditioning. I still do interval running about once a week, even though what I really enjoy is long continuous runs. These are personal preferences.

Walk/runs or interval runs are the advised methods of training early in your conditioning program. After you're well conditioned you'll have to decide what type of running you enjoy the most. Just be sure that your training includes a long sequence in which the aerobic system predominates. Remember it takes about three minutes to switch into the aerobic phase. It also takes about two minutes to replenish the ATP-PC system after it has been depleted. So whether your interval of running is 440 yards or one mile, two minutes of resting-walking-flexing is the appropriate period of recovery before running again.

Another way to avoid the unpleasantness of lactic acid accumulating in your blood is to increase the intensity of your exercise slowly. As I mentioned earlier, it's inadvisable for someone less than a highly trained young athlete to go abruptly into intense exercise that will be prolonged for a matter of minutes. In fact, even reasonably well conditioned young men abruptly stepping on a treadmill going up a slight grade at nine miles per hour can show abnormalities in their electrocardiograms. Those of you who have stress tests will start off slowly and will increase your work (speed and grade of treadmill) only every one to three minutes (depending on the protocol). This is a good thing to bear in mind when you're exercising—even after you've become reasonably well conditioned. If your cardiologist isn't inclined to take a chance of driving you abruptly into vigorous exercise, you might be well advised to be equally cautious.

## Heart-Rated Exercise and Aerobics

The type of conditioning you will want for good cardiovascular health and pleasant relaxation is aerobic. Aerobic conditioning starts after about three minutes of sustained heart rate between 70 and 85 percent of your maximal heart rate. The beauty of heart-rated exercise and aerobic training is that it takes into account your physical condition. Say you're in terrible shape. You have all you can do to push the elevator button or twist the knob of your TV set. What does it take to start getting you in condition? Actually very little. Brisk walking will probably take you above 70 percent of maximal heart rate—right into the aerobic range. Well then, say you've been training regularly for two months or are starting off in pretty good condition. What does it take now to reach a level of conditioning? Probably only running will get your rate up to an aerobic level. And what does it take to get the heart rate of a marathon runner into the 70 to 85 percent range? Something like seven- or eight-minute miles.

Table 10–1 has some key information for you. It gives you the range of heart rate for your age that you should sustain for successful aerobic conditioning. For beginners and for warm-up, aim for 60 percent of maximal heart rate. After you've progressed to the point of entering aerobic training, stay closer to the 70 percent column; then as you progress comfortably, you may get closer to the 85 percent limit. However, you should achieve conditioning as long as you get above 70 percent. Conditioning, predictably, takes place sooner for higher training heart rates and for longer periods of time at those higher rates. Thus, 10 minutes at 70 percent, three days a week, will provide some conditioning experience. However, 30 minutes daily at a sustained 85 percent would provide a higher level of conditioning sooner. And of course competitive distance runners perform at a level beyond the 85 percent limit. But beyond 85 percent you cross the anaerobic threshold. And that's where lactic acid pain starts. The dedicated and addicted runners talk about "crashing through the wall of pain." Maybe you'll become an addict, too. However, this presentation has as its only goal cardiovascular health through nonpunishing exercise. What you do and where you go after you achieve satisfactory conditioning is your business.

I went through the little routine in the previous paragraph just to catch those Type A individuals who have been thinking ahead trying to figure out how to speed up the process, if not beat the system. It took you a long time to get into lousy shape. The program being suggested here, or the exercise prescription you may receive from a cardiologist, is designed for gradual and safe conditioning. And gradual as it is, it doesn't really take very long at all. But please don't rush it. There's no one to compete with. Your goal is health, not the achievement of a given time or a given distance.

Now just look at Table 10–1. You'll notice that your maximal heart rate slows with age, as does your resting pulse. So the training heart rate that is recommended also decreases with age. However, these numbers are not engraved in stone. They're based on surveys of "normal" individuals and on such simple arithmetic approximations as subtracting your age from 220 to obtain a predicted maximal rate. But those of you who have stress tests will find out what your own maximal rate actually is. Your personal exercise prescription can then be based on 70 to 85 percent of that specific rate. My maximal rate turns out to be considerably higher than the formula predicts for me. And because I maintain a reasonable level of conditioning, my resting heart rate is much lower than the American average.

For those of you who can control your competitiveness and wish just to have an idea of how you do in 12-minute and 1.5-mile tests, you may take the tests every month or two. Someday you may get up and feel great and know you're going to have a good run. Well, look at your watch when you start and again when you reach the end of 1.5 miles. See how you did—*if* you feel that you ran well. If you feel you didn't run well, don't bother checking. It really doesn't matter that much. I don't time myself more than three or four times a year. But I do take my heart rate after almost every run.

# Pre-Enrollment Information and Regulations

Although I'm extremely anxious to get on with the sections on running, I feel I have to emphasize a few points, some of which have been discussed before and some of which will be discussed again (and again).

**1**   *Don't* enter an exercise program without medical clearance if your risk profile or age and stage require such clearance. Why? Because severe and sudden exertion in the poorly conditioned individual can place a serious stress on the cardiovascular system.

**2**   *Don't* expect that exercise can be taken as an isolated activity rather than as a component of an entire life-style to reduce your risk of coronary heart disease. Most marathon runners are by the requirements of their avocation committed to a healthy life-style. Someone like Walter Stack could personify the marathon ideal. Mr. Stack, at age 71, runs 17 miles and swims one-half mile every day before going to work at the physically taxing job of hod carrier. For recreation in his 72nd year he has scheduled five marathon runs. So when a marathoner has a heart attack it's so rare as to be newsworthy in the sense of man-bites-dog. But it occurs. And when it does I believe it reflects severe genetic and/or environmental factors. I also believe that most runners who get into trouble *do not* approach their exercise as only one component of an overall commitment to healthful living. They are not sufficiently in touch with themselves to recognize when they are doing something unphysiologic, punishing, and damaging. Two examples should suffice. In the 1978 New York Marathon, a runner began having chest pains at 8 kilometers but ran 5.6 kilometers more before collapsing. Another runner training for this same event died a month before the marathon after a hard run. As a sign of his obsession with running, one week before his death he had emblazoned on his t-shirt: "You haven't really run a good marathon until you drop dead at the finish line.—Pheidippides." So the word is: *Do not undertake serious aerobic exercise unless you embrace a full health program in a nonobsessive way.*

**3**   *Don't* do vigorous exercise when you have an acute infection. Believe me, I've tried it, and it's counterproductive and risky.

**4**   *Do* look for *variety* as well as *regularity* in your exercise and running. Make it fun. Repeating exactly the same routines in exactly the same way at the same time every day can become a drag. That isn't to say that you shouldn't adhere to the general principles of habit formation, but once you've formed the habit and stated the theme, develop your own variations and inventions. We've decided that about 30 minutes a day must be set aside for exercise. But it doesn't have to be the same routine day after day, as long as a basic minimum is achieved.

After aerobic exercise, the cornerstone of the basic minimum, the next block is stretching, flexibility, and strength for the major muscle groups and large joints—what I called the 10-20-30 exercises in Chapter 9. Please look at Table 10–2 for a typical program that should provide optimal cardiovascular-pulmonary health for most of us. But then look at Table 10–3 to see how such a program may be translated into practice for someone who has made exercise a habit and is reasonably well conditioned. Actually, the events recorded could easily represent my own exercise journal for the past ten days. Exercise some days lasted about 30 minutes, other days less, other days more. But it averaged out so that the basic minimum was accomplished. An 85 percent heart rate was not considered necessary, nor was it always achieved. However, an aerobic goal of 70 percent or better was always fulfilled. As you'll also note, the exercise is not confined to weekends, although weekends offer more time for long slow distance running, hiking, climbing, skiing, swimming, tennis, and other recreational exercise.

An exercise program must be faithfully followed on weekdays when the demands of the job are maximal. Aerobic exercise confined to weekends may be counterproductive. As a rule of thumb it has been suggested that deconditioning starts after about three days of layoff. If you've had three days without aerobic exercise you should restart at a lower level and build up reasonably rapidly to your conditioned maintenance level. It follows that if you don't exercise during the workweek you are unlikely ever to get satisfactorily conditioned on the weekends alone.

Your exercise program will also benefit if you exploit your own biorhythms. I'm a morning person, so I feel my best when I run early. Late evening is my next best time—and right after work, around the supper hour, is absolutely my worst. Find your best time of day and unless it's unavoidable, don't select a time to run that is incompatible with your personal biological cycles.

# Introduction to Running 101

Here's where the fun begins. Decide what stage you belong to for entry into running from Table 9–2 (page 171). Carry it to the point where medical clearance is mandated. If you don't require medical clearance or if you do and have obtained clearance, you're ready to proceed. Since I think that the majority of adults reading this book will fall into Stages III or IV, we'll take Stage IV as our example and reference point. Those in other stages can pick up their program as we go along. The sequences of conditioning are outlined in Tables 10–4 through 10–8.

The difference between the stages arises mainly at the points when medical clearance is required and when aerobic training may begin. Those in Stage IV who have been in the heart-rated walking program for a minimum of three weeks at 60 to 70 percent of maximal heart rate (see Table 9–3), who are walking comfortably for 1.5 miles each day in 20 minutes or less and have been doing regular flexibility and stretching exercises, may proceed to a walk/run program. As shown in Table 9–3, the first one to four weeks should be 1-mile walks, but starting at the fifth week at the latest (or the second week at the earliest) the walking distance should be 1.5 miles. Anyone at any age, under 65, who does not have a serious disability should be able to walk 1.5 miles in 20 minutes within two months of starting training. The 20 minutes is put in only as a guide to distinguish between a strolling pace and a walking pace. But if you find you're having trouble reaching even this minimal goal within two months, don't rush it. Exercise faithfully and regularly until you achieve this level. Then you may proceed.

From here on, for everyone except the competitive runner, how fast a rate you achieve for your walk/run and run is of no real interest. What's of interest is how fast your heart rate is. *It's not how fast your legs go but how fast your heart goes.* So the next step is to increase your heart rate to the aerobic range of 70 to 85 percent of maximal and to keep it there for 10 to 12 minutes by a rhythmic combination of slow running and brisk walking.

Now let's back up for a moment to look briefly at the Stage V conditioning sequence. It really shouldn't be necessary for you to read each of the sequences—only the one in which you fall. And you made this decision by studying Table 9–2. So don't waste your time or allow yourself to be intimidated by all the tables, when only one of them applies to you. But there are a few points to be made. Stage V conditioning may be very slow or may not. If you're older than 60, you may not ever progress beyond walking, stretching, and flexibility exercises *if* you're just beginning to exercise after many years or decades of sedentary behavior. But you'll also note something in Table 10–4 that applies to all ages and stages. If you're already aerobically trained, you're not expected to regress when you reach a certain age. Walter Stack, at 71, can probably run the legs off me and a lot of other people my age and younger who think of themselves as runners. So I've put a qualifier in Table 10–4: *if you are not currently in aerobic conditioning*. It's hardly necessary to point out that for the maintenance levels in Table 10–8, your performance in the 1.5-mile run is not expected to drop by two minutes when you celebrate your fiftieth birthday. It's also possible that if you're starting a program at age 45, you may find that your comfortable level is that recommended for a 50-year-old. Don't worry about it. Just follow your heart rate.

To look at the other end of the age spectrum, you may wonder if kids really can get into aerobic conditioning. Table 9–3 suggests that 6-year-olds are candidates for an exercise program. Believe me, if handled right, the early-school-age child has the physical capacity to perform marvelously well. But there are special problems for the younger ages, so a chapter is devoted to them.

However, when you add running to walking, you add the need for running gear. Running shorts, a jogging suit, and heavy gym socks are useful, but well-cushioned running shoes that fit properly are essential. You can do all your running in jeans and an old T-shirt, but please shop around and get quality shoes before you ever start running seriously. There are fads and a bit of a "running-shoe chic." Ignore them. Just look critically at the shoes for cushioning and fit to save your feet and legs.

When running, start at a very slow pace and slow to a walk if you become uncomfortable. As you run, notice how your feet hit the ground. Consciously strive to have them hit as lightly as possible. *Don't* run on your toes or land on your heels. The impact can be damaging to muscles and joints, as well as painful. When running, your foot strikes with a force of about three times your body weight. An average male of 165 pounds slams his foot on the ground with 500 pounds of force 1,000 times in just a mile. That's 250 tons of crunching stress on each foot, ankle, and knee for every mile you run. So pay attention when you're starting out. Be sure your feet are striking as lightly and smoothly as possible. You'll note that it's the outer edge of the foot that touches first, then the whole foot, before pushing off with the front of the foot and the toes. This is really the natural way to run. But just check yourself and make sure that you're not establishing an unnatural gait.

Now just run or walk/run for about a half-mile, being sure that you feel comfortable all the way. Then you may let yourself increase your rate slightly, challenge yourself a little, but don't push too hard. You should run the last mile in such a way that when you complete 1.5 miles, you'll feel like you want to go farther.

The criteria of a successful conditioning run at any level of training are: maintaining the aerobic range of 70 to 85 percent of maximal, and feeling at the end of the run that you want to run more.

That's it for the beginner.

## Intermediate Running 201

When you enroll in this course you join 25 million Americans—probably many more than that by the time this is published. You may consider yourself a runner if you invest a minimum of 60 minutes per week in aerobic running, run at least six miles per week, and do your running on weekdays as well as weekends.

An intermediate runner may have running as his or her sole aerobic exercise or the program may be varied with swimming, cycling, rowing, cross-country skiing, or some suitable rhythmic exercises during which a fast heart rate can be sustained for more than ten minutes. The intermediate runner will also want some variety in his running program. Long-distance days alternating with short-distance days. Speed-play, in which short, fast runs alternate with longer runs. The runner in this class usually enjoys running a great deal, but is not hopelessly hooked—and so he can happily do other things. If the weather is miserable he doesn't suffer from a compulsion that takes him out into a foot of snow, a driving rainstorm, or a wind chill of −50°F.

## Advanced Running 301

This is a limited enrollment seminar for those who have reached something approaching a mystical level in their running. It's also for the marathoners and mini-marathoners. Running is no longer merely for health but has become equated with being (as Dr. George Sheehan has observed). You don't have to be reminded to get in your minimal 60 minutes of aerobic running per week or your 6 miles. More likely your total distance run may be 16 or 60 miles a week.

Every now and then I feel I'm crossing the threshold into the realm of the advanced. One sign is when I'm going to work knowing full well that I've just completed a three-mile run, yet I see the runners still out on the mall—and I want to get back and join them. And when I have time for long slow distance running, more than three miles, and start getting a runner's high, and can almost sense my brain waves shifting from beta to alpha or even theta—a new level of consciousness—that's a sign. When these things happen the experience can be exhilarating to anyone.

But as I've indicated, 301 is a limited enrollment seminar. It's beyond the scope and intent of our Whole Heart Program. Those of you who may eventually become hopeless running-junkies won't need references to reading material on the subject.

## Special Problems in Getting Aerobic Exercise

The fundamental aerobic exercise is running, but lap-swimming is also an excellent aerobic exercise for those who have the opportunity. You'll have to find a swimming pace that increases your heart-rate to the recommended level (see Table 10–1, page 186) and maintain that pace for 10 to 15 minutes to achieve your aerobic workout. Climbing stairs is another good exercise—10 to 15 minutes of climbing is something I've resorted to on occasions when traveling and unable to do anything better.

Those who don't care to run outside in foul weather or in overwhelming air pollution can do rope-jumping or running in place. But if you're going to jump rope, you have to start gradually and do a little of it regularly (say, three minutes three times a week). Starting gradually and always continuing to jump rope even during periods of running will keep your feet and legs accustomed to the different stresses that jumping and running in place entail. If you haven't jumped rope for months and decide to use this exercise for a full aerobic workout on a rainy day, you may regret it. Your sore feet and ankles may wash you out of running for a few days.

Careless and poorly prepared exercisers have to give up running entirely or for prolonged periods of time and switch to swimming, cycling, or rowing because they haven't trained to handle the full range of stress. Ex-football players and skiers who've had repeated injuries may not be able to obtain an adequate aerobic workout because of the pain of running. Your best assurance for successful pain-free running will be your 10-20-30 exercises and cushioned, well-fitting running shoes.

If you're sufficiently affluent, high-quality stationary cycles, rowing machines, and treadmills will provide a good workout. A cycle that combines a handlebar rowing option offers more exercise than a cycle alone. I personally favor this type of equipment. But a word of caution: Don't buy a "cheapo." Some chain stores and discount stores offer what appear to be real bargains. I tried one, and it was a lemon. My advice would be to get heavy-duty, high-quality equipment from a reputable sporting goods or exercise equipment store—or forget it and run in the rain. Be prepared to pay a minimum of $400 for a single piece of equipment.

Finally, many of you who remember back to physical education classes and the army or navy should know that you can get an aerobic workout from calisthenics, sustaining an appropriately high rate going from one routine to another. From burpees to straddle hops to squat jumps to push-ups. I won't spell it out. I rate such routines somewhere between a hernia repair and a root canal job in desirability. But those who don't object are welcome to this alternative. And some of you may also want to do a little more with strength exercises: pull-ups, rope climbs, and even weight lifting in the context of weight training rather than "body sculpture."

There is one problem in obtaining aerobic exercise that affects women more than men: how to run at times other than during daylight hours. For married women, running with their husbands is an answer totally compatible with the family commitment to exercise. But for women living alone there's the despicable threat of attack. In the absence of a male running companion, and if it is absolutely not possible to run during the daytime, then only well-lighted, well-populated streets should even be considered. To my mind, running in the dark (early morning or evening) is not a desirable option for women. Jumping rope or using exercise equipment in the home is to be preferred. The requirement for these exercises is the same as for running: to get the heart rate up to between 70 and 85 percent of maximum, and keep it there for 10 to 15 minutes. Another alternative is exercise classes at the Y or some such facility. Of special appeal to many women are the aerobic dance classes. Unfortunately, exercise classes designed for women are frequently held in the daytime—which restricts the participation of working women.

TABLE
**10–1**

# Heart Rates at Rest and with Exercise

*The aerobic training range is 70 to 85 percent of maximal rate. Beginners and those warming up should aim at 60 percent.*

| Age | Average at Rest Male | Average at Rest Female | Maximal | Beginner + Warm-up 60 % | Training Range 70 % to | Training Range 85 % |
|-----|------|--------|---------|------|------|------|
| 6–10 | 85 | 90 | 205 | 123 | 146 | 174 |
| 11–15 | 80 | 85 | 210 | 126 | 147 | 179 |
| 16–20 | 75 | 80 | 200 | 120 | 140 | 170 |
| 21–25 | 75 | 80 | 195 | 117 | 137 | 166 |
| 26–30 | 75 | 80 | 190 | 114 | 133 | 162 |
| 31–35 | 75 | 80 | 185 | 111 | 130 | 157 |
| 36–40 | 75 | 80 | 180 | 108 | 126 | 153 |
| 41–45 | 75 | 80 | 175 | 105 | 123 | 149 |
| 46–50 | 75 | 80 | 170 | 102 | 119 | 145 |
| 51–55 | 75 | 80 | 165 | 99 | 116 | 140 |
| 56–60 | 75 | 78 | 160 | 96 | 112 | 136 |
| 61–65 | 73 | 76 | 155 | 93 | 109 | 132 |
| 66+ | 70 | 74 | 150 | 90 | 105 | 128 |

TABLE
**10–2**

# Satisfactory Weekly Exercise Routines

## Variety Schedule

**Day 1**   Full 10-20-30 exercises for 6–10 minutes
Aerobic run for 10–15 minutes
Cool down for 2 minutes optional

**Day 2**   Flexibility and stretching for 3 minutes
Aerobic run for 20–25 minutes
Cool down for 2 minutes

**Day 3**   Full 10-20-30 exercises for 6–10 minutes
Aerobic run for 10–15 minutes
Cool down for 2 minutes optional

**Day 4**   Recreational exercise or no exercise

**Day 5**   Flexibility and stretching for 3 minutes
Aerobic run for 20–25 minutes
Cool down for 2 minutes

**Day 6**   Full 10-20-30 exercises for 6–10 minutes
Aerobic run for 10–15 minutes
Cool down for 2 minutes optional

**Day 7**   Flexibility and stretching for 3 minutes
Aerobic run for 20–25 minutes
Cool down for 2 minutes

## Minimal Schedule Would Be:

3 days of the full 10-20-30 exercises
3 days of aerobic run for 20 minutes preceded by flexibility and
   stretching
1 day of recreational exercise or no exercise

| TABLE 10-3 | **Sample Exercise Journal for Ten Days** |
|---|---|

**Friday**

Traveling away from home (Chicago). Morning: 10-20-30 exercises and 20-minute run along Lake Michigan. Distance unknown. Heart rate at end of run 168. Felt great.

**Saturday**

Back home in Denver. Morning: stretching and flexibility warm-up for 3 minutes. Slow first half-mile, good tempo 2-mile run. Heart rate 176. Afternoon—took cub scout pack rock climbing in the mountains at 8,500 feet for 3 hours. Felt great.

**Sunday**

Decided on no exercise, blaming knee bruised in climbing. (But the real problem may have been that the cub scouts wore me out.)

**Monday**

Early evening: 10-20-30 exercises. Ran only 1 mile, felt terrible till almost the end. Couldn't establish a comfortable pace. Heart rate 152 at the end. Total exercise time less than 15 minutes.

**Tuesday**

Morning: 10-20-30 exercises. Ran 2 miles. Heart rate 172. Felt good. Exercise time about 20 minutes. Evening did 10 minutes of weight lifting.

**Wednesday**

Morning: stretching and flexibility before running 2 miles. Didn't want to stop, I felt so good. Heart rate 176. Before supper completed 10-20-30 exercises. Total exercise time for the day about 25 minutes.

**Thursday**

Morning: 10-20-30 exercises. Lousy day at work. Ran 2.5 miles in the evening to clear head. Heart rate 160. Felt so-so. Lifted weights for about 10 minutes.

**Friday**

Morning: flexibility and 1.5-mile run. Heart rate 164. Felt reasonably good, but ran out of time.

**Saturday**

10-20-30 and 3-mile run. About 30 minutes exercise time. Heart rate 180. Felt great. Hiking in mountains about 2 hours.

**Sunday**

10-20-30 and 2.5-mile run. Heart rate 172. Felt good. About 30 minutes exercise time. Two hours of yard work. Lifted weights for about 10 minutes.

TABLE
10-4

# Sequence of Stage V Conditioning

**1. Over 60:** Physical examination, stress test, and individualized exercise prescription from your physician are required. If you are not currently in aerobic conditioning, the exercise programs here are not suitable for you without medical consultation.

**2. 50-59:** Have physical examination, stress test, and medical clearance as soon as possible. Begin:

    **a** Weight normalization.

    **b** Physical life-style.

    **c** Daily stretching and flexibility exercises.

    **d** Start heart rate record.

    **e** Daily 1-mile strolls as slowly as desired.

    **f** *Do not proceed beyond this point without medical clearance.*

    **g** After medical clearance, heart-rated walking program may begin and progress according to guidelines in Table 9-3 through Level 2.

    **h** After 8-12 weeks have another medical examination to obtain clearance for aerobic conditioning.

    **i** If aerobic conditioning is not recommended, continue with walking program at Level 2 as your maintenance program, but you may increase the time you spend walking (at 60-70 percent rate) to as long as your time and your physician will allow.

    **j** If aerobic conditioning is recommended, you may go to the Stage IV sequence and begin with item 3.

TABLE
10–5
# Sequence of Stage IV Conditioning

1   Have a physical examination, stress test, and medical clearance for conditioning as soon as it can be scheduled.

2   Begin:

    **a**   Weight normalization.
    **b**   Physical life-style.
    **c**   Daily stretching and flexibility exercises.
    **d**   Heart rate record.
    **e**   Heart-rated walking program at 60 to 70 percent of maximal heart rate (through Level 2).
    **f**   *Do not proceed beyond this point until you have medical clearance.*

3   After following a physical life-style, and briskly walking 1.5 miles per day, with comfort, at a 60 to 70 percent heart rate, the following may be added:

    **a**   Strength and flexibility exercises.
    **b**   Recreational cycling and swimming.
    **c**   Interval training for running (walk/run) and swimming (lap and rest, lap and rest).

4   A full program of exercises may begin when:

    **a**   You are less than 20 percent overweight.
    **b**   You are able to sustain with comfort a heart rate of 70 to 85 percent of maximum for 10 minutes per day (at least 3 days per week) by any combination of walking, interval running, interval swimming, or cycling.
    **c**   Your resting heart rate is less than 80.
    **d**   Your recovery heart rate is less than 100, 10 minutes after aerobic exercise for a minimum period of 10 minutes.

5   Your maintenance level is:

    **a**   Heart rate of 70 to 85 percent for 60 minutes per week achieved in 3 to 6 exercise periods spaced throughout the week as well as on the weekend (e.g., running, swimming, cycling, rowing, jumping rope, cross-country skiing, or other aerobic exercise).
    **b**   10-20-30 exercises: full program for stretching, flexibility, and strength—at least 3 times per week spaced throughout the week.

6   As a monitor of your maintenance level:

    **a**   Your heart rate on rising in the morning will probably be less than 60 and, with quiet activity, less than 70.
    **b**   Periodically check your recovery heart rate to be certain that 10 minutes after exercise it is less than 100. If it is *not,* consult with your doctor.
    **c**   Some of you may also wish to periodically check your performance in running by the 12-minute test or the 1.5-mile test. Men may be able to maintain the following:

|  | 12 Minutes | 1.5 Miles |
|---|---|---|
| Age 35–50 | 1.5 miles | 12 minutes |
| Age 50–60 | 1.3 miles | 14 minutes |

Women may achieve similar times but generally aim for a 10 percent lower level.

**d** *What you achieve on the performance tests is of relatively little significance. Your heart rate is your guide and monitor, not your running time. If you're very competitive DON'T take the tests.*

<br>

| TABLE<br>**10–6** | **Sequence of Stage III Conditioning** |
|---|---|

**1** All those over 35 and those under 35 who have risk factors specified in Table 9–1 should have a physical examination, stress test, and medical clearance for conditioning as soon as it can be scheduled. It is assumed that those who are currently participating in aerobic exercise have had prior medical clearance as mandated by their age and risk factors.

**2** Begin:
  **a** Weight normalization.
  **b** Physical life-style.
  **c** Full 10-20-30 exercises.
  **d** Recreational cycling and swimming.
  **e** Heart rate record.
  **f** Heart-rated walking program through Level 2 in Table 9–3.
  **g** *Do not proceed beyond this point without medical clearance.*

**3** After following a physical life-style and walking briskly for 1.5 miles per day, with comfort, at a heart rate of 60 to 70 percent of maximal, interval training may begin with Level 3 walk/run in Table 9–3. Interval training for swimming may also be utilized.

Those who have entered their heart program at a stage where they were already aerobically trained would just continue with a maintenance program as noted below.

**4** A full program of exercises may begin when:

  **a** You are less than 20 percent overweight.
  **b** You are able to sustain with comfort a heart rate of 70 to 85 percent of maximum for 10 minutes per day (at least 3 days per week) by any combination of walking, interval running, interval swimming, or cycling.
  **c** Your resting heart rate is less than 80.
  **d** Your recovery heart rate is less than 100, 10 minutes after aerobic exercise for a minimum period of 10 minutes.

**5**    Your maintenance level is:

    **a**  Heart rate of 70 to 85 percent for 60 minutes per week achieved in 3 to 6 exercise periods spaced throughout the week as well as on the weekend (e.g., running, swimming, cycling, rowing, jumping rope, cross-country skiing, or other aerobic exercise).

    **b**  10-20-30 exercises: full program for stretching, flexibility, and strength—at least 3 times per week spaced throughout the week.

**6**    As a monitor of your maintenance level:

    **a**  Your heart rate on rising in the morning will probably be less than 60 and, with quiet activity, less than 70.

    **b**  Periodically check your recovery heart rate to be certain that 10 minutes after exercise it is less than 100. If it is *not,* consult with your doctor.

    **c**  Some of you may also wish to periodically check your performance in running by the 12-minute test or the 1.5-mile test. Men may be able to maintain the following:

|            | 12 minutes | 1.5 Miles  |
| ---------- | ---------- | ---------- |
| Age 35–50  | 1.5 miles  | 12 minutes |
| Age 50–60  | 1.3 miles  | 14 minutes |

Women may achieve similar times but generally aim for a 10 percent lower level.

    **d**  *What you achieve on the performance tests is of relatively little significance. Your heart rate is your guide and monitor, not your running time. If you're very competitive DON'T take the test.*

| TABLE 10–7 | **Sequence of Stage II Conditioning** |

**1**   It is assumed that those who are currently participating in aerobic exercise have had prior medical clearance as mandated by their age ( > 35) or risk factors in Table 9–1.

**2**   Those under 35 *with risk factors* may progress as follows:

    **a**   Weight normalization program.
    **b**   Physical life-style.
    **c**   Full 10-20-30 exercises.
    **d**   Recreational cycling and swimming.
    **e**   Heart rate record.
    **f**   Heart-rated walking program through Level 2 (Table 9–3).
    **g**   *Those over 25 do not proceed beyond this point without medical clearance.*

**3**   Those under 25 *with risk factors* may enter Level 3 walk/run and other interval training while awaiting clearance.

**4**   A full program of exercises may begin when:

    **a**   You are less than 20 percent overweight.
    **b**   You are able to sustain with comfort a heart rate of 70 to 85 percent of maximum for 10 minutes per day (at least 3 days per week) by any combination of walking, interval running, interval swimming, or cycling.
    **c**   Your resting heart rate is less than 80.
    **d**   Your recovery heart rate is less than 100, 10 minutes after aerobic exercise for a minimum period of 10 minutes.

**5**   Your maintenance level is:

    **a**   Heart rate of 70 to 85 percent for 60 minutes per week achieved in 3 to 6 exercise periods spaced throughout the week as well as on the weekend (e.g., running, swimming, cycling, rowing, jumping rope, cross-country skiing, or other aerobic exercise).
    **b**   10-20-30 exercises: full program for stretching, flexibility, and strength—at least 3 times per week spaced throughout week.

**6**   As a monitor of your maintenance level:

    **a**   Your heart rate on rising in the morning will probably be less than 60, and with quiet activity, less than 70.
    **b**   Periodically check your recovery heart rate to be certain that 10 minutes after exercise it is less than 100. If it is *not,* consult with your doctor.
    **c**   Some of you may also wish to periodically check your performance in running by the 12-minute test or the 1.5-mile test. Men may be able to maintain the following:

|  | 12 Minutes | 1.5 Miles |
|---|---|---|
| Age 35–50 | 1.5 miles | 12 minutes |
| Age 50–60 | 1.3 miles | 14 minutes |

    Women may achieve similar times but generally aim for a 10 percent lower level.

    **d**   *What you achieve on the performance tests is of relatively little significance. Your heart rate is your guide and monitor, not your running time. If you're very competitive DON'T take the tests.*

TABLE
**10–8** | **Sequence of Stage I Conditioning**

**1**   Medical clearance should not be necessary.

**2**   By definition you should already be in reasonably good condition. You may wish to spend 1 week at Level 2 walking, and 1 week at Level 3 walking while accommodating to the 10-20-30 exercise program—or maintaining whatever balanced program you currently follow (e.g., Royal Canadian Air Force, West Point, etc.).

**3**   If your present program is doing what it should for you, don't make any changes, but you may wish to make comparisons and check performances.

**4**   If you've been training regularly you should:

   **a**   Easily sustain with comfort a heart rate between 70 percent and 85 percent of maximum for 20 minutes per day at least 3 days per week by aerobic exercise.
   **b**   Your resting heart rate, if you're over 15 years old, is less than 64 for males and less than 70 for females.
   **c**   Your recovery heart rate is less than 100, 5 minutes after a minimum period of 10 minutes of aerobic exercise.
   **d**   If these criteria are not met, you probably are not in Stage I, and you may wish to go back to Stage II and work your way up to maintenance level.

**5**   Your maintenance level is:

   **a**   Heart rate of 70 to 85 percent for 60 minutes per week achieved in 3 to 6 exercise periods spaced throughout the week as well as on the weekend (e.g., running, swimming, cycling, rowing, jumping rope, cross-country skiing, or other aerobic exercise).
   **b**   10-20-30 exercises: full program for stretching, flexibility, and strength—at least 3 times per week spaced throughout the week.

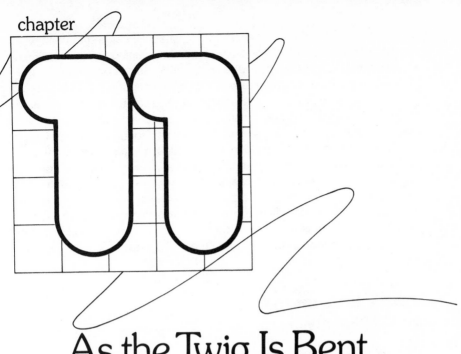

# As the Twig Is Bent

his may be the most important chapter in *The Whole Heart Book*. Preventive programs are valuable for adults, but if they are started in childhood the potential effect is enormous.

In 1972, a conclusion was reached from a well-known epidemiologic study, the Framingham study, that started cardiologists and pediatricians scurrying up unfamiliar and untraveled paths. Their conclusion: Atherosclerosis, the basis of heart attacks in adults, is really a pediatric problem.

Of course it is! Logically, what we are is the product of all that has gone before in our heredity and environment. And childhood is that first quarter of life into which is compressed most of our growth, development, and habit formation. But doctors are still not used to looking at 4-year-olds within the perspective of what will happen to them when they're 40. Although medical orientation is changing, it is happening all too slowly. Coronary heart disease is still too often perceived as a disease of adults, not as a disease beginning in childhood. Childhood? We can take it back further than that—to infancy and even to what the mother does during pregnancy.

Let's now take the risk factors that we've found to be important in adults and apply this knowledge to children to see if we can discover what the early influences are in the eventual development of coronary heart disease. And what can be done early—in infancy and childhood—to change the course of disease. A better way to say it might be: What can be done early in life to promote lasting good health? The latter formulation is more consistent with our interest in health maintenance rather than in the crisis treatment of disease.

## Genetic Risk and Family History

Here we go again. It's unavoidable. Heart disease runs in families. Our study of adults with early heart attacks showed that the heritability of heart attacks was 56 to 63 percent. That is, more than half of the total contribution to heart attacks comes from heredity. Yet few of us would be inclined to insist on the medical screening of prospective mates. So given this initial genetic handicap, we can certainly try to identify those families and individuals within families who are at increased risk, and toward whom an aggressive program of preventive care should be directed. One problem with identifying the infant or child at genetic risk is that there are no sizeable studies that have followed risks evident in childhood through adult life to the actual event of a heart attack. The best one can do is select risk factors that are associated with heart attacks in adults and see if they are present in children. There are a couple of problems with this approach, because risk factors such as smoking and high blood pressure don't enter into consideration in infancy and early childhood when, ideally, you'd like to begin your program.

Well, what can you identify in the infant or child? You have to stress the genetic factors. The family history of heart attack, high blood pressure, and stroke. The factor of highest risk discovered in adults is that of heart attack before age 55 in a first-degree relative (parent, sibling, or child). The problem with this is that most parents of infants and young children are relatively young. So even if they themselves are candidates for heart attack, they aren't likely to have them until they're in their forties or fifties. And by that time their kids are likely to be grown, so all the precious years of preventive programs in childhood have been lost. If the parents are older, or have heart attacks at very early ages, then the genetic risk is clearly evident for the child.

But it's not necessary to depend entirely on the knowledge of disease in first-degree relatives. The risk is greatest if the relative is close, but there is a familial risk that can be calculated on the basis of disease in more distant relatives. Grandparents, uncles, and aunts are second-degree relatives, and we have data that approximate the amount of risk that occurs if there have been heart attacks in these relatives, and in even more distant ones.

# Genetic Risk and Cholesterol, Triglycerides, and Lipoproteins

This is an area for screening that applies to infants and children and will help define those children at very high risk from blood fat abnormalities caused by the large effects of a single major gene mutation. Screening for cholesterol and triglycerides will also help discover the less serious abnormalities caused by the addition of small effects of many genes (polygenes). We have proposed that at 1 to 2 years of age, infants and young children who are at increased risk of having a heart attack when they become adults may be identified by physicians by obtaining a careful family history of heart attacks and strokes and by taking a fasting specimen of blood for cholesterol and triglycerides, usually before the child has eaten breakfast. Children who have not had such a study done at this early age may have it done at any age—but the earlier the better.

Most, but not all, individuals with a significant genetic risk of heart attack have an abnormality in the area of cholesterol, triglycerides, and lipoproteins. Conversely, many individuals and families may have moderate elevations of these factors without a discernible increase in risk of cardiovascular disease. In Chapter 12 you'll be given risk scales for children, which take into account the additive effects of these risks.

But there are families who are at unusually high risk—the single mutant gene (or monogenic) disorders. These can best be identified by family studies in which not only is there evidence of early heart disease but the affected family members also clearly have much higher levels of cholesterol and/or triglycerides than the unaffected members of the family. The disorders are transmitted directly from one of the parents, and the chances are one in two that a child will be affected. This is called autosomal dominant inheritance, and there are three forms that are seen relatively frequently.

Children with these inherited disorders require much more than the low-risk strategy of healthful living. They may require very strict diet and medication. Although the event is rare, sometimes two individuals with the same single mutant gene disorder (hypercholesterolemia type IIa) marry, and the chances are one in four that a child of that marriage will have the disastrous homozygous (double-dose) form of the disease. You were introduced to such a family in Chapter 5. These children, who fortunately represent perhaps no more than one per million in America, are subject to heart attacks before they reach 10 years of age—and rarely survive to the age of 20. If you or a member of your family has an extremely high level of cholesterol, you may need to discuss this problem with a clinical geneticist or a cardiologist who has a strong interest in the genetics of heart disease.

Although I have some misgivings about going into detail regarding how to identify children at highest risk, I feel that the guidelines must be offered. So here are some clinical profiles.

## Type IIa Hypercholesterolemia

The infant or child over 1 year of age and less than 20 years who has the heterozygous (single-dose) form will have a cholesterol level that is frequently over 300 and almost always over 240. The child will not have high triglycerides and will not have some associated disease, such as hypothyroidism, to explain the high cholesterol. The key to the diagnosis is the family study. About half of the family members, going back through whichever side of the family the disease was transmitted, will have very high cholesterol, and the other half will be normal. Examples of cholesterol levels in the family would be: father, 325 (affected); mother, 180 (normal); patient, 280 (affected); sister, 160 (normal). Children with this problem will need not only a lifetime commitment to prudent diet, exercise, no smoking, and stress control, but will in most cases require a very strict diet and probably medication. The extremely rare double-dose form of the disease (coming from both sides of the family) may require a special operation called portacaval shunt. In children with a double-dose homozygous problem, cholesterol levels are usually near 1,000 and they develop skin growths (called xanthomas) on their knuckles, elbows, heels, and knees.

**Other single gene types** ○ Other single gene types follow the same guidelines; they must be diagnosed by family studies showing that affected individuals have much higher levels of triglycerides alone, cholesterol alone, or both cholesterol and triglycerides than unaffected family members. And there must not be some other underlying disease to account for the high levels. In some cases, strict diet may not be sufficient, and medication may be required.

**Polygenes and environmental triggers** ○ Elevations of cholesterol and/or triglycerides caused by the small effects of many genes interacting with environmental triggers such as diet, medication, and other diseases are more common and more manageable. In these families the blood fat levels are lower and similar in all family members. That is, if one child has a cholesterol of 220, his brother may have 210, his sister 235, his father 250, and his mother 215 (cholesterols being relatively higher in adults than in children). In these families, medication should not be necessary. Prudent diet, exercise, commitment against smoking, and encouraging stress control—a healthful life-style is all that should be needed. A similar commitment is desirable for individuals and families *without* high levels of cholesterol or triglycerides, because heart attacks may also occur in families without high blood fats (by American norms). That's the ringer. "Normal" cholesterol in America and northern Europe is incredibly high by Japanese standards. And the Japanese have heart attacks much less frequently than Americans.

The optimistic conclusion I would like to propose based on what has been discussed in this section is that for most Americans and Europeans a healthful life-style is the prescription for heart attack prevention. For those at high risk, the commitment must be more profound—the diet may have to become more typically Japanese than American in fat and cholesterol content. And medication may be needed. With these additional prescriptions, especially when starting as early as childhood, there can be reason to hope for a normal life and something approaching a normal life expectancy.

## Dietary Management for Kids

Kids eat what's available to eat at home, and what they've learned to eat at early ages. The second half of that sentence is just as important as the first, because a lot of the calories that older children consume are taken outside of the home—school lunches and snacks. If they have developed habits of blowing their allowances or earnings on junk foods, there will be a problem in behavior modification. So the earlier good habits are established, the better.

**Infants** ○   Much of what we eat is in response to acquired tastes. How many of you who enjoy beer now could honestly say you liked that first sip? There are hundreds of similar examples from onions to oysters. The baby food industry has until recently loaded baby foods with salt and sugar—not because babies have a taste or need for these additives, but because mommies taste the food they feed the young ones. And mommies have an acquired taste for these items. The Japanese, who are so good about maintaining low fat, low cholesterol diets, load up on salt to the extent that Americans and Europeans may find their soups unpalatable. We've got our own acquired taste for salt, but it's set lower than that of the Japanese. There are other cultures whose people do fine on one-tenth the salt intake of Americans. Salt is discussed at length in the chapter on high blood pressure, but the point here is that much of our appetite for salt is culturally determined. And our taste for salt is acquired as early as infancy.

The next problem related to infant feeding is of equal if not greater importance. Fat babies can become fat children and fat adults. Although there is some debate concerning fat cell size and fat cell number in obesity, there is general agreement that infancy is a critical period for the development of fat cells. Overfed babies appear to develop more fat cells *(which will be with them the rest of their lives)*, and these individuals become capable of accumulating more fat than infants who have normal nutrition. So the groundwork for obesity is laid by the loving mother who stuffs her baby. This is not to say that anyone is advocating that mothers underfeed babies. Doctors have growth charts and curves for babies, and the weight should be appropriate for the length. This is one reasonable monitor of adequate caloric nutrition.

One practice that is still prevalent, and is incomprehensible to me, is feeding egg yolks to babies. Needless to say, it is not recommended for families in which there is a problem with high cholesterol. And I find difficulty justifying feeding egg yolks even to completely normal babies. Ostensibly it's to give them iron. But it's a pinch of iron in a bucket of cholesterol and fat. And giving a 15-pound baby only one egg yolk is equivalent on a weight basis to cramming ten eggs into a 150-pound adult.

Strict dietary control of fats and cholesterol is generally not advocated in the first year of life, even in families with single gene disorders. But a prudent diet, avoiding obvious excess of cholesterol (such as egg yolk) and foods that clearly have a high saturated fat content, is a reasonable approach to the dietary management of infants from high-risk families.

**200**

**The remainder of the first decade** ○ Fat cells continue to increase in number until a child is 8 to 10 years old. And the fat content of a given cell depends on how many calories are made available for storage as fat. Here's where the "starving Armenians" and parental admonitions to clean the plate do uncalculated damage to the dietary habits of children.

I'm a plate-cleaner. As a child of the Depression it would be hard for me to be otherwise. So a solution for me and for my family is to be sure that the portions on the plate are small. Small portions to begin with and caution regarding the size of second portions will assuage the parental conscience regarding waste. For parents without such hang-ups, the family members should be encouraged to leave a little food on the plate.

In preschool and young school age children, snack foods must be looked at critically, because they represent 30 percent of the caloric intake, and are usually either heavily salted or are heavy in sugar and fat. Make available nutritious snacks: fruits, vegetables, grains, skim milk. The hungry kid coming in from school can really be just as happy with a bowl of shredded wheat and skim milk as with a handful of cookies and a bottle of pop. It all depends on what's available and what he gets used to having. Remember, bad habits will have to be "unlearned"—often more difficult to accomplish than learning.

A prudent diet is a desirable goal for most kids. Some additional restrictions may be required for high-risk children. Table 11–1 provides some general guidelines. Details on diet are to be found in Chapters 4 and 5. Salt restriction is discussed in Chapter 7. One key point to remember is that the major source of both protein *and cholesterol* in the school age child is whole milk. By the simple tactic of substituting skim milk for whole milk you can ensure that your child receives the benefit of protein without paying the penalty of cholesterol and saturated fat.

**The second decade** ○ Adolescence with all its stress and distress occupies much of this period. Bad dietary patterns, already established, may be changed, but they require the full commitment of the young person. Parental dictums, as such, are often counterproductive. This is a dangerous period in many ways, a time when young people, especially girls, gain weight prodigiously. Fat cells may no longer increase in number, but they can increase greatly in size. This is also a time when fad diets may compete with junk diets to make sound nutrition run a poor third in the emerging teenager's priorities.

But the same principles still prevail. Good nutrition is a family responsibility, and children in both the first and second decades can be caught up in the family's commitment. Our children, sometimes to our discomfort, delight in pointing out any real or imagined dietary indiscretions in their parents. (In fact, our youngest is prepared to wrestle me to the ground to prevent me from indulging. She was raised on principles of good nutrition, so it's easy for her. What does she know about the yearnings of a recovered junk-food junkie?)

But that's an obvious digression. The two main problems in this age period relate to the previous experience of the child. If he (or she) was on a prudent diet in the first decade of life, there's not much of a problem. Snack foods and school lunches are the only concerns, if family meals and the household food supply conform to the concept of the prudent diet. For the child at low risk, the school lunch may be consumed even if it includes common items such as "greaseburgers" and whole milk. For the child at high risk, if the school will not stock nonfat or low fat milk and persists in high fat and high cholesterol menus, a sack lunch will have to be used. Many school systems are enlightened, however. The chief dietician for the Denver public schools took the initiative to get low fat milk into the school lunch program. Rather than my going to her with the suggestion, she came to me to ask for support for this proposal.

Junk foods for snacks become more of an issue the older the child gets and the more he's inclined to spend his money on such items. If the pantry at home is kept well-stocked with palatable alternatives that are nutritious, this is a controllable problem. The low-risk adolescent can take a reasonable amount of junk food without much hazard. The high-risk teenager must be well informed and fully committed. The diet must be maintained much more rigorously. A physician or nutritionist may have to provide added support.

The more serious problem comes in families trying to start a new dietary program when there are teenagers who have already established dietary preferences. There's no point in telling them that you have many more years of bad dietary experiences than they do, and that if *you* can break the bad habits, *they* can. Their habits are just as real as yours. They've lasted a lifetime—just like yours. A program of behavior modification and commitment is just as necessary in this age group as it is in adults. The principles of these topics discussed in previous chapters apply to children in the second decade of life. Some kids will embrace the new ideas with enthusiasm. Some will even develop a fervor that may be so intense that it will need to be tempered. And some will stubbornly resist every step you try to take, even though they've recently witnessed their father (or mother) almost die of a heart attack at age 40.

**Weight reduction** ○ If you have an overweight child (greater than 10 percent above weight for height on your doctor's standard growth charts), and if this child is ten years of age or younger, careful attention to meal planning, quantity of food eaten, and foods made available in the context of the entire family being committed to weight normalization and prudent diet is all that is likely to be necessary. Very slow weight loss or merely holding the weight constant while allowing the child's height to catch up is often sufficient when accompanied by a good exercise program. The input of a physician or dietician should not be necessary if a well-balanced diet is provided.

The obese child (greater than 20 percent overweight) will have to lose at a little faster pace in order to see some early rewards of diet and exercise. Medical assistance may be necessary. And for the older child, in particular the rebellious teenager, the wisest course may be to turn the problem over to your physician. The most a wise parent may be able to do with this age group is make the right foods available in the appropriate quantity and get off the kid's back.

For those of you who may want to make your own calculations as to how much overweight your child may be for his height, in the Appendix you've been supplied with the growth charts we use at the University of Colorado together with instructions for use.

## Exercise

Exercise can easily become habit-forming. And failure to exercise can just as easily become a way of life. You usually don't have to encourage the preschool child to exercise (unless you've allowed television to rule his or her life). The young child, by nature, is constantly active, exploring, and testing muscles and skills and coordination. Children readily devote the entire day to what would correspond to interval exercise training in adults. Try following the 3- to 10-years-olds around and duplicate their movements and energy expenditure. It's a revealing workout.

So where do we go wrong? For openers, let's look briefly at three problems: the television set, the automobile, and sports programs.

Television is a marvelous baby-sitter. Kids will sit in front of the tube for hours, enchanted, enthralled, and stupefied. We won't go into the potentially deleterious psychological and intellectual impact of unrestricted television here, but will confine ourselves to the physical impact. Kids who need the opportunity to blow off steam and challenge their developing bodies may sit drugged for hours before that insidious electronic tranquilizer.

The solution is not difficult to perceive (but may be more than a little difficult to implement). Restrict television watching to a specified number of hours per week agreed on by the family.

The automobile is another problem for youngsters as well as adults. The American dream of having a piece of land away from the congestion of the central city has been achieved for many families since World War II in the suburbs and through the good offices of the automobile. But we've had too much of a good thing when kids are chauffeured constantly over distances that could easily be negotiated on foot or by bicycle. Ironically, the children are often *driven* to gymnastics lessons, Little League, and other putative physical activities. Obviously, if the gym or the game is located several miles away, there's a limit to how much time can be invested in slower forms of transit. But I think we must all look hard at the automobile and the exercise deprivation that can be associated with abusing it. The energy crunch may turn into a blessing for the national health.

Finally, there's the concept of sports programs for kids. Little League baseball, Pop Warner football, and the spectrum of competitive sports that emphasize skills with balls and "winning is everything" have come under scrutiny lately. The adoption of soccer to the North American scene may be taken as a good sign. Winning can still be everything for those who find that orientation appealing, but some aerobic conditioning is possible in soccer if you're a halfback. Running, rowing, jumping rope, swimming, and cross-country skiing are good aerobic sports for kids to learn early. All of these sports carry well through adult years.

I believe parents should take an active interest in the school's program of physical education for their children. They should use the gentle persuasion of parent-teachers' organizations to see that aerobic conditioning has a central position in their school program, and that physical conditioning for strength and flexibility is promoted as a rewarding activity, not as a punishment. Finally, they should request that sports that can be used for a lifetime are taught.

We noted in Chapter 9 that a 6-year-old can undertake an exercise program. At this age running is fun for many, and a hassle for just a few. Jumping rope is enough of a challenge that most boys and girls take to it eagerly. It's an excellent rainy day substitute for running. A time should be selected for the children to devote, as a routine, at least ten minutes to aerobic conditioning each day. This can be in the early morning for the genetic larks in the family, or before or after supper for the owls. It's best accomplished if a parent is involved. This is more for habit formation, especially if there is an adequate physical education program at school. But it can also represent a little bit of family togetherness on the way to developing a life-style. The key is to make it fun.

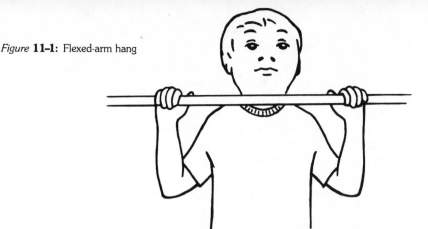

*Figure* **11–1:** Flexed-arm hang

As for warm-up and strength and flexibility exercises, children can perform the same ones as are recommended for men and women. Some of these exercises may be greeted by unrestrained laughter, because kids need warming up about as much as Nevada needs more desert. However, flexibility exercises, to gain and maintain maximal range of motion of joints, are useful. Gymnastics training is particularly valuable in this regard.

Exercises for strength can also begin at age 6. Both boys and girls take particular pride in these types of activities: sit-ups, push-ups, pull-ups, rope-climbs, pole-climbs, straight- and flexed-arm hangs, and hand-over-hand on overhead ladders. If you have the space, a $50 investment in a piece of gym equipment (with overhead ladder) is well spent. But playground equipment in parks and schoolyards may be even more challenging, if not as convenient. A bar with rubber friction ends may be wedged into a doorway for chinning indoors.

Table 11–2 gives some expectations for physical performance for healthy boys and girls at various ages. The goals of the 12- to 13-year-olds are reasonable to maintain into adult life, although some kids will go much higher. This is especially true for running, where one would expect that the older teenager and young adult (of either sex) would be able to run 1.5 miles in little more than ten minutes. How to do push-ups and sit-ups has been described in Chapter 9. Girls can do regular push-ups as easily as boys. The straight-arm hang is self-explanatory; the child merely hangs from a bar with arms straight and feet off the ground. The flexed-arm hang is achieved by holding the standard pull-up position with the arms flexed, backs of the hands to the face, the chin over the bar, but not resting on it, and the feet off the ground. The pull-up or chin is accomplished with the feet always off the ground, pulling the chin over the bar and allowing the body to return to the straight-arm hang before pulling up again.

The standing long jump is also self-explanatory: measuring how far the child can jump from a standing position rather than from a run.

The youngster just starting training may have very poor performance to begin with, but it's nothing less than remarkable how rapidly almost every child progresses through regular exercise. From the straight-arm hang to the flexed-arm hang to ten pull-ups may take a slim 8-year-old no more than a few months of training. The heavier children will not do as well in events where their extra weight is a handicap. But presumably, attention will be addressed to diet in those children who require it at the same time that exercise programs are being undertaken.

One thing that's really valuable about having your child exercise at home and gain in skill under the supervision of parents is that it can (and should) be a completely nonpunishing and rewarding experience. The physically slower child doesn't have to feel threatened or be ridiculed by unsympathetic classmates, as may happen at school. He may develop at his own pace with encouragement and private tutoring by parents and sibs. Even kids who appear to be totally without physical aptitude may flourish under these conditions. Needless to say, the confidence they gain from experiencing the burgeoning of their physical skills has a very positive effect. No table is offered for advancing levels of physical performance for kids. The aerobic walk/run routine suggested for adults in Chapter 9 is easily adaptable to children. The exercises for strength are merely started at a level at which kids can perform initially and are increased at their own pace to the minimal physical performance goals in Table 11–2. Most kids go sailing past those goals in short order. The only exercise that may benefit from sequencing is the straight-arm hang followed by flexed-arm hang, before starting pull-ups. But lots of kids don't even need this sequence.

For parents who may desire more illustrations and narrative on physical performance achievements, for both boys and girls, I would suggest the *Webelos Scout Book* published by the Boy Scouts of America or *The West Point Fitness and Diet Book*. The Webelos book, which is only $1.50 and may be purchased at any department store that has Scouting supplies in its children's department, has some good short sections on physical performance for kids. To put in an additional plug for Scouting, it really is a good way for boys and girls to gain competence in many areas as well as in physical abilities. The West Point book, $3.95 in paperback, is useful for the whole family.

A final couple of points on exercise. Heart rates (see Table 10–1 on page 186) throughout the childhood age range are higher than in adults, and are usually higher in girls (80–90) than in boys (75–85). Paradoxically some fairly well-conditioned children may have relatively fast resting heart rates until they reach their early teens. But these kids are capable of high rates with exertion and have a very fast recovery time.

A problem that children have more than adults is the "stitch in the side." This pain in the side of the lower chest or upper abdomen is probably related to our old acquaintance, lactic acid accumulation, but as far as I know, its exact etiology has not been carefully studied. The stitch becomes less of a problem as the child becomes better conditioned and is quite rare in the reasonably well-conditioned child or adult.

And as a last caution, vigorous exercise in the presence of an infection (a cold, flu, etc.) is as undesirable and counterproductive in the child as in the adult.

## High Blood Pressure

High blood pressure in childhood is often produced by definable causes such as kidney disease or a narrowing (coarctation) of the major artery of the body (aorta). The high blood pressure that afflicts perhaps 24 million American adults and becomes most noticeable in the third, fourth, and fifth decades of life is a primary disorder, familial in nature, and interacting with a number of factors such as salt intake, stress, and obesity.

Can predisposition to this type of high blood pressure be readily detected in infants and children? Unfortunately, not as easily as one would wish by just taking casual blood pressure readings. Those children who will develop high blood pressure at 30 or 40 may have "normal" pressures throughout childhood. Conversely, those who are in a higher percentile for blood pressure at one age may be in a lower percentile at a later age. The epidemiologic jargon for this phenomenon is that blood pressure "doesn't track well" through childhood and early adult life.

The genetics of high blood pressure is a complex subject and is hotly disputed. But that's really not important to the lay person or to the practicing physician. What's important is to know whether high blood pressure is present in the family. Some children in these families will have pressures that stay in the higher percentiles and will continue to progress to true hypertension when they're adults. Certain stress tests may help identify those who will need special attention. At about 12 years of age a child with a blood pressure reading of 140/90 represents the ninety-fifth percentile—that is, a child with such a reading has a higher pressure than 95 percent of children his age. Any child with a pressure that remains at 140/90 on repeated visits should be considered to have high blood pressure requiring medical attention. Please refer to Chapter 7, Figures 7–1 and 7–2, for blood pressure graphs in children.

As was pointed out in the chapter on high blood pressure, experimental evidence suggests that early intervention is necessary in the course of high blood pressure to prevent it from becoming irreversible. But until you can tell exactly which child is at high risk, what do you do? Here is where a "low-risk strategy" is valid. If there is a positive family history for high blood pressure, salt intake should be restricted in kids—whatever their casual blood pressures may be—to between 3 and 5 grams per day (i.e., between 1,200 and 2,000 milligrams of sodium per day). The taste for salt is not hard to modify in children. And there is much potential benefit to be gained from moderate salt restriction with no hazard that I can see. For the child who is persistently above the ninety-fifth percentile in blood pressure readings and does not have secondary high blood pressure due to kidney disease or some other definable cause, I would recommend holding salt intake to a maximum of 3 grams per day.

A 10-year-old, for example, gets his largest amount of daily salt from added salt. Then comes bread, followed by snack foods. If added salt and snack foods are monitored and consciously lowered, this should be sufficient to achieve moderate reduction.

## Smoking

This topic has been discussed in detail in Chapter 6 as it relates to the newborn infant, child, and teenager. For this chapter, a few points will be repeated because they are so important.

The first reason kids smoke is because their parents do. The next is because their older brothers and sisters do. These people are their first-line role models. Then comes the peer group, and if they don't have a strong, well-prepared defense, they effortlessly slide into smoking. By age 18, one-third of all American kids smoke regularly. While it may be hard for an adult to understand it, *addiction* to smoking is a real phenomenon among teenagers. And the addicted adult quite likely acquired his addiction as a teenager.

Smokers may be divided into two categories, even in adolescence: the beginners and the dependent smokers. Children in the beginner category are much easier to deal with through health education. And, indeed, if they don't see smoking in their homes, and if they are actively participating in a general program of family health, smoking is unlikely to begin. On the other hand, the dependent smoker at age 15 must be approached in the same way as the dependent smoker at age 40 or 50. Dependent smoking requires psychological intervention.

## Type A and Stress Control

Kids with Type A behavior? While there has not been a scale designed specifically to define Type A behavior for children, many of the features of the Type A adult discussed in Chapter 8 are recognizable in the child. If you as a parent have Type A behavior or are married to such an individual, you can recognize the signs.

The study that needs to be performed after a Type A scale is developed for kids is one on the heritability of this behavior. Does this mean that Type A behavior is inherited? Probably. At least it tends to be familial, and how much is inherited versus how much is due to living in a Type A environment remains to be sorted out. You should know that there is a very active branch of genetics, called behavioral genetics, that looks into problems like this.

Well, what can you do with your child to prevent him from becoming an uptight, Type A adult—especially if the problem has an important genetic component? First, start looking for clues. Is he or she *almost* always well-organized and prompt? (No kid is *always* well-organized.) That's a good sign in many ways. Maybe he'll be organized enough to get through school and hold down a regular job. *But* is he often impatient and intolerant of the lack of organization and promptness in other family members? When a 10-year-old becomes distraught while waiting for the rest of the family to get into the car, or acutely anxious at the thought of not getting to school 15 minutes early, start paying attention.

Table 8–1 on page 148 gives a number of adult Type A characteristics, many of which, when you stop to think about them, can be extended to children. But as I've said, there's been no study validating childhood manifestations of Type A behavior. Common sense should help bridge that particular gap. Parents sensitive to their children can recognize if they're stressed, uptight, and anxious without the benefit of a table or formal training in pediatrics or child psychology.

All right, say you recognize some telltale signs; what next? It's back to habit formation. You'll have to help your child develop ways to cope with this common affliction. And it is common. The investigators who proposed the behavior types feel that Type A behavior is present in more Americans than Type B is. Thus, it really may come down to a matter of degree. If you and your children are by nature (by heredity and environment) Type A, you can strive for constructive control. Channel that behavior into productivity and curb the potentially self-defeating and self-damaging aspects of Type A-ness. It appears to be a matter of degree. In our epidemiologic study there was a higher risk of heart attack when comparing extreme Type A (4+) with least Type A (1+). There was no difference if moderate degrees were included.

Two things need emphasis. You don't want to try to make a Type B out of a Type A (even if you could). Your somewhat aggressive straight-A student may get under people's skins now and then, but you don't want to try to convert him into a dropout, wandering aimlessly through life. Your goal is to help him smooth out those jagged edges that sometimes injure others, but most often injure only himself. The second point that needs emphasis is that your help has to be fairly subtle. A Type A kid doesn't need someone on his back all the time. Gentle molding and shaping are what is required. An aggressive Type A parent constantly pointing out the Type A flaws in the character of his Type A offspring is counterproductive at best.

When the younger child gets uptight, soothe him out of it. Show him the alternative responses that are better for him. The older child, the teenager, is ready for more definitive instruction in life orientation. This is a time when kids are likely to become deeply religious or equally deeply committed to something they conceive of as being greater than themselves. This is a time when meditation can be taught and readily adopted into the life-style of the young person.

Children can and should be taught productive ways to handle stress, whether they're at high risk of coronary heart disease or not. But for the child who is at high risk, it is a parental obligation to provide guidance in this important area of disease prevention. The habits for a lifetime are established in childhood.

# A Risk Index for Children _____

When we started out to develop methods of discovering infants and children who might be candidates for coronary heart disease as adults, we concentrated on the newborn infant. This was a convenient time to get blood (from the umbilical cord) and a family history—since family members tend to congregate to welcome the new addition. We found problems with this approach. The family history may certainly be obtained at this time, but other risk factors are not optimally found in the newborn period. Cholesterol and triglycerides taken from the cord blood do not "track" well throughout infancy and early childhood. By 1 to 2 years of age, however, the blood findings become quite reliable and reproducible at examinations through subsequent years of childhood.

Now please direct your attention to Table 11–3. As you remember, in Chapter 2 (Table 2–2) a risk questionnaire was presented with the promise that after you obtained the needed information you would be shown how to calculate your risk index in Chapter 12. This questionnaire was distilled from a much more comprehensive protocol that we've used in our genetic-epidemiologic studies of patients who had experienced heart attacks before 55 years of age.

Then we looked at children in these families to try to decide how many of the risks could be identified at early ages. Table 11–3 shows the information you will need to obtain in collaboration with your child's physician to determine your child's potential risk of having a heart attack as an adult. In parentheses are the ages when this information can be gathered. What was surprising was that most of the crucial data could be obtained in the 1- and 2-year-olds: positive family history of cardiovascular disease, cholesterol and triglycerides, diabetes (a history of diabetes in a first-degree relative appeared to be as strong a risk factor as diabetes in the patient himself), and relative weight (fat babies are on their way to becoming fat adults).

All of the remaining risks could be assessed later in childhood, but all of them were relevant for pediatric patients. For example, hypertension (high blood pressure) is a familial disease, and we've observed that more than half of the risk of heart attack comes from heredity. Therefore, we feel that it's reasonable to use a family history of high blood pressure as a potential early indicator of risk, and as a basis for caution in the use of salt in the diet. The risk factor of hypertension may be initially assigned to a child (subject to later revision) if any or all of these criteria are met: (1) positive family history of high blood pressure; (2) blood pressure equal to or greater than 140/90 (by the time a child reaches 10 to 12 years of age 140/90 represents the ninety-fifth percentile—that is, 140/90 is higher than 95 percent of blood pressures in children of this age group); (3) blood pressure reading in the ninety-fifth percentile for children younger than 10 to 12 years of age (see Figures 7–1 and 7–2).

An exercise history and an effort to judge the developing behavior pattern of the child are relevant: the habits formed in childhood carry on into adult life. This isn't to say that anyone is going to predict a heart attack for a sedentary 9-year-old who gets uptight about being late for school. The point of the risk index is not to be able to say: "See, I told you so." Rather it's to say: "These are factors that may represent risks, and it's prudent to attempt to reduce these risks."

The final points come from smoking: Of all the environmental risk factors that have roots in childhood, this may be the most critical. In presenting this sort of material, I used to dismiss smoking as being a risk factor that is not relevant to childhood. But one-third of teenagers in the United States smoke regularly. And one child in eight between the ages of 12 and 14 is a regular smoker. The addicted adult smoker frequently became addicted as a teenager. Smoking is a pediatric problem that must be recognized as such and treated as such.

In Chapter 12, we'll put the risks together to make up a risk index for each member of the family, adults and children.

| TABLE 11-1 | **Dietary Guidelines for Children at Risk** |
|---|---|

| **Children at low risk** | **Children at high risk** |
|---|---|
| Prudent diet | Prudent diet |
| | plus |
| | **1** *only* skim milk (drinking and cooking) |
| | **2** limit: 1 egg yolk per week |
| | **3** more rigorous salt restriction (3 grams per day) |
| | **4** further recommendations from physician |
| | **5** possible medication |

TABLE
11-2 **Physical Performance Goals for Boys and Girls**

|  | Boys and Girls | | | Boys | Girls |
|---|---|---|---|---|---|
|  | **6-7** | **8-9** | **10-11** | **12-13** | **12-13** |
| Straight-arm hang | 60 sec. | 60 sec. | 90 sec. | 120 sec. | 90 sec. |
| Flexed-arm hang | 20 sec. | 30 sec. | 40 sec. | 60 sec. | 40 sec. |
| Pull-ups | 2 | 4 | 6 | 10 | 6 |
| Push-ups | 10 | 15 | 20 | 30 | 20 |
| Bent-leg sit-ups | 20 | 35 | 50 | 60 | 50 |
| Standing long jump | 4 ft. | 5 ft. | 6 ft. | 7 ft. | 6 ft. |
| 50-yard dash | 9 sec. | 8.5 sec. | 7.5 sec. | 7 sec. | 7.5 sec. |
| 600-yard walk/run | 2 min. 30 sec. | 2 min. 15 sec. | 2 min. | 2 min. | 2 min. |
| 1.5 miles | — | 16 min. | 14 min. | 12 min. | 12 min. |

TABLE
11–3

## Suggested Parent-Physician Collaboration to Identify Children at Risk of Early Heart Attack as Adults

1   Obtain family history for heart attacks in first- and second-degree relatives before age 55 and before age 65 (age 1–2).

2   Obtain family history of high blood pressure (essential hypertension) in first-degree relatives (age 1–2).

3   Obtain family history for juvenile diabetes in first-degree relatives (age 1–2).

4   Cholesterol and triglycerides on fasting specimen. Repeat with lipoproteins if abnormality is evident (age 1–2).

5   If lipids and lipoproteins are abnormal, obtain blood studies on available first-degree relatives (age 1–2).

6   Begin to "track" blood pressure annually—a minimum of 3 readings at a visit (age 1–2).

7   Plot height and weight on growth curves. If overweight for height, calculate percent overweight (age 1–2).

8   Obtain exercise history (age 5–10).

9   Assess behavior type (age 5–10).

10   Obtain smoking history (age 12–    ).

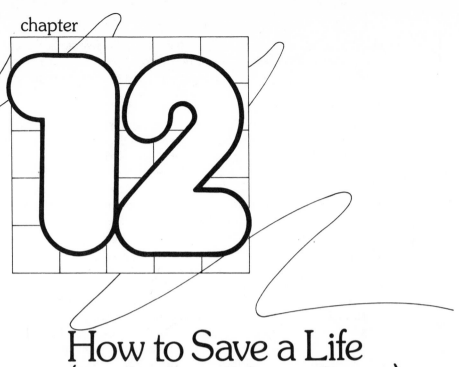

# How to Save a Life (Including Your Own)

This is where we get it all together. We're going to try to decide what your risks are, whether they're low or high. And we're going to look at some suggestions that just might help lessen those risks.

Let me tell you a little bit more about the risk formulas in this chapter, how they were derived, and how they were tested (and continue to be tested). All of the risks that appear in the questionnaires have long been suspected of playing a role in the development of atherosclerosis leading to heart attacks. These questionnaires, by the way, appear as Table 12–1 for adults and Table 12–2 for children. Table 12–1 was introduced in Chapter 2.

But if these were just "suspected" risks or "possible" risks, one would have to be extremely cautious about reaching conclusions. So let me add the assurance that studies of the environmental risks have been repeated many times by many investigators, and the great weight of opinion (despite the potential for disagreement in epidemiologic studies) supports these risks as being important.

Now for the genetic risks. There has been almost a century of recognition that heredity is important in heart attacks. There also have been many family studies over the years that have shown the role of inheritance in various aspects of atherosclerosis, lipoproteins, and heart attacks. But I must make it clear that the data on how important heredity is, and what its relative role is as compared with environment, come from my own studies of data that I and my co-workers have personally collected or have analyzed from epidemiologic studies conducted by other investigators.

We used a variety of methods to weigh the genetic and environmental risks, including some fairly powerful computer techniques. Then we put the weighted risks into a risk formula and tested it on patients who had heart attacks at early ages and compared these patients with their age-matched controls. Thus, the test itself was tested to determine how accurate the formula was in discriminating between individuals who have heart attacks and those who don't. Finally, another mathematical device was used to predict how much the risk of heart attack was increased for a given level of risk score.

I would be the first to acknowledge that as one gets away from patients and into mathematical models the numbers become less real than they first appeared to be. Don't be dazzled by these numbers or numbers from anyone else, but accept them only as approximations consistent with our present state of knowledge.

## Calculating Risks for Adults

Table 12–3 tells you how many points you are assessed for the risks you recorded in the questionnaire, Table 12–1.

**Family history** ○ Through no fault of your own, if you have a first-degree relative (parent, sibling, child) who has had a heart attack before age 55, you have 3 risk points against you. A second-degree relative (grandparent, uncle, aunt) with a heart attack before 65 costs 1 point, and so on. In this section you select only the single highest value. If your father had a coronary at 54, your mother a stroke at 63, and your grandfather a coronary at 61, your point score is still only the single highest value: 3 points for the coronary in your father—*not* 6.5 points for all the cardiovascular events in your family.

**Lipids**  ○  This section is the most complicated the scoring system gets. The most points you can have charged against you for what your blood cholesterol and triglycerides reveal is 2. If your cholesterol is 275 it costs you 2 points. If your cholesterol is 250 it costs 1 point. And if your triglycerides are elevated to above 200, it may or may not cost you, because the highest total you can get in this section is 2. Therefore, triglycerides of 230 and cholesterol of 210 give you only .5 points, because the cholesterol isn't high enough to score. If the triglycerides of 230 occur together with the cholesterol of 275, 2 points is still the maximum score for this section. However, if you pair the triglycerides of 230 (.5 points) with the cholesterol of 250 (1 point), you are assessed 1.5 points. Please reread this section and Table 12–3 if my description has failed to make it clear on the first reading.

**Other Risks**  ○  These risk factors *all* add to the total. If you smoke, don't get adequate aerobic exercise (as defined in Table 12–1), have a blood pressure greater than 140/90, and are greater than 20 percent overweight (relative weight > 1.20), your point total for this section is 3.5. The question on diabetes deserves some comment. You are assessed one point if you have diabetes *or* if a first-degree relative has juvenile-onset diabetes (i.e., diabetes starting at an early age and requiring insulin).

As you can see, the opportunities you have to reduce your personal risk come under the Lipids and Other Risks sections. You can lower your cholesterol. You can also exercise and stop smoking and reduce both your weight and your blood pressure. We'll talk about these implications a little later.

Do you have all the information to add up your risk score? Let's assume you do. What does the score mean? This is where the mathematical manipulations enter the picture, and where a great deal of caution must be exercised in interpretation. Table 12–3 also shows how much your risk is increased for various scores from 3 to 5. (At 5.5 the risk probability falls victim to the methodology and the curve becomes asymptotic. Our present methods don't permit us to give risks for scores of 5.5 and above.)

All right, say you added up your score and found you had 5.5 points, and 3 irreducible points were from your heredity. Does that mean you might as well throw in the towel? Your risk is so high, what's the use? Not at all. The assumption I make in dealing with high-risk patients and families is that the increased risk (whether it's twofold or fifteenfold) exists in those *not* actively trying to reduce their risks. This is a legitimate assumption. The patients in our study who had heart attacks at early ages were not, with two exceptions, following anything resembling a serious and balanced program for cardiovascular health. We had some people who were, for example, getting good exercise, but diet, weight, cholesterol, smoking, or other risk factors were not being aggressively attacked. The two who did have premature coronary disease had extremely serious genetic predispositions plus the damage of many years of high environmental risk factors. The changes they made were appropriate, but would have been much more effective if started earlier.

But as I've mentioned, there's a preventive program for any age or stage of your disease—including the period following a heart attack. The earlier you start your program, the better. And the lower you get your risk score, the better.

Let's take another example—a somewhat (23 percent) overweight, sedentary, Type A cardiologist, with a cholesterol of 290 and triglycerides of 380. Both of his parents had coronary heart disease; one had an onset before age 55. All he seemed to have going for him was that he didn't smoke, didn't have a diabetic risk, and had normal blood pressure. Our overweight (it really didn't show that much) cardiologist scored 7 points. So high he was "off the curve."

So what could be done for someone at apparently extremely high risk? Weight reduction, subtract .5 points. Regular exercise, subtract 1 point. Behavioral stress control, subtract .5 points. Cholesterol and triglyceride reduction through strict diet. Not much effect. The cholesterol dropped to 260, but despite his reduction to desirable weight (actually looking a little skinny), the triglycerides stayed high. In fact, the count went up to 390. Medications were required, which reduced the cholesterol to 215 and the triglycerides to 220. Our 7-point walking disaster is down to 3.5 points.

Does this mean he still has three times the risk of an early coronary that someone with no points has? Possibly. But we can't get hung up on the exact number. What's important is how much his risk has been reduced. He is still at increased risk because of an unfortunate heredity. But he's doing everything possible to lower his risk—and, in fact, is now in better cardiovascular health from the point of view of standard epidemiologic (not genetic) risks than the average American male of his age.

## Calculating Risks for Children

Here we must make it clear that we are taking risk factors known to be associated with early-onset coronary heart disease in adults and seeing if these same risk factors can be identified in children. This absolutely is not to say that the risk factors you see in children have to lead to an unfortunate outcome.

On the contrary, what we're saying is: "Look, positive family history, high cholesterol, high blood pressure, smoking, and other factors are the current top suspects as causes of coronary disease and stroke—no matter at what age they're discovered. Therefore if you can identify these factors in children, even young children, these factors are the ones to do something about, today. This is the direction for a rational preventive program at our present state of knowledge."

We don't want to see every kid on a severely restrictive diet. But we do want those at high risk to have optimal dietary management compatible with the level of their risk. As for recommending that kids refrain from starting to smoke, get plenty of exercise, maintain ideal weight, blood pressure, and stress control, there is only benefit to be gained at no risk that I can discern.

Fill out your children's questionnaires (Table 12–2), or if they're old enough, have them fill them out. Then turn your attention to Table 12–4. You'll see that, except for cholesterol and triglyceride levels, the risk points are the same as in adults. Children tend to run lower levels than adults, so the numbers are commensurately reduced.

Say we have a 12-year-old boy whose 57-year-old father had a sudden heart attack (2.5 points). The anxious family comes in for counseling. The boy is found to have a cholesterol of 230 (2 points) and triglycerides of 70. He's a scholarly, sedentary type who has not been encouraged to exercise by his scholarly, sedentary, older parents (1 point). At 12 years and 2 months of age, he is 59 inches tall (fiftieth percentile). The fiftieth percentile for weight is 90 pounds at 12 years, but our boy unfortunately weighs 118 pounds (118/90 = 1.31; his relative weight is 1.31). This costs another .5 points. (You can do these weight calculations for kids using the growth standard curves supplied in the Appendix.) The boy tried a couple of cigarettes at age 11, but not since, and he states that he does not intend to smoke.

This youngster has 6 risk points against him. However, by diet, exercise, and reorientation of his life-style, he has been able to reduce his risk points to 2.5. And the beauty of it is that he's begun to reduce the risk before his blood vessels have sustained significant damage.

## Additional Factors

Our risk formulas include some items that we haven't discussed in detail. There are also other factors that are now known to be important but don't as yet appear in the risk formulas. And there will certainly be more factors entering the picture as our knowledge increases. Let's pick out a few entities for a quick once-over.

**HDL (high-density lipoprotein)** ○  HDL has received considerable attention recently. When we do a risk factor analysis today we look at HDL. However, our data on HDL was incomplete for a sizeable segment of our genetic-epidemiologic study, so I've been unable to include this very important factor in our risk formula. (We estimated HDL by looking only at alpha lipoprotein.) When we accumulate enough data it certainly will be included. The interesting point about HDL as compared with other lipoproteins is that the *more* you have of it the *lower* your risk. It appears that if your blood cholesterol is attached to HDL rather than LDL (low-density lipoprotein) your blood vessels are protected rather than harmed. Exercise and perhaps some dietary programs (including alcohol in moderation) may contribute to raising your level of HDL. However, genetics rears its head again. Some of your HDL level depends on your sex (higher in women), your race (e.g., apparently higher in Blacks), and your family (some families have higher levels than others). HDL is, in epidemiologic studies, turning out to be a highly important factor in resistance to coronary disease (when it's high) and susceptibility to heart attacks (when it's low).

**Diabetes** ○  This is a devastating risk factor, and one that could command an entire volume for discussion. Relegating it to a couple of paragraphs of descriptive material does not reflect its importance, but rather mirrors our inability to have a positive impact on the problem.

Diabetics, especially those whose disease starts in childhood or young adulthood (juvenile or insulin-dependent diabetics), may sometimes experience a very rapid decline in the health of their blood vessels. This decline often appears to be unrelated to how well controlled their diabetes is. That's the discouraging part. Because if we could say that the blood vessel disease could be prevented by superb control, we'd be following the thesis of this book to the letter. Our pitch has been that we have something in prevention for any age, stage, or cause of cardiovascular disease. I believe that this may someday be true in diabetic vascular disease, as well. But I would be less than candid if I suggested that a preventive is clearly available right now.

A curious finding has appeared in our studies that may eventually illuminate this problem. Having a first-degree relative with juvenile diabetes appears to be as great a cardiovascular risk as actually having diabetes. This, on the surface, appears to make little biologic sense and I'm not confident that the observation will hold up. However, if it is confirmed, there may be a common basis in tissue and clotting factor differences that seems to exist not only in diabetics, but in their families.

**Blood Clotting** ○ There has been intensive investigation into this area of potential risk. The most prominent clotting risk appears to be related to small elements in the blood called platelets. Patients who have heart attacks seem to have platelets that don't circulate for as long a lifetime as those who don't have heart attacks. Other clotting factors may also play roles and are being investigated.

**Tissue Type** ○ This takes us back to heart transplantation. The first patient we did a heart transplant on received the heart of a teen-aged girl (with absolutely no coronary disease). Yet in eight months the heart revealed coronary arteries that were almost completely plugged up. We knew that the tissue types of the donor and recipient were different for one specificity, and we could see that anti-heart antibodies had been formed to reject the heart. The question we asked ourselves was: Could heart attacks have as a component, a rejection process? And could those who have heart attacks have certain tissue types that make them vulnerable to heart attacks, and could a process akin to rejection be playing a role? Only just now as we're able to study a large number of different tissue types are we in a position to attack this question. If forced to give an answer to the question now, I would say, *very cautiously,* that certain tissue types may be emerging as more common in early heart attack victims than in those who don't have early-onset coronary disease. Obviously, this area will require more work.

**Hormones** ○ One reason often given in the past for women not having early heart attacks as frequently as men was that they were protected until menopause by abundant female hormone. Then a study was done that suggested that *men* who have early heart attacks have *higher* levels of *female* hormone than those who don't. And women who receive additional synthetic female hormones as oral contraceptives (the Pill) are at greater risk of heart attack and stroke than those who don't. At this time the interactions between levels of hormones and heart attacks and strokes must be subjected to further investigation.

**Factors Discovered and Yet to Be Discovered** ○ Certainly there are many things we still don't understand about the causes of heart attacks and strokes. Every few months we may expect new information to be added to our fund of knowledge, which will make it possible to be more accurate in our identification of those at risk, and more precise in our programs of prevention.

What you've been given up to this point is a great deal of the most up-to-date information that goes into determining whether you and your family are at low risk or high risk—or some intermediate risk—of early-onset coronary heart disease. In the next section we'll wrestle with the question of what exactly is low risk, and what is high risk. Then in subsequent sections we'll review what the steps are to follow for the level of risk you may have.

## How High Is Your Personal Risk?

This question turns out to be a little harder than it looks. For openers, if you have no points against you it would appear that your risk is minimal. And if you have 3 points against you, your risk is twice as high for having coronary disease as someone with no risk points. And if you have 5 points your risk is increased fifteenfold.

But what if you've got 1 or 2 points? Or have 6 points and can only lower your risk to 2.5 points? Or maybe you do everything possible and still can't lower your risk below 4 points.

I would define minimal risk as no points (or by working at your Whole Heart Program until you achieve no points against you).

I would initially define a person potentially at high risk as anyone who has early-onset coronary disease or stroke in his family and who has not eliminated all possible risks within his control, or anyone scoring 3 points or above on our risk index.

But there are obvious problems with that. And for these we'll have to resort to accommodation and the art of the possible. We must create a category called intermediate risk. If you're doing everything that can be done to reduce your risk and still have 3 points or more, I don't believe most of you in that position should still be assigned high risk. Since I come under that description, I'm doubly inclined to accept the concept of intermediate risk and to appreciate the potential value of dedicated risk reduction. So for those who have between 0 and 3 points or who have maximally reduced their risks to the lowest achievable level, intermediate risk is a reasonable classification. And for those at intermediate risk the preventive program is the same as for those at high risk: all out.

Finally, there are some risks that are strong enough to stand by themselves without even being incorporated into a risk index. These risks are smoking, cholesterol greater than 240, blood pressure greater than 160/100, and diabetes. I believe that anyone who has one of these risks and *who is not doing everything possible* to achieve optimal cardiovascular health is at significant risk even if the total risk score is less than 3.

# The Low-Risk Strategy of Prevention

This is the direction of prevention appropriate for an entire community or state or country—across the board: the dietary goals of the U.S. Senate Select Committee, and the Surgeon General's report, *Smoking and Health*. It's what many millions of Americans have embraced. Healthful life-style.

If your genetic risk is not high, cessation (or avoidance) of smoking, aerobic exercise, stress control, weight normalization, maintenance of normal blood pressure, and a prudent diet are the components of the healthful life-style. This life-style will not only keep your risk of cardiovascular disease low, but will reduce your risks of many other causes of early death and disability. The risk-benefit ratio of this strategy appears to be entirely in favor of benefit.

And I would add, as a personal approach, that I believe that those who are not at high risk are entitled to considerable dietary flexibility and moderate flexibility in exercise requirements. Just because my family needs a strict low cholesterol diet doesn't mean that everyone else should be subjected to the same restrictions. If you as an adult have blood cholesterol lower than 200 and triglycerides lower than 100 on your present diet, I would find it hard to justify imposing a stricter diet on you. If your kids have cholesterols below 150 and triglycerides below 80, let them go to McDonald's (within reason).

If you're not at high risk and are quite trim despite an inch of pinch, I don't think you have to worry that much. Certainly, if you are less than 10 percent over desirable weight without even having an inch of pinch, I wouldn't advocate your losing weight by wasting muscle.

If you're not at high risk and get regular aerobic exercise, but prefer to substitute tennis a couple of times a week during the summer, do it. Even a *walking* round of golf in place of an aerobic workout is acceptable occasionally. A round of golf in a golf cart is not an acceptable substitute, however, for anything except watching television.

# The High-Risk (and Intermediate-Risk) Strategy

The goal here is to lower your risk points as far as possible. Preferably this should be done without medications, but medications and even surgery may be required in some cases.

Your diet has to be strict and your weight should be on the low side of the desirable weight range. You can have as much recreational exercise as you want *in addition to* (not instead of) the full required time with aerobics.

Any individual with risk points would benefit from consulting with a physician interested in preventive care. This includes anyone who needs a diet more restrictive than the prudent diet—and certainly anyone who needs medication.

There are also obvious reasons for being under the regular care of a physician. Certainly if you've had a heart attack or have congenital heart disease, rheumatic heart disease, high blood pressure, or diabetes, you already must be receiving regular medical attention. In addition, I'd advise that any adult with a cholesterol above 240, any child with a cholesterol above 190, and anyone with a first-degree relative having a heart attack before age 55 should have regular medical input designed to maintain the lowest possible risk score.

As I've already asserted, if you're at high risk, it's really essential that you have an established relationship with a physician knowledgeable in the diagnosis and treatment of cardiovascular diseases and attuned to preventive measures. There will be many issues that will arise requiring his knowledge and your confidence in his knowledge and concern.

Most of you reading this account who are at high risk will not have symptoms, but if you suspect something more is wrong than some points against you on a risk scale, you need a doctor. If you, like Matthew Arnold, are experiencing chest pain, you're in no better position to treat it than he was. But your physician is. There are reliable diagnostic studies to determine the cause of the pain. And there are some significant new opportunities for treatment.

Those of you who have risk factors requiring an exercise stress test before starting aerobic training will be exposed to a valuable diagnostic device in standard practice today that helps your physician evaluate the condition of your heart. As with all diagnostic tools, stress testing is not 100 percent reliable, but it provides answers in which a high degree of confidence can be placed. If you're having symptoms that concern your physician, he'll most likely evaluate you first with a resting electrocardiogram followed by taking an electrocardiogram while you're challenging your heart with well-controlled, well-monitored exercise.

If it turns out that your heart is compromised, there are medications to use, such as nitroglycerin and related compounds, which allow an increase in the flow of blood through the coronary arteries. Nitroglycerin-type drugs relieve the chest pain that occurs when the circulation to the heart muscle is deficient. Another group of drugs relieve chest pain by decreasing the amount of work the heart muscle performs (and thus the requirements of blood that the coronary arteries must supply). The generic prototype of these drugs is called propranolol. Propranolol-type drugs have an additional benefit in prevention of disturbances of the rhythm of the heart. A common complication in patients with coronary disease (and a common cause of death) is that the heart rhythm becomes abnormal.

Some chest pain from coronary disease becomes so severe and so intractable to medical management that coronary bypass surgery is recommended. In this operation a section of vein is commonly taken from the leg and hooked up between the main blood vessel coming from the heart (the aorta) and the heart muscle, thus "bypassing" the point where a coronary artery is obstructed. This in effect provides a new "coronary blood vessel." There is still some debate as to whether the coronary bypass operation provides anything more than relief of chest pain. Obviously it is hoped that the "new blood vessel" will greatly improve the circulation to the heart muscle, and with it improve survival.

My present bias is that coronary bypass surgery *does* do a little more than relieve chest pain. And if the patients who receive the bypass embrace a stage-specific preventive program, including careful diet and smoking cessation, the operation is beneficial beyond the relief of pain. Epidemiologists and many cardiologists are concerned about the so-called risk/benefit ratio of the operation. On a population basis, the enormous expense (over a billion a year) is not remotely cost-effective for the small amount of benefit gained. On an individual basis, the story may be quite different.

What options are available to the high-risk patient who shows no evidence of heart disease? First, of course, is the Whole Heart Program. Then the diet (as strict as required), and even medication for lowering cholesterol and triglycerides. Blood pressure control (including medication if needed). Smoking abrogation. Stress control. Aerobic exercise (after stress testing to be sure the patient enters the program at an appropriately monitored level). Then comes the need to know symptoms, signs, and what to do to save a life (including your own).

## Saving Lives

Various estimates have been made, but most of the data suggests that about 60 percent of deaths among heart attack victims occur before they ever reach a hospital. Yet there is much evidence to suggest that many, if not most, of these lives could be saved if people—including the victims, their family members, co-workers, and bystanders—had a little basic knowledge. This knowledge is readily available. It is clear from many studies throughout the industrialized world that delay in recognizing and promptly treating heart attack victims is responsible for the high incidence of preventable deaths. While a mobile coronary care unit arriving within minutes of a coronary event is ideal, there is much that the individual can do in the interim or in the absence of such a unit.

A patient at high risk should become familiar with the symptoms of coronary disease, angina, and heart attack—and what to do should they occur. These symptoms and signs should be discussed with a physician. The American Heart Association distributes information on this subject, and a modification of their material is reproduced here in Table 12–5. The purpose of printing this information is only to introduce you to the subject. Any physician who has worked extensively with patients with heart problems knows how difficult it sometimes is to evaluate the symptoms of coronary disease—angina or frank heart attack. But knowing some general facts will help the patient at high risk to be able to discuss the problem more knowledgeably with his or her physician. And having an understanding of the symptoms could possibly prove to be lifesaving.

**Cardiopulmonary resuscitation** ○ CPR is another topic for the high-risk *family* to be well informed about; and I believe that all family members of appropriate age should be trained in this skill. Not that if you have a heart attack requiring resuscitation (i.e., you stop breathing and your heart slows or stops beating) you can do anything for yourself. But the people most often around you are family members, and these will be the ones who can and must do something. And an individual trained in CPR can of course be in a position to help anyone in need. The steps of CPR are given in Table 12–6, and again are adapted from material from the American Heart Association. It's unlikely that your physician would have the time to do anything more than discuss this with you briefly and refer you to a CPR training course. And in fact physicians not often exposed to these problems will themselves have to take regular refresher courses in CPR.

Work with your local heart association, Red Cross, hospital volunteer group, fire department, or whatever. In fact, members of high-risk families should take the lead in this area, and maintain their own skills by being teachers in CPR training programs.

**Medications** ○ The use of medications for high-risk patients not having evidence of heart disease is clearly a controversial topic that can' only be resolved by close collaboration with your physician. If you're entering the age when high-risk patients most often have coronary events, would it be useful for you to carry on your person a nitroglycerin preparation and also, possibly, a propranolol-type drug? There are advantages to this approach. Recent evidence suggests that a class of drugs called calcium antagonists may prevent the sudden death associated with spasm of the coronary arteries. It also appears that one or two aspirin a day may not only help prevent clotting but may also reduce spasm by acting through the complex system of prostaglandins. Other anti-clotting drugs that act on platelets are also being used. I believe that there is a valid option here, but the course you follow should be carefully thought out and arrived at after weighing the merits of the alternatives in your own case with your own physician.

## The Golden Mean

Although I've given you some approaches and methods that have proved effective in the preventive management of various groups of people, this doesn't mean you will find that everything I've offered will be applicable to you—or effective for you.

I've usually given the *maximal* behavior modification approaches (where behavior modification is what is indicated) so you will have all the tools you may need available to you. The optimal program for the majority of people will be less than a maximal approach, but more than a minimal recommendation, such as: "Eat half as much and exercise twice as much."

Your dietary orientation need not be as rigid and unbending as that of a Javert. Your exercise program must certainly offer more rewards than pain. The life-style you adopt, if it is to become firmly established, will have to be clearly recognizable as providing a superior and more gratifying approach to your well-being than the life-style you are forsaking.

Be flexible in everything. Even the one modification I support most—that is, stopping smoking before undertaking the rest of the Whole Heart Program—is subject to negotiation. Diet, flexibility exercises, and the walking pre-aerobic phase of conditioning may precede smoking cessation in some cases. However, in good conscience, I still can't recommend aerobic training for smokers over 35 who have other risk factors.

The narrative ends with this chapter, but I commend to you the reference materials, charts, questionnaires, tables, and data in the Appendix. As a demonstration of flexibility, I've even provided a food composition table for what you may purchase at fast food franchises.

You may find it enlightening and/or horrifying (e.g., McDonald's fish filet sandwich has more calories, more fat, and more cholesterol than the hamburger because of all the stuff you get in addition to the fish). You will also find a table telling you how many calories you burn with various activities. If you didn't already know it, it takes a lot of exercise to burn up a few extra calories. If you're normally active you burn calories at the rate given in Tables 4–6 and 4–7. If you weigh 175 pounds and run four miles a day (doing ten-minute miles) and are on the 1-pound-a-week weight-loss diet, you'll lose 2 pounds a week rather than 1.

## The Decision

There's much that we don't know about heart attack prevention, but much that we do know. I've shared with you some of my understanding of the subject with the hope that it will reach out and touch you, and perhaps contribute to the health and well-being of you and your family.

If you're at low risk, there may be very few changes to make in your life-style to keep your risk low. If you're at high risk you may have to devote a great deal of attention to your personal health prescription. But whatever your risk and whatever your prescription, the benefits appear to be very great.

What I must stress again is that there is enormous potential for preventing heart attacks. Data from Finland and the United States confirm that heart attacks and death rates from heart attacks are declining. In *most* cases heart attacks are preventable at the ages of the thirties through the sixties. What also should be stressed is that *deaths* from heart attacks may be dramatically reduced. The patient with heart disease, at any stage before or after a heart attack, may look forward to a program that may restore him to as high a level of physical performance as is compatible with the damage already sustained.

Heart attacks don't have to take a person by surprise. Those at high risk may be identified. And heart attacks don't have to kill you. There's much that can be done during those critical minutes before reaching a hospital: recognizing what's happening to a victim, instituting emergency measures, and mobilizing a rescue service. In histories of heart attacks the theme occurs again and again. Delays. Delays from failure to recognize the symptoms and signs (even when the patient is a doctor). Delays before lifesaving actions are started. You possess in this book information on how to identify those at risk, how to avoid delays—and information on prompt actions for survival.

And even for those whose disease has progressed to the point of a heart attack, there is increasing opportunity to limit the damage done and to restore the patient to a full and active life.

There is progress. More progress than I would ever have believed possible just a decade ago. You have the opportunity—the right—to share in this progress.

The decision is now up to you.

| TABLE 12-1 | **Questionnaire for Adults to Use in Heart Attack Risk Formula** |
|---|---|

1   Has a first-degree relative (parent, sibling, child) had a heart attack or developed coronary heart disease before age 55?

2   Has a first-degree relative (parent, sibling, child) had a heart attack or developed coronary heart disease before age 65?

3   Has a second-degree relative (grandparent, uncle) had a heart attack or developed coronary heart disease before age 65?

4   Has a first-degree relative had a stroke before age 55?

5   Has a first-degree relative had a stroke before age 65?

6   Is your blood cholesterol greater than 270?

7   Is your blood cholesterol greater than 240?

8   Is your blood cholesterol greater than 220?

9   Is your level of triglycerides greater than 200?

10   Do you smoke more than half a pack of cigarettes per day?

11   Do you have diabetes?

12   Does a first-degree relative have diabetes that started before adulthood and requires the use of insulin?

13   Do you get regular aerobic exercise, sustain an exercise heart rate greater than 150 for at least 10 consecutive minutes, with no more than two days between exercise periods, and totaling a minimum of 60 minutes per week?

14   Is your blood pressure greater than 140/90 without treatment? (Note: either a systolic, upper reading, of 140 or a diastolic, lower reading, of 90 is sufficient.)

15   Is your relative weight greater than 1.20? That is, are you more than 20 percent overweight? (See page 48 for method of calculating relative weight.)

16   Do you get 14 or more points on the Type A behavior scale? (See page 148.)

TABLE
12-2

## Questionnaire for Children and Adolescents Aged 1-19 Years

*To Use in Heart Attack Risk Formula*

**A**    The following information can be obtained when a child is as young as 1-2 years.

**1**   Has a first-degree relative (parent or sibling) had a heart attack or coronary disease with onset before age 55?

**2**   Has a first-degree relative had a heart attack or coronary disease with onset before age 65?

**3**   Has a second-degree relative (grandparent, uncle, aunt) had a heart attack or coronary disease with onset before age 65?

**4**   Is the cholesterol level greater than 220 on two tests?

**5**   Is the cholesterol level greater than 190 on two tests?

**6**   Are the triglycerides higher than 120 on two tests?

**7**   Does the child *or* a first-degree relative have juvenile-onset diabetes?

**8**   Is the relative weight greater than 1.20?

**B**    The following information will be obtainable at later ages throughout childhood and adolescence, as early as 5 years and as late as 19 years.

**1**   Is the blood pressure "tracking" at the ninety-fifth percentile, or 140/90 or higher?

**2**   Does the child show excessive Type A behavior?

**3**   Does the child get daily, vigorous exercise, some of which is aerobic?

**4**   Does the youngster smoke?

TABLE
12–3

# Risk Index for Early-onset Coronary Heart Disease

*(Maximum Score = 10)*

| Circle and Add Your Points | **Family History** *(Select the single highest value. The maximum score for this section is 3.)* |
|---|---|
| 3.0 | Coronary disease in first-degree relative before age 55. |
| 2.5 | Coronary disease in first-degree relative before age 65. |
| 1.0 | Coronary disease in second-degree relative before age 65. |
| 1.0 | Stroke in first-degree relative before age 55. |
| 0.5 | Stroke in second-degree relative before age 65. |
| | **Cholesterol and Triglycerides** *(Select the single highest cholesterol value. Select the triglyceride value—if elevated. The maximum score for this section is 2.)* |
| 2.0 | Cholesterol greater than 270. |
| 1.0 | Cholesterol greater than 240. |
| 0.5 | Cholesterol greater than 220. |
| 0.5 | Triglycerides greater than 200. |
| | **Other Risks** *(Add all values. The maximum score for this section is 5.)* |
| 1.5 | Smoking—more than $1/2$ pack per day. |
| 1.0 | Diabetes in patient or juvenile diabetes in first-degree relative. |
| 1.0 | No regular aerobic exercise. |
| 0.5 | Blood pressure greater than 140/90. |
| 0.5 | Relative weight greater than 1.20. |
| 0.5 | Type A. |

## Risk Scores and Increased
## Risks of Early-onset Coronary Heart Disease

| Risk Score | Increased Risk |
|------------|----------------|
| 3 | 2× |
| 3.5 | 3× |
| 4 | 5× |
| 4.5 | 6× |
| 5 | 15× |
| 5.5 | not calculable by present methods |

*This material is repeated for you to fill out in the Tear-Out Appendix.*

TABLE
12-4

# Risk Index for Children and Adolescents*

| Circle and Add Your Points | Family History (Same as for adults—single highest value.) |
|---|---|
| 3.0 | Coronary disease in first-degree relative before age 55. |
| 2.5 | Coronary disease in first-degree relative before age 65. |
| 1.0 | Coronary disease in second-degree relative before age 55. |
| 1.0 | Stroke in first-degree relative before age 55. |
| 0.5 | Stroke in second-degree relative before age 65. |

| | Cholesterol and Triglycerides (Score as for adults. Maximum score is 2.) |
|---|---|
| 2.0 | Cholesterol greater than 220. |
| 1.0 | Cholesterol greater than 190. |
| 0.5 | Triglycerides greater than 120. |

| | Other Risks (Add all values.) |
|---|---|
| 1.5 | Smoking regularly. |
| 1.0 | Diabetes in patient or juvenile diabetes in first-degree relative. |
| 1.0 | No regular aerobic exercise. |
| 0.5 | Blood pressure greater than 140/90, or systolic (upper number) or diastolic (lower number) pressure greater than ninety-fifth percentile. |
| 0.5 | Relative weight greater than 1.20 ( > 20 percent overweight). |
| 0.5 | Type A. |

*See Risk Scores and Increased Risks, Table 12–3.

TABLE
**12-5**

# Heart Attack

## Some Signals

1    Pressure, squeezing, fullness, or pain in the center of the chest behind the breastbone, which may spread to the shoulders, upper abdomen, neck, jaws, back, or arms (more often to the left shoulder and arm, but either or both sides may be involved).

2    The pain may *not* be severe *or* it may be crushing.

3    Shortness of breath.

4    Feeling of weakness.

5    Sweating.

6    Nausea.

## Actions for Survival

1    Recognize the signals (as described above).

2    Stop activity and sit down or lie down.

3    If pain lasts for more than two minutes call your mobile coronary care unit or emergency rescue service or go to the nearest hospital emergency room with 24-hour service.

4    For those under a doctor's care:

    a   If the doctor has prescribed nitroglycerin, place a tablet under the tongue. If the pain is typical angina it should disappear within three minutes. If it is "prolonged ischemia" or a heart attack (or some other condition), it is not as likely to "respond" to nitroglycerin within three minutes.

    b   If a physician has suggested a propranolol-type drug, swallow a tablet with a sip of water if nitroglycerin has not relieved the pain within three minutes.

    c   Immediately follow through with emergency rescue service or hospital emergency room.

    d   Have a family member or co-worker notify physician of where patient will be.

TABLE
12-6

# Steps in Cardiopulmonary Resuscitation (CPR)

*A-B-C for Airway, Breathing, Circulation. (You need a training course and periodic refresher courses in CPR.)*

## A  Airway

1  Look—at the chest and stomach for movement.

2  Listen—for sounds of breathing.

3  Feel—for breath on your cheek.

4  Open the airway (mouth).

    a  Tilt the head back.
    b  Pull the chin down.

## B  Breathing (mouth-to-mouth)

1  One hand under victim's neck or pulling chin to hold mouth open.

2  Other hand pushing on forehead (to keep head tilted back). Fingers of this hand should pinch the nose shut.

3  Four quick full breaths mouth-to-mouth.

## C  Circulation

1  Check the carotid pulse (you learned to locate this in Chapter 2) to see if heart is beating. If you can't find a pulse, proceed to:

2  Cardiac compression. With the victim flat on his back on a hard surface, press the heel of one hand on the lower half of the breastbone, with the other hand on top. Depress the breastbone about $1\frac{1}{2}$ to 2 inches (in an adult) by bringing your shoulders and body weight over the victim's chest, locking your elbows, and pushing with your arms straight. (This takes a fairly good push.) Take the pressure off the breastbone completely—then repeat the pressure.

3  One-person technique. If there is no one to help, the breathing and cardiac compression must be performed by the same person—two quick breaths for every 15 compressions (at a rate of about 80 compressions per minute).

4  Two-person technique. One rescuer breathes for every 5 compressions performed by the other rescuer at about 60 compressions per minute.

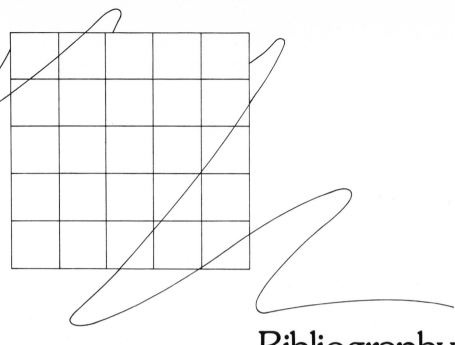

# Bibliography

## Low Fat, Low Cholesterol Cookbooks

Bennett, Ira, and Simon, Martin. **The Prudent Diet.** New York: David White, 1973.

Cavainani, Mabel. **The Low Cholesterol Cookbook.** Chicago: Henry Regnery Company, 1972.

Cutler, Carol. **Haute Cuisine for Your Heart's Delight.** New York: Clarkson N. Potter, Inc., 1973.

Eshleman, Ruthe, and Winston, Mary. **The American Heart Association Cookbook.** New York: David McKay, 1975.

Guerard, Michel. **Cuisine Minceur.** New York: William Morrow and Co., Inc., 1976.

**125 Favorite Low-Fat, Low-Cholesterol Recipes.** Good Housekeeping Institute, 1968.

## Weight Reduction Books

Davis, Helen A. **The No Willpower Diet.** New York: Dell, 1969.

Glenn, Morton B. **How to Get Thinner Once and for All.** Greenwich, Connecticut: Fawcett Crest, 1965.

Jolliffe, Norman. **Reduce and Stay Reduced on the Prudent Diet.** 2d ed. New York: Simon and Schuster, 1957.

Mayer, Jean. **Overweight: Causes, Cost, and Control.** Englewood Cliffs, New Jersey: Prentice-Hall, 1968.

## Exercise Books

Anderson, James L., and Cohen, Martin. **The West Point Fitness and Diet Book.** New York: Avon Books, 1978.

Cooper, Kenneth. **The New Aerobics.** New York: Bantam Books, 1976.

Cooper, Mildred, and Cooper, Kenneth. **Aerobics for Women.** New York: Bantam Books, 1973.

**Royal Canadian Air Force Exercise Plans for Physical Fitness.** New York: Pocket Books, Inc., 1962.

## Books on Behavior, Stress, and Meditation

Benson, Herbert, and Klipper, Miriam Z. **The Relaxation Response.** New York: Avon Books, 1976.

Friedman, Meyer, and Roseman, Ray. **Type A Behavior and Your Heart.** Greenwich, Connecticut: Fawcett Publications, Inc., 1975.

# A Note on the Appendixes

This book contains both a Permanent Appendix and a Tear-Out Appendix. The Permanent Appendix contains new information for general reference, including a comprehensive food composition table. The Tear-Out Appendix contains charts that have appeared elsewhere in the book. Here you can remove them from the book and fill them out as part of the program. We have included only one copy of each chart in the Tear-Out Appendix, so you may want to have several copies made after tearing the sheet out of the book. The material in the Tear-Out Appendix follows its sequence of presentation in the chapters. Tables found only within the text can be located through the Index or the list of tables in the beginning of the book.

permanent

# Appendix

| | Quantity or Amounts | Calories | Protein (g) | Total Fat (g) | Saturated Fat (g) | Unsaturated Fat (g) | Cholesterol (mg) | Carbohydrates (g) | Sodium (mg) |
|---|---|---|---|---|---|---|---|---|---|
| **Baby Food** (Commercially prepared) | | | | | | | | | |
| Cereals, precooked, dry, nutrients added | | | | | | | | | |
| Barley | 100 g | 348 | 13.2 | 1.2 | — | — | — | 73.6 | — |
| | 1 oz. | 102 | 3.1 | .7 | — | — | — | 21.5 | — |
| | 1 T. | 8 | .2 | .1 | — | — | — | 1.7 | — |
| High-protein | 100 g | 357 | 35.2 | 3.7 | — | — | — | 48.1 | — |
| | 1 oz. | 101 | 9.9 | 1.3 | — | — | — | 13.2 | — |
| | 1 T. | 9 | .9 | .1 | — | — | — | 1.2 | — |
| Oatmeal | 100 g | 375 | 16.5 | 5.5 | — | — | — | 66.0 | — |
| | 1 oz. | 109 | 4.0 | 2.0 | — | — | — | 19.1 | — |
| | 1 T. | 8 | .3 | .2 | — | — | — | 1.5 | — |
| Rice | 100 g | 371 | 6.6 | 1.6 | — | — | — | 80.0 | — |
| | 1 oz. | 108 | 2.0 | .6 | — | — | — | 21.7 | — |
| | 1 T. | 10 | .2 | .1 | — | — | — | 2.1 | — |
| Desserts | | | | | | | | | |
| Custard pudding, all flavors | 100 g | 100 | 2.3 | 1.8 | — | — | — | 18.6 | — |
| | 1 oz.=2 T. | 28 | .7 | .5 | — | — | — | 5.3 | — |
| Fruit pudding | 100 g | 96 | 1.2 | .9 | — | — | — | 21.6 | — |
| | 1 oz.=2 T. | 27 | .3 | .3 | — | — | — | 6.1 | — |
| Dinners (2–4% protein) | | | | | | | | | |
| Beef noodle | 100 g | 48 | 2.8 | 1.1 | — | — | — | 6.8 | — |
| | 1 oz.=2 T. | 14 | .8 | .3 | — | — | — | 1.9 | — |
| Cereal, egg yolk, bacon | 100 g | 82 | 2.9 | 4.9 | — | — | — | 6.6 | — |
| | 1 oz.=2 T. | 23 | .8 | 1.4 | — | — | — | 1.9 | — |
| Chicken noodle | 100 g | 49 | 2.1 | 1.3 | — | — | — | 7.2 | — |
| | 1 oz.=2 T. | 14 | .6 | .4 | — | — | — | 2.0 | — |
| Macaroni, tomato, meat, cereal | 100 g | 67 | 2.6 | 2.0 | — | — | — | 9.6 | — |
| | 1 oz.=2 T. | 19 | .7 | .6 | — | — | — | 2.7 | — |
| Split peas, vegetables, ham | 100 g | 80 | 4.0 | 2.1 | — | — | — | 11.2 | — |
| | 1 oz.=2 T. | 23 | 1.1 | .6 | — | — | — | 3.2 | — |
| Vegetables, chicken, cereal | 100 g | 52 | 2.1 | 1.4 | — | — | — | 7.7 | — |
| | 1 oz.=2 T. | 15 | .6 | .4 | — | — | — | 2.2 | — |
| Vegetables, liver, cereal | 100 g | 47 | 3.1 | .4 | — | — | — | 7.8 | — |
| | 1 oz.=2 T. | 13 | .9 | .1 | — | — | — | 2.2 | — |
| Vegetables, lamb, cereal | 100 g | 58 | 2.2 | 2.0 | — | — | — | 7.7 | — |
| | 1 oz.=2 T. | 16 | .6 | .6 | — | — | — | 2.2 | — |

| | Quantity or Amounts | Calories | Protein (g) | Total Fat (g) | Saturated Fat (g) | Unsaturated Fat (g) | Cholesterol (mg) | Carbohydrates (g) | Sodium (mg) |
|---|---|---|---|---|---|---|---|---|---|
| **Dinners, 6–8% protein** | | | | | | | | | |
| Beef with vegetables | 100 g | 87 | 7.4 | 3.7 | — | — | — | 6.0 | — |
| | 1 oz.=2 T. | 23 | 2.1 | 1.0 | — | — | — | 1.7 | — |
| Chicken with vegetables | 100 g | 100 | 7.4 | 4.6 | — | — | — | 7.8 | — |
| | 1 oz.=2 T. | 28 | 2.1 | 1.3 | — | — | — | 2.0 | — |
| Turkey with vegetables | 100 g | 86 | 6.7 | 3.2 | — | — | — | 7.6 | — |
| | 1 oz.=2 T. | 24 | 1.9 | .9 | — | — | — | 2.2 | — |
| Veal with vegetables | 100 g | 63 | 7.1 | 1.6 | — | — | — | 5.1 | — |
| | 1 oz.=2 T. | 18 | 2.0 | .5 | — | — | — | 1.4 | — |
| **Fruit and fruit products** | | | | | | | | | |
| Applesauce | 100 g | 72 | .2 | .2 | — | — | — | 18.6 | — |
| | 1 oz.=2 T. | 20 | .1 | .1 | — | — | — | 5.3 | — |
| Bananas, strained | 100 g | 84 | .4 | .2 | — | — | — | 21.6 | — |
| | 1 oz.=2 T. | 24 | 1 | .1 | — | — | — | 6.1 | — |
| Fruit dessert with | 100 g | 84 | .3 | .3 | — | — | — | 21.5 | — |
| tapioca | 1 oz.=2 T. | 24 | .1 | .1 | — | — | — | 6.1 | — |
| Peaches | 100 g | 81 | .6 | .2 | — | — | — | 20.7 | — |
| | 1 oz.=2 T. | 23 | .2 | .1 | — | — | — | 5.9 | — |
| Pears | 100 g | 66 | .3 | .1 | — | — | — | 17.1 | — |
| | 1 oz.=2 T. | 19 | .1 | — | — | — | — | 4.8 | — |
| Prunes with tapioca | 100 g | 86 | .3 | .2 | — | — | — | 22.4 | — |
| | 1 oz.=2 T. | 24 | .1 | .1 | — | — | — | 6.4 | — |
| **Meat, poultry, eggs** | | | | | | | | | |
| Beef, strained | 100 g | 99 | 14.7 | 4.0 | — | — | — | 0 | — |
| | 1 oz.=2 T. | 28 | 4.1 | 1.1 | — | — | — | 0 | — |
| Beef, junior | 100 g | 118 | 19.3 | 3.9 | — | — | — | 0 | — |
| | 1 oz.=2 T. | 33 | 5.5 | 1.1 | — | — | — | 0 | — |
| Chicken | 100 g | 93 | 13.5 | 3.8 | — | — | — | 0 | — |
| | 1 oz.=2 T. | 36 | 3.9 | 2.2 | — | — | — | 0 | — |
| Egg yolks, strained | 100 g | 210 | 10.0 | 18.4 | — | — | — | .2 | — |
| | 1 oz.=2 T. | 60 | 2.8 | 5.2 | — | — | — | .1 | — |
| Lamb, strained | 100 g | 107 | 14.6 | 4.9 | — | — | — | 0 | — |
| | 1 oz.=2 T. | 30 | 4.1 | 1.4 | — | — | — | 0 | — |
| Lamb, junior | 100 g | 121 | 17.5 | 5.1 | — | — | — | 0 | — |
| | 1 oz.=2 T. | 34 | 5.0 | 1.4 | — | — | — | 0 | — |
| Liver, strained | 100 g | 97 | 14.1 | 3.4 | — | — | — | 1.5 | — |
| | 1 oz.=2 T. | 27 | 4.0 | 1.0 | — | — | — | .4 | — |
| Pork, strained | 100 g | 118 | 15.4 | 5.8 | — | — | — | 0 | — |
| | 1 oz.=2 T. | 33 | 4.4 | 1.6 | — | — | — | 0 | — |

| | Quantity or Amounts | Calories | Protein (g) | Total Fat (g) | Saturated Fat (g) | Unsaturated Fat (g) | Cholesterol (mg) | Carbohydrates (g) | Sodium (mg) |
|---|---|---|---|---|---|---|---|---|---|
| Veal, strained | 100 g | 91 | 15.5 | 2.7 | — | — | — | 0 | — |
| | 1 oz.=2 T. | 26 | 4.4 | .8 | — | — | — | 0 | — |
| **Vegetables** | | | | | | | | | |
| Beans, green | 100 g | 20 | 1.4 | .1 | — | — | — | 5.1 | — |
| | 1 oz.=2 T. | 6 | .4 | — | — | — | — | 1.4 | — |
| Beets | 100 g | 37 | 1.4 | .1 | — | — | — | 8.3 | — |
| | 1 oz.=2 T. | 10 | .4 | — | — | — | — | 2.4 | — |
| Carrots | 100 g | 29 | .7 | .1 | — | — | — | 6.8 | — |
| | 1 oz.=2 T. | 8 | .2 | — | — | — | — | 1.9 | — |
| Peas | 100 g | 54 | 4.2 | .2 | — | — | — | 9.3 | — |
| | 1 oz.=2 T. | 15 | 1.2 | .1 | — | — | — | 2.6 | — |
| Spinach | 100 g | 43 | 2.3 | .7 | — | — | — | 7.5 | — |
| | 1 oz.=2 T. | 12 | .7 | .2 | — | — | — | 2.1 | — |
| Squash | 100 g | 25 | .7 | .1 | — | — | — | 6.2 | — |
| | 1 oz.=2 T. | 7 | .2 | — | — | — | — | 1.8 | — |
| Sweet potatoes | 100 g | 67 | 1.0 | .2 | — | — | — | 15.5 | — |
| | 1 oz.=2 T. | 19 | .3 | .1 | — | — | — | 4.4 | — |

## Beverages, alcoholic

| | Quantity or Amounts | Calories | Protein (g) | Total Fat (g) | Saturated Fat (g) | Unsaturated Fat (g) | Cholesterol (mg) | Carbohydrates (g) | Sodium (mg) |
|---|---|---|---|---|---|---|---|---|---|
| Beer, 4.5% alcohol | 100 g | 42 | .3 | 0 | — | — | — | 3.8 | 7 |
| (standard) | 1 fl. oz. | 12 | .1 | 0 | — | — | — | 1.0 | 2 |
| | 12 fl. oz. | 151 | 1.2 | 0 | — | — | — | 13.7 | 25 |
| Beer, low carbohydrate | 100 g | — | — | — | — | — | — | — | — |
| (light) | 1 fl. oz. | 6–8 | — | — | — | — | — | .1 | — |
| | 12 fl. oz. | 70–100 | — | — | — | — | — | 1.4 | — |
| Distilled liquors (gin, rum, whiskey) | | | | | | | | | |
| 80 proof | 100 g | 231 | — | — | — | — | — | tr | 1 |
| | 1 fl. oz. | 65 | — | — | — | — | — | — | — |
| 86 proof | 100 g | 249 | — | — | — | — | — | tr | 1 |
| | 1 fl. oz. | 70 | — | — | — | — | — | — | — |
| 90 proof | 100 g | 263 | — | — | — | — | — | tr | 1 |
| | 1 fl. oz. | 74 | — | — | — | — | — | — | — |
| 94 proof | 100 g | 275 | — | — | — | — | — | tr | 1 |
| | 1 fl. oz. | 77 | — | — | — | — | — | — | — |
| 100 proof | 100 g | 295 | — | — | — | — | — | tr | 1 |
| | 1 fl. oz. | 83 | — | — | — | — | — | — | — |

| | Quantity or Amounts | Calories | Protein (g) | Total Fat (g) | Saturated Fat (g) | Unsaturated Fat (g) | Cholesterol (mg) | Carbohydrates (g) | Sodium (mg) |
|---|---|---|---|---|---|---|---|---|---|
| **Mixed drinks** | | | | | | | | | |
| Collins | 10 fl. oz. | 200 | — | — | — | — | — | — | — |
| Daiquiri | 3½ fl. oz. | 200 | — | — | — | — | — | 13.0 | — |
| Gin gimlet | 4 fl. oz. | 160 | — | — | — | — | — | 10.8 | — |
| Manhattan, sweet | 3½ fl. oz. | 200 | — | — | — | — | — | 4.5 | — |
| Martini, dry | 3½ fl. oz. | 150 | — | — | — | — | — | .6 | — |
| Screwdriver | 8 fl. oz. | 288 | — | — | — | — | — | 25.6 | — |
| Wine, sweet, | 100 g | 137 | .1 | 0 | — | — | — | 7.9 | 4 |
| 18% alcohol | 1 fl. oz. | 39 | — | — | — | — | — | 2.3 | 1 |
| | 3½ fl. oz. | 141 | .1 | 0 | — | — | — | 7.9 | — |
| Wine, dry, 12% alcohol | 100 g | 85 | .1 | 0 | — | — | — | 4.2 | 5 |
| | 1 fl. oz. | 25 | — | — | — | — | — | 1.2 | 1 |
| | 3½ fl. oz. | 87 | .1 | 0 | — | — | — | 4.2 | 5 |

## Beverages, nonalcoholic

| | Quantity or Amounts | Calories | Protein (g) | Total Fat (g) | Saturated Fat (g) | Unsaturated Fat (g) | Cholesterol (mg) | Carbohydrates (g) | Sodium (mg) |
|---|---|---|---|---|---|---|---|---|---|
| Carbonated | | | | | | | | | |
| Club soda | 100 g | 0 | — | — | — | — | — | 0 | — |
| Cola type soda | 100 g | 39 | — | — | — | — | — | 10.0 | — |
| | 1 fl. oz. | 12 | — | — | — | — | — | 3.2 | — |
| | 12 fl. oz. | 144 | — | — | — | — | — | 39.4 | — |
| Cream type soda | 100 g | 43 | — | — | — | — | — | 11.0 | — |
| | 1 fl. oz. | 13 | — | — | — | — | — | 3.5 | — |
| | 12 fl. oz. | 156 | — | — | — | — | — | 42.6 | — |
| Fruit type soda | 100 g | 46 | — | — | — | — | — | 12.0 | — |
| | 1 fl. oz. | 14 | — | — | — | — | — | 3.7 | — |
| | 12 fl. oz. | 168 | — | — | — | — | — | 27.6 | — |
| Ginger ale | 100 g | 31 | — | — | — | — | — | 8.0 | — |
| | 1 fl. oz. | 9 | — | — | — | — | — | 2.4 | — |
| | 12 fl. oz. | 108 | — | — | — | — | — | 26.8 | — |
| Quinine soda | 100 g | 31 | — | — | — | — | — | 8.0 | — |
| | 1 fl. oz. | 9 | — | — | — | — | — | 2.4 | — |
| | 12 fl. oz. | 108 | — | — | — | — | — | 26.8 | — |
| Root beer | 100 g | 41 | — | — | — | — | — | 10.5 | — |
| | 1 fl. oz. | 13 | — | — | — | — | — | 3.2 | — |
| | 12 fl. oz. | 156 | — | — | — | — | — | 38.4 | — |
| Soda, diet, | | | | | | | | | |
| less than 1 cal./oz. | 12 fl. oz. | 1 | — | — | — | — | — | .2 | — |

**245**

# Nutritional Guide

| | Quantity or Amounts | Calories | Protein (g) | Total Fat (g) | Saturated Fat (g) | Unsaturated Fat (g) | Cholesterol (mg) | Carbohydrates (g) | Sodium (mg) |
|---|---|---|---|---|---|---|---|---|---|
| Noncarbonated | | | | | | | | | |
| Coffee, plain | 100 g | 0 | — | — | — | — | — | — | — |
| Kool-Aid, sugar sweetened | 9 fl. oz. | 91 | — | — | — | — | — | 23.0 | — |
| Tea, plain | 100 g | 0 | — | — | — | — | — | — | — |

## Breads, Cereals, Grains, Pasta
Breads (check pkg.— slices vary)

| | Quantity or Amounts | Calories | Protein (g) | Total Fat (g) | Saturated Fat (g) | Unsaturated Fat (g) | Cholesterol (mg) | Carbohydrates (g) | Sodium (mg) |
|---|---|---|---|---|---|---|---|---|---|
| Bagel | 3″—2 oz. | 165 | — | — | — | — | — | 29.0 | — |
| Biscuits, baking powder | 100 g | 369 | 7.4 | 17.0 | 4.0 | 11.0 | — | 45.8 | 626 |
| | 1 oz.—2″ | 104 | 2.1 | 4.8 | 1.1 | 3.1 | — | 12.9 | 178 |
| Boston brown bread | 100 g | 211 | 5.5 | 1.3 | 1.0 | 2.0 | — | 45.6 | 251 |
| | 1 oz. | 60 | 1.5 | .3 | .3 | .6 | — | 12.9 | 71 |
| 1 slice | 1.7 oz. | 102 | 2.5 | .5 | .5 | .9 | — | 21.9 | 120 |
| Corn bread | 100 g | 233 | 6.1 | 8.4 | 1.0 | 2.0 | 69 | 32.9 | 744 |
| | 1 oz. | 66 | 1.7 | 2.4 | .3 | .6 | 20 | 9.4 | 212 |
| 1 slice | 4 oz. | 264 | 6.8 | 9.6 | 1.2 | 2.2 | 80 | 37.3 | 844 |
| Cracked wheat bread | 100 g | 263 | 8.7 | 2.2 | 1.0 | 2.0 | — | 52.1 | 529 |
| | 1 oz. | 75 | 2.5 | .6 | .3 | .6 | — | 14.8 | 150 |
| 1 slice | .8 oz. | 66 | 2.2 | .6 | .2 | .4 | — | 13.0 | 132 |
| Crescent dinner roll | 1.2 oz. | 127 | — | — | — | — | — | 15.2 | — |
| French or Vienna bread | 100 g | 290 | 9.1 | 3.0 | 1.0 | 2.0 | — | 55.4 | 580 |
| | 1 oz. | 82 | 2.5 | .9 | .3 | .6 | — | 15.7 | 165 |
| 1 slice | 1.8 oz. | 102 | 3.2 | 1.1 | .2 | .4 | — | 19.4 | 203 |
| French roll (hoagie or sub) | 11×3″ | 392 | 12.3 | 4.1 | — | — | — | 74.8 | 783 |
| Hamburger bun | 100 g | 311 | 8.5 | 5.4 | 1.0 | 4.0 | — | 56.0 | 560 |
| | 1 oz. | 88 | 2.4 | 1.5 | .3 | 1.1 | — | 16.0 | 159 |
| 1 bun | 1.4 oz. | 123 | 3.3 | 2.1 | 1.4 | 5.6 | — | 22.4 | 222 |
| Hard roll (Kaiser) | 1 roll | 156 | 4.9 | 1.6 | .4 | 1.1 | — | 29.8 | 313 |
| Italian bread | 100 g | 276 | 9.1 | .8 | — | — | — | 56.4 | 585 |
| | 1 oz. | 78 | 2.6 | .2 | — | — | — | 16.0 | 166 |
| 1 slice | 1.4 oz. | 83 | 2.7 | .2 | — | — | — | 16.9 | 176 |
| Muffins, blueberry | 100 g | 281 | 7.3 | 9.3 | — | — | — | 41.9 | 632 |
| | 1 oz. | 80 | 2.1 | 2.6 | — | — | — | 11.9 | 179 |
| 1 muffin | 1.4 oz. | 112 | 2.9 | 3.6 | — | — | — | 16.8 | 251 |
| Muffin, English | 2 oz. | 140 | — | — | — | — | — | 28.4 | — |
| Pancakes | 100 g | 225 | 7.2 | 7.3 | 3.0 | 5.0 | 60 | 32.4 | 564 |
| | 1 oz.=4″ | 64 | 2.0 | 2.0 | .9 | 1.4 | 28 | 9.2 | 160 |

# Nutritional Guide

| | Quantity or Amounts | Calories | Protein (g) | Total Fat (g) | Saturated Fat (g) | Unsaturated Fat (g) | Cholesterol (mg) | Carbohydrates (g) | Sodium (mg) |
|---|---|---|---|---|---|---|---|---|---|
| Popover, home recipe | 1 pop. | 90 | 3.5 | 3.7 | 1.2 | 2.0 | 59 | 10.3 | 88 |
| Raisin bread | 100 g | 262 | 6.6 | 2.8 | 1.0 | 2.0 | — | 53.6 | 365 |
| | 1 oz. | 74 | 1.8 | .8 | .3 | .6 | — | 15.2 | 103 |
| 1 slice | .9 oz. | 66 | 1.6 | .7 | .3 | .5 | — | 13.4 | 93 |
| Rye bread | 100 g | 243 | 9.1 | 1.1 | 1.0 | 2.0 | — | 52.0 | 557 |
| 1 slice | 1 oz. | 69 | 2.6 | .3 | .3 | .6 | — | 14.7 | 158 |
| Tortilla, corn or flour | .7 oz.=5" | 42 | — | — | — | — | — | 9.7 | — |
| Waffles, 7" round | 1 waffle | 209 | 7.0 | 7.4 | 3.0 | 5.0 | 60 | 28.1 | 356 |
| White bread | 100 g | 270 | 8.7 | 3.2 | 1.0 | 2.0 | — | 50.5 | 507 |
| | 1 oz. | 76 | 2.4 | .9 | .3 | .6 | — | 14.3 | 144 |
| 1 slice | .8 oz. | 63 | 2.1 | .9 | .2 | .4 | — | 11.5 | 114 |
| Whole wheat bread | 100 g | 243 | 10.5 | 3.0 | 1.0 | 2.0 | — | 47.7 | 527 |
| | 1 oz. | 69 | 2.9 | .8 | .3 | .6 | — | 13.5 | 149 |
| 1 slice | .9 oz. | 62 | 2.6 | .8 | .2 | .5 | — | 12.5 | 134 |
| Zwieback | 100 g | 423 | 10.7 | 8.8 | — | — | — | 74.3 | 250 |
| | 1 oz. | 120 | 3.0 | 2.5 | — | — | — | 21.1 | 71 |
| | | | | | | | | | |
| Cereal, Grains, Pasta | | | | | | | | | |
| Barley, dry | 100 g | 348 | 9.6 | 1.1 | — | — | — | 77.2 | — |
| | 1 oz. | 99 | 2.7 | .3 | — | — | — | 22.0 | — |
| Bran flakes, 40% | 100 g | 303 | 10.2 | 1.8 | — | — | — | 80.6 | 925 |
| | 1 oz.=¾ c. | 86 | 2.8 | .5 | — | — | — | 22.9 | 263 |
| Bulgur, cooked | 100 g | 182 | 6.2 | 3.3 | .5 | 2.0 | — | 32.8 | 460 |
| | 1 oz.=¼ c. | 48 | 1.7 | .9 | — | — | — | 10.0 | 131 |
| Corn flakes or Chex | 100 g | 386 | 7.9 | .4 | — | — | — | 85.3 | 1005 |
| | 1 oz.=1 c. | 110 | 2.2 | .1 | — | — | — | 24.7 | 286 |
| Corn flakes, | 100 g | 386 | 4.4 | .2 | — | — | — | 91.3 | 775 |
| sugar-coated | 1 oz.=1 c. | 110 | 1.3 | — | — | — | — | 26.0 | 220 |
| Corn grits, cooked | 100 g | 51 | 1.2 | .1 | — | — | — | 11.0 | 205 |
| | 1 oz. | 14 | .3 | — | — | — | — | 3.1 | 58 |
| | 1 cup | 120 | 2.5 | .2 | — | — | — | 27.0 | 499 |
| Farina, cooked | 100 g | 42 | 1.3 | .1 | — | — | — | 8.7 | 144 |
| | 1 oz. | 12 | .3 | — | — | — | — | 2.5 | 41 |
| | 1 cup | 103 | 2.6 | .2 | — | — | — | 21.8 | 353 |
| Macaroni, cooked | 100 g | 148 | 5.0 | .5 | — | — | — | 30.1 | 1 |
| | 1 oz. | 42 | 1.4 | .1 | — | — | — | 8.5 | — |
| | 1 cup | 192 | 6.4 | .7 | — | — | — | 39.1 | 1 |
| Noodles, chow mein | 100 g | 489 | 13.2 | 23.5 | — | — | 12 | 58.0 | — |
| | 1 oz. | 140 | 3.8 | 6.7 | — | — | 4 | 16.6 | — |
| | 1 cup | 224 | 6.1 | 10.7 | — | — | 5 | 26.1 | — |

| | Quantity or Amounts | Calories | Protein (g) | Total Fat (g) | Saturated Fat (g) | Unsaturated Fat (g) | Cholesterol (mg) | Carbohydrates (g) | Sodium (mg) |
|---|---|---|---|---|---|---|---|---|---|
| Noodles, egg, cooked | 100 g | 125 | 4.1 | 1.5 | — | — | — | 23.3 | 2 |
| | 1 oz. | 36 | 1.1 | .4 | — | — | — | 23.3 | 1 |
| | 1 cup | 200 | 6.1 | 2.2 | — | — | — | 37.3 | 2 |
| Oat flakes, dry | 100 g | 397 | 14.9 | 5.7 | 1.0 | 4.1 | — | 70.7 | 1200 |
| | 1 oz. = $\frac{2}{3}$ c. | 107 | 4.3 | 1.6 | — | — | — | 19.0 | 343 |
| Oatmeal, cooked | 100 g | 55 | 2.0 | 1.0 | .2 | .8 | — | 9.7 | 218 |
| | 1 oz. | 15 | .5 | .2 | — | — | — | 2.7 | 62 |
| | 1 cup | 132 | 4.3 | 2.4 | — | — | — | 23.3 | 523 |
| Rice, brown, cooked | 100 g | 119 | 2.5 | .6 | .2 | .4 | — | 25.5 | 282 |
| | 1 oz. | 34 | .7 | .2 | — | — | — | 7.3 | 80 |
| | 1 cup | 232 | 4.9 | 1.2 | — | — | — | 49.7 | 550 |
| Rice cereal, puffed | 100 g | 399 | 6.0 | .4 | — | — | — | 89.5 | 2 |
| | 1 oz. | 114 | 1.7 | .1 | — | — | — | 25.6 | — |
| | 1 cup | 60 | .9 | .1 | — | — | — | 13.4 | 1 |
| Rice, white, cooked | 100 g | 109 | 2.0 | .2 | .1 | .1 | — | 24.2 | 374 |
| | 1 oz. | 31 | .6 | — | — | — | — | 6.9 | 107 |
| | 1 cup | 223 | 4.1 | .2 | .1 | .1 | — | 49.6 | 767 |
| Spaghetti, cooked | 100 g | 148 | 5.0 | .5 | — | — | — | 30.1 | 79 |
| | 1 oz. | 42 | 1.4 | .1 | — | — | — | 8.6 | 23 |
| | 1 cup | 192 | 6.5 | .7 | — | — | — | 39.1 | 90 |
| Wheat bran | 100 g | 238 | 10.8 | 1.8 | — | — | — | 78.8 | 490 |
| | 1 oz. | 68 | 3.0 | .5 | — | — | — | 21.1 | 140 |
| Wheat germ | 100 g | 391 | 30.0 | 11.5 | 2.0 | 9.0 | — | 49.5 | 9 |
| | 1 oz. = $\frac{1}{4}$ c. | 111 | 8.5 | 3.3 | .6 | 2.6 | — | 14.0 | 3 |
| Wheat, rolled, cooked | 100 g | 75 | 2.2 | .4 | — | — | — | 16.9 | 295 |
| | 1 oz. | 21 | .6 | .1 | — | — | — | 4.8 | 84 |
| | 1 cup | 180 | 5.3 | 1.0 | — | — | — | 40.6 | 708 |
| Wheat, shredded | 100 g | 354 | 9.9 | 2.0 | .3 | 1.5 | — | 79.9 | 4 |
| biscuits, plain | 1 oz. = 1 c. | 124 | 3.5 | .7 | — | — | — | 28.0 | 1 |

## Cakes, Candy, Cookies, Desserts, Pies

Cakes, made from
home recipes

| | | | | | | | | | |
|---|---|---|---|---|---|---|---|---|---|
| Angel food cake, plain | 100 g | 269 | 7.1 | .2 | — | — | — | 60.2 | 283 |
| | 1 oz. | 77 | 2.0 | .1 | — | — | — | 17.2 | 81 |
| $\frac{1}{12}$ of 10×4 cake | 1 piece | 161 | 4.3 | .1 | — | — | — | 36.1 | 170 |
| Boston cream pie, with | | | | | | | | | |
| custard and | 100 g | 302 | 5.0 | 9.4 | — | — | — | 49.9 | 186 |
| powdered sugar | 1 oz. | 86 | 1.4 | 2.7 | — | — | — | 14.3 | 53 |
| $\frac{1}{8}$ of 8×3$\frac{1}{2}$ pie | 1 piece | 311 | 5.2 | 9.7 | — | — | — | 51.4 | 192 |

# Nutritional Guide

| | Quantity or Amounts | Calories | Protein (g) | Total Fat (g) | Saturated Fat (g) | Unsaturated Fat (g) | Cholesterol (mg) | Carbohydrates (g) | Sodium (mg) |
|---|---|---|---|---|---|---|---|---|---|
| Chocolate sheet cake, | 100 g | 366 | 4.8 | 17.2 | 4.0 | 9.0 | — | 52.0 | 294 |
| plain | 1 oz. | 105 | 1.4 | 4.9 | 1.1 | 2.6 | — | 14.8 | 84 |
| 3×3×2 size | 1 piece | 322 | 4.2 | 15.1 | 3.8 | 8.0 | — | 45.8 | 259 |
| Chocolate, 2-layer, | 100 g | 369 | 4.5 | 16.4 | 5.0 | 7.0 | 43 | 55.8 | 235 |
| chocolate icing | 1 oz. | 105 | 1.3 | 4.7 | 1.4 | 2.0 | 13 | 15.9 | 67 |
| $\frac{1}{12}$ of 8×3 layer | 1 piece | 288 | 3.5 | 12.8 | 4.9 | 6.8 | 32 | 43.5 | 183 |
| | 1 cupcake | 162 | 2.0 | 7.2 | 2.0 | 3.0 | 19 | 24.6 | 103 |
| Fruitcake, dark, loaf | 100 g | 379 | 4.8 | 15.3 | 3.3 | 10.5 | 45 | 59.7 | 158 |
| | 1 oz. | 108 | 1.4 | 4.8 | 1.0 | 3.3 | 13 | 17.0 | 45 |
| | $\frac{1}{2}×2×1\frac{1}{2}$ | 114 | 1.4 | 4.6 | 1.0 | 3.2 | 14 | 18.0 | 49 |
| Gingerbread | 100 g | 317 | 3.8 | 10.7 | 3.0 | 8.0 | — | 52.0 | 237 |
| | 1 oz. | 91 | 1.0 | 3.1 | .1 | 2.3 | — | 14.8 | 68 |
| | 2×3×3 | 371 | 4.4 | 12.5 | 3.2 | 8.7 | — | 60.8 | 277 |
| Pound cake, | 100 g | 473 | 5.7 | 29.5 | 7.0 | 20.0 | — | 47.0 | 110 |
| old-fashioned | 1 oz. | 135 | 1.6 | 8.4 | 2.0 | 5.7 | — | 13.4 | 31 |
| | $3\frac{1}{2}×3×\frac{1}{2}$ | 142 | 1.7 | 8.9 | 2.3 | 6.2 | — | 14.1 | 33 |
| Sponge cake | 100 g | 297 | 7.6 | 5.7 | 2.0 | 2.0 | 246 | 54.1 | 167 |
| | 1 oz. | 85 | 2.2 | 1.6 | .6 | .6 | 71 | 15.5 | 48 |
| $\frac{1}{12}$ of 10″ tube cake | 1 piece | 196 | 5.0 | 3.8 | 1.2 | 1.8 | 162 | 35.7 | 110 |
| White cake, 2-layer, | 100 g | 375 | 4.6 | 16.0 | 4.0 | 9.0 | — | 54.0 | 323 |
| plain | 1 oz. | 107 | 1.3 | 4.8 | 1.1 | 2.6 | — | 15.4 | 93 |
| $\frac{1}{12}$ of 8″, 2-layer | 1 piece | 207 | 2.5 | 8.8 | 6.0 | 11.0 | — | 29.8 | 179 |
| with coconut icing | 1 piece | 301 | 3.0 | 10.8 | 3.9 | 6.1 | — | 49.2 | 208 |
| with uncooked | | | | | | | | | |
| white icing | 1 piece | 308 | 2.7 | 10.6 | 3.1 | 6.6 | — | 51.6 | 192 |
| Yellow cake, plain, | 100 g | 363 | 4.5 | 12.7 | 4.0 | 9.0 | — | 58.2 | 258 |
| 2-layer | 1 oz. | 104 | 1.3 | 3.6 | 1.1 | 2.6 | — | 16.6 | 74 |
| $\frac{1}{12}$ of 8″ cake | 1 piece | 206 | 2.6 | 7.2 | 6.0 | 11.0 | — | 33.0 | 146 |
| with carmel icing | 1 piece | 308 | 3.4 | 9.9 | 2.9 | 6.1 | — | 52.1 | 192 |
| with chocolate icing | 1 piece | 288 | 3.3 | 10.3 | 3.4 | 5.8 | 33 | 47.7 | 164 |
| Cakes, made from | | | | | | | | | |
| bought mixes | | | | | | | | | |
| Angel food, plain | 100 g | 259 | 5.7 | .2 | — | — | 0 | 59.4 | 146 |
| | 1 oz. | 74 | 1.6 | .1 | — | — | 0 | 16.9 | 48 |
| $\frac{1}{12}$ of 10″ tube cake | 1 piece | 137 | 3.0 | .1 | — | — | 0 | 31.5 | 77 |
| Coffee cake 8×5$\frac{1}{2}$×1$\frac{1}{2}$ | 100 g | 322 | 6.3 | 9.6 | — | — | — | 52.4 | 431 |
| | 1 oz. | 92 | 1.8 | 2.7 | — | — | — | 14.9 | 123 |
| $\frac{1}{6}$ of size above | 1 piece | 232 | 4.5 | 6.9 | — | — | — | 37.7 | 310 |
| Cupcakes, white, 2$\frac{3}{4}$ in., | | | | | | | | | |
| plain | 1 cupcake | 116 | 1.6 | 4.0 | — | — | — | 18.4 | 149 |

| | Quantity or Amounts | Calories | Protein (g) | Total Fat (g) | Saturated Fat (g) | Unsaturated Fat (g) | Cholesterol (mg) | Carbohydrates (g) | Sodium (mg) |
|---|---|---|---|---|---|---|---|---|---|
| Cupcakes, white, chocolate icing | 1 2¾″ | 172 | 2.2 | 6.0 | — | — | — | 28.4 | 161 |
| Devil's food, chocolate | 100 g | 339 | 4.4 | 12.3 | 5.0 | 7.0 | 48 | 58.3 | 262 |
| icing | 1 oz. | 97 | 1.3 | 3.5 | 1.4 | 2.0 | 14 | 16.6 | 75 |
| 1⁄12 of 8″, 2-layer | 1 piece | 312 | 4.0 | 11.3 | 4.3 | 5.5 | 33 | 53.6 | 241 |
| | 1 cupcake | 156 | 2.0 | 5.7 | 2.5 | 3.5 | 18 | 26.8 | 121 |
| Honey spice with | 100 g | 352 | 4.1 | 10.8 | 3.5 | 6.0 | — | 60.9 | 245 |
| caramel icing | 1 oz. | 101 | 1.2 | 3.1 | 1.0 | 1.7 | — | 17.4 | 70 |
| 1⁄12 of 8″, 2-layer | 1 piece | 363 | 4.2 | 11.1 | 3.5 | 6.0 | — | 62.7 | 252 |
| Yellow with chocolate | 100 g | 337 | 4.1 | 11.3 | 4.0 | 6.0 | 48 | 57.6 | 227 |
| icing | 1 oz. | 96 | 1.2 | 3.2 | 1.1 | 1.7 | 14 | 16.5 | 65 |
| 1⁄12 of 8″, 2-layer | 1 piece | 310 | 3.8 | 10.4 | 3.4 | 5.4 | 36 | 53.0 | 209 |
| | 1 cupcake | 155 | 1.9 | 5.2 | 1.7 | 2.7 | 18 | 26.5 | 79 |
| **Candy** | | | | | | | | | |
| Caramels, plain | 100 g | 399 | 4.0 | 10.2 | 5.6 | 4.2 | — | 76.6 | 226 |
| | 1 oz. | 113 | 1.1 | 2.9 | 1.6 | 1.2 | — | 21.7 | 64 |
| Chocolate chips, | 100 g | 507 | 4.2 | 35.7 | 20.0 | 14.0 | — | 57.0 | 2 |
| semisweet | 1 oz. | 144 | 1.2 | 10.1 | 5.7 | 3.9 | — | 16.2 | 1 |
| | 1 cup = 6 oz. | 862 | 7.1 | 60.7 | 34.0 | 23.7 | — | 96.9 | 3 |
| Chocolate, milk, plain | 100 g | 520 | 7.7 | 32.3 | 20.0 | 14.0 | — | 56.9 | 94 |
| | 1 oz. | 147 | 2.2 | 9.2 | 5.1 | 3.5 | — | 16.1 | 27 |
| Chocolate, milk, | 100 g | 543 | 14.1 | 38.1 | 15.7 | 20.0 | — | 44.6 | 66 |
| with nuts | 1 oz. | 154 | 4.0 | 10.8 | 4.5 | 5.7 | — | 12.6 | 19 |
| Chocolate coated candy | | | | | | | | | |
| Almonds | 100 g | 569 | 12.3 | 43.7 | 7.0 | 35.0 | — | 39.6 | 59 |
| | 1 oz. (6–8) | 161 | 3.5 | 12.4 | 2.1 | 9.8 | — | 11.2 | 17 |
| Coconut | 100 g | 438 | 2.8 | 17.6 | 10.0 | 6.6 | — | 72.0 | 197 |
| | 1 oz. | 124 | .8 | 5.0 | 2.9 | 1.9 | — | 20.4 | 56 |
| Fudge, caramel, | 100 g | 433 | 7.7 | 18.1 | 6.0 | 9.0 | — | 64.1 | 204 |
| peanuts | 1 oz. | 123 | 2.2 | 5.1 | 1.4 | 3.5 | — | 18.2 | 58 |
| Hard peanut butter | 100 g | 463 | 6.6 | 19.6 | 6.0 | 13.0 | — | 70.6 | 163 |
| center | 1 oz. | 131 | 1.9 | 5.5 | 1.6 | 3.7 | — | 20.0 | 46 |
| Mints, large, 2½ × ⅜ | 1 mint | 144 | .6 | 3.7 | 1.0 | 2.1 | — | 28.4 | 65 |
| Nougat and caramel | 100 g | 416 | 4.0 | 13.9 | 4.2 | 9.5 | — | 72.8 | 173 |
| | 1 oz. | 118 | 1.1 | 3.9 | 1.2 | 2.7 | — | 20.6 | 49 |
| Raisins | 100 g | 425 | 5.4 | 17.1 | 10.0 | 6.0 | — | 70.5 | 64 |
| | 1 oz. = 50 r. | 120 | 1.5 | 4.8 | 2.7 | 1.9 | — | 20.0 | 18 |
| Fondant, candy corn | 100 g | 364 | .1 | 2.0 | .4 | 1.4 | — | 89.6 | 212 |
| | 1 oz. = 20 | 103 | — | .6 | .1 | .4 | — | 25.4 | 60 |

| | Quantity or Amounts | Calories | Protein (g) | Total Fat (g) | Saturated Fat (g) | Unsaturated Fat (g) | Cholesterol (mg) | Carbohydrates (g) | Sodium (mg) |
|---|---|---|---|---|---|---|---|---|---|
| Fudge, chocolate | 100 g | 400 | 2.7 | 12.2 | 5.0 | 6.0 | — | 75.0 | 190 |
| | 1 oz. | 113 | .8 | 3.5 | 1.2 | 2.1 | — | 21.3 | 54 |
| Fudge, chocolate with | 100 g | 426 | 3.9 | 17.4 | 6.0 | 11.0 | — | 69.0 | 171 |
| nuts | 1 oz. | 121 | 1.1 | 4.9 | 1.2 | 4.3 | — | 19.6 | 48 |
| | 1 cu. in. | 89 | .8 | 3.7 | .9 | 2.5 | — | 14.5 | 36 |
| Hard candy | 100 g | 386 | 0 | 1.1 | — | — | — | 97.2 | 32 |
| | 1 oz. | 109 | 0 | .3 | — | — | — | 27.6 | 9 |
| Jelly beans | 100 g | 367 | — | .5 | — | — | — | 93.1 | 12 |
| | 1 oz. = 10 | 104 | — | .1 | — | — | — | 26.4 | 3 |
| Marshmallows | 100 g | 319 | 2.0 | — | — | — | — | 80.4 | 39 |
| | 1 oz. | 90 | .6 | — | — | — | — | 22.8 | 11 |
| | 1 c. sm. | 147 | .9 | — | — | — | — | 37.0 | 18 |
| Peanut brittle | 100 g | 421 | 5.7 | 10.4 | 2.0 | 7.0 | — | 81.0 | 31 |
| | 1 oz. | 119 | 1.6 | 2.9 | .6 | 2.2 | — | 23.0 | 9 |
| **Cookies** | | | | | | | | | |
| Brownies, with nuts, | 100 g | 485 | 6.5 | 31.3 | 7.0 | 22.0 | 83 | 50.9 | 251 |
| home recipe | 1 oz. | 139 | 1.9 | 8.9 | 2.0 | 6.3 | 24 | 14.5 | 72 |
| $1\frac{3}{4} \times 1\frac{1}{8}$ | 1 brownie | 97 | 1.3 | 6.3 | 1.4 | 4.4 | 17 | 10.2 | 50 |
| Butter cookie, $2\frac{1}{2} \times \frac{1}{4}$ | 100 g | 457 | 6.1 | 16.9 | — | — | — | 70.9 | 418 |
| | 1 oz. | 131 | 1.7 | 4.8 | — | — | — | 20.3 | 119 |
| | 10 cookies | 229 | 3.1 | 8.5 | — | — | — | 35.5 | 209 |
| Chocolate chip, | 100 g | 516 | 5.4 | 30.1 | 8.0 | 20.0 | — | 60.1 | 348 |
| home recipe, $2\frac{1}{2}''$ | 1 oz. | 147 | 1.5 | 8.6 | 2.3 | 5.7 | — | 17.0 | 99 |
| | 4 cookies | 206 | 2.2 | 12.0 | 3.4 | 7.9 | — | 24.0 | 139 |
| Fig bars | 100 g | 358 | 3.9 | 5.6 | 1.0 | 3.0 | — | 75.4 | 252 |
| | 1 oz. | 102 | 1.1 | 1.6 | .3 | .9 | — | 22.0 | 72 |
| | 4 cookies | 200 | 2.2 | 3.1 | .9 | 2.1 | — | 42.2 | 141 |
| Gingersnaps, $2 \times \frac{1}{4}$ | 100 g | 420 | 5.5 | 8.9 | 1.0 | 3.0 | — | 79.8 | 571 |
| | 1 oz. | 120 | 1.6 | 2.5 | .3 | .9 | — | 23.0 | 163 |
| | 10 cookies | 294 | 3.9 | 6.2 | 1.6 | 4.3 | — | 55.9 | 400 |
| Ladyfingers, | 100 g | 360 | 7.8 | 7.8 | 1.0 | 3.0 | 356 | 64.5 | 71 |
| $3\frac{1}{4} \times 1\frac{3}{8} \times 1\frac{1}{8}$ | 1 oz. | 103 | 2.2 | 2.2 | .3 | .9 | 100 | 18.4 | 21 |
| | 4 cookies | 158 | 3.4 | 3.4 | 1.1 | 1.8 | 157 | 28.4 | 31 |
| Macaroons, $2\frac{3}{4} \times \frac{1}{4}$ | 100 g | 457 | 5.3 | 23.2 | 16.0 | 6.0 | — | 66.1 | 34 |
| | 1 oz. | 136 | 1.5 | 6.6 | 4.6 | 1.7 | — | 19.0 | 10 |
| | 2 cookies | 181 | 2.0 | 8.8 | 5.2 | 2.6 | — | 25.1 | 13 |
| Oatmeal with raisins, | 100 g | 451 | 28.0 | 15.4 | 4.0 | 11.0 | — | 73.5 | 162 |
| $2\frac{5}{8} \times \frac{1}{4}$ | 1 oz. | 129 | 1.7 | 4.4 | 1.1 | 3.1 | — | 21.0 | 46 |
| | 4 cookies | 235 | 3.2 | 8.0 | 2.1 | 5.6 | — | 38.2 | 84 |

**251**

# Nutritional Guide

| | Quantity or Amounts | Calories | Protein (g) | Total Fat (g) | Saturated Fat (g) | Unsaturated Fat (g) | Cholesterol (mg) | Carbohydrates (g) | Sodium (mg) |
|---|---|---|---|---|---|---|---|---|---|
| Peanut butter sandwich, $1\frac{3}{4} \times \frac{1}{2}$ | 100 g | 473 | 10.0 | 19.1 | — | — | — | 67.0 | 173 |
| | 1 oz. | 135 | 2.9 | 5.5 | — | — | — | 19.0 | 49 |
| | 4 cookies | 232 | 4.9 | 9.4 | — | — | — | 32.8 | 85 |
| Sandwich type, chocolate, Oreo | 100 g | 495 | 4.8 | 22.5 | 4.0 | 11.0 | — | 69.3 | 483 |
| | 1 oz. | 141 | 1.4 | 6.4 | 1.1 | 3.1 | — | 19.6 | 138 |
| | 4 cookies | 198 | 1.9 | 9.0 | 2.4 | 6.3 | — | 27.7 | 193 |
| Shortbread, $1\frac{5}{8} \times 1\frac{5}{8} \times \frac{1}{4}$ | 100 g | 498 | 7.2 | 23.1 | 4.0 | 11.0 | — | 65.1 | 60 |
| | 1 oz. | 142 | 2.1 | 6.6 | 1.1 | 3.1 | — | 18.6 | 17 |
| | 10 cookies | 374 | 5.4 | 17.3 | 4.3 | 12.4 | — | 48.8 | 45 |
| Sugar cookies, home recipe, $2\frac{1}{4} \times \frac{1}{4}$ | 100 g | 444 | 6.0 | 16.8 | 4.0 | 11.0 | — | 68.0 | 318 |
| | 1 oz. | 127 | 1.7 | 4.8 | 1.1 | 3.1 | — | 19.4 | 91 |
| | 10 cookies | 355 | 4.8 | 13.4 | 3.6 | 9.3 | — | 54.4 | 254 |
| Vanilla wafers, $1\frac{3}{4} \times \frac{1}{4}$ | 100 g | 462 | 5.4 | 16.1 | 4.0 | 11.0 | — | 74.4 | 252 |
| | 1 oz. | 132 | 1.5 | 4.6 | 1.1 | 3.1 | — | 21.2 | 72 |
| | 10 cookies | 185 | 2.2 | 6.4 | — | .9 | — | 29.8 | 101 |
| **Desserts** | | | | | | | | | |
| Apple brown betty | 100 g | 151 | 1.6 | 3.5 | 1.0 | 1.0 | — | 29.7 | 153 |
| | 1 oz. | 43 | .5 | 1.0 | .3 | .3 | — | 8.5 | 44 |
| | 1 cup | 325 | 3.4 | 7.5 | 3.2 | 3.3 | — | 63.9 | 329 |
| Bread pudding with raisins | 100 g | 187 | 5.6 | 6.1 | 3.0 | 2.0 | — | 28.4 | 201 |
| | 1 oz. | 53 | 1.6 | 1.7 | .9 | .6 | — | 8.1 | 57 |
| | 1 cup | 496 | 14.8 | 16.2 | 7.7 | 6.9 | — | 75.3 | 533 |
| Charlotte russe | 100 g | 286 | 5.9 | 14.6 | 7.0 | 6.0 | — | 33.5 | 43 |
| | 1 oz. | 82 | 1.7 | 4.2 | 2.0 | 1.7 | — | 9.5 | 12 |
| | 1 serving | 326 | 6.7 | 16.6 | 8.3 | 6.4 | — | 38.2 | 49 |
| Chocolate syrup, thin | 100 g | 245 | 2.3 | 2.0 | 1.0 | 1.0 | — | 62.7 | 52 |
| | 1 oz.=2 T. | 92 | .9 | .8 | .4 | .3 | — | 23.5 | 20 |
| Cream puffs with custard filling | 100 g | 233 | 6.5 | 13.9 | 4.0 | 9.0 | 144 | 20.5 | 83 |
| | 1 oz. | 66 | 1.9 | 3.9 | 1.1 | 2.6 | 41 | 5.9 | 24 |
| | 1 puff | 303 | 8.5 | 18.1 | 5.6 | 11.2 | 188 | 26.7 | 108 |
| Custard, baked | 100 g | 115 | 5.4 | 5.5 | 3.0 | 2.0 | 105 | 11.1 | 79 |
| | 1 oz. | 33 | 1.5 | 1.6 | .9 | .6 | 30 | 3.2 | 23 |
| | 1 cup | 305 | 14.6 | 14.3 | 6.8 | 6.1 | 278 | 29.4 | 209 |
| Doughnut, cake type | 100 g | 391 | 4.5 | 18.6 | 4.0 | 13.0 | — | 51.4 | 501 |
| | 1 oz. | 112 | 1.3 | 5.3 | 1.1 | 3.7 | — | 15.0 | 143 |
| | 1=2 oz. | 227 | 2.7 | 10.8 | 2.7 | 7.6 | — | 29.8 | 291 |
| Doughnut, raised type | 100 g | 414 | 6.3 | 26.7 | 6.0 | 19.0 | — | 37.7 | 234 |
| | 1 oz. | 118 | 1.8 | 7.6 | 1.7 | 5.4 | — | 10.7 | 67 |
| | 1=1$\frac{1}{2}$ oz. | 176 | 2.7 | 11.3 | 2.8 | 8.1 | — | 16.0 | 99 |

# Nutritional Guide

| | Quantity or Amounts | Calories | Protein (g) | Total Fat (g) | Saturated Fat (g) | Unsaturated Fat (g) | Cholesterol (mg) | Carbohydrates (g) | Sodium (mg) |
|---|---|---|---|---|---|---|---|---|---|
| Eclair with custard and chocolate icing | 100 g | 239 | 6.2 | 13.6 | 4.0 | 8.0 | — | 23.2 | 82 |
| | 1 oz. | 68 | 1.7 | 3.9 | 1.1 | 2.3 | — | 6.6 | 23 |
| | 1 eclair | 239 | 6.2 | 13.6 | 4.4 | 8.3 | — | 23.2 | 82 |
| Gelatin dessert, plain | 100 g | 59 | 1.5 | 0 | — | — | — | 14.1 | 51 |
| | 1 oz. | 17 | .4 | 0 | — | — | — | 4.0 | 15 |
| | 1 cup | 142 | 3.6 | 0 | — | — | — | 33.8 | 122 |
| Ice cream, plain, 10% fat | 100 g | 193 | 4.5 | 10.6 | 7.0 | 4.0 | 40 | 20.8 | 63 |
| | 1 oz. | 55 | 1.3 | 3.0 | 2.0 | 1.1 | 11 | 5.9 | 18 |
| | 1 cup | 257 | 6.0 | 14.1 | 7.8 | 5.1 | 53 | 27.7 | 84 |
| Ice cream, frozen French custard, soft | 100 g | — | — | — | — | — | — | — | — |
| | 1 cup | 334 | 7.8 | 18.3 | 10.1 | 6.7 | 97 | 36.0 | 109 |
| Ice milk, 5.1% fat | 100 g | 152 | 4.8 | 5.1 | 3.0 | 2.0 | 20 | 22.4 | 69 |
| | 1 oz. | 43 | 1.4 | 1.5 | .9 | .6 | 6 | 6.4 | 19 |
| | 1 cup | 199 | 6.3 | 6.7 | 3.7 | 2.4 | 26 | 29.3 | 89 |
| Pudding, chocolate, home recipe | 100 g | 148 | 3.1 | 4.7 | 3.0 | 2.0 | — | 25.7 | 56 |
| | 1 oz. | 42 | .9 | 1.3 | .9 | .6 | — | 7.3 | 16 |
| | 1 cup | 385 | 8.1 | 12.2 | 6.7 | 4.9 | — | 66.8 | 146 |
| Pudding, chocolate, from mix, cooked with milk | 100 g | 124 | 3.4 | 3.0 | 2.0 | 1.0 | 12 | 22.8 | 129 |
| | 1 oz. | 35 | 1.0 | .9 | .6 | .3 | 3.4 | 6.5 | 37 |
| | 1 cup | 322 | 8.8 | 7.8 | 4.3 | 2.8 | 30 | 59.3 | 335 |
| Pudding, chocolate, from mix, instant, made with milk | 100 g | 125 | 3.0 | 2.5 | 1.0 | 1.0 | — | 24.4 | 124 |
| | 1 oz. | 36 | .9 | .7 | .3 | .3 | — | 6.9 | 35 |
| | 1 cup | 325 | 7.8 | 6.5 | 3.6 | 2.5 | — | 63.4 | 322 |
| Pudding, vanilla (blancmange) | 100 g | 111 | 3.5 | 3.9 | 2.0 | 1.0 | 14 | 15.9 | 65 |
| | 1 oz. | 32 | 1.0 | 1.1 | .6 | .3 | 4 | 4.5 | 19 |
| | 1 cup | 283 | 8.9 | 9.9 | 5.5 | 3.6 | 35 | 40.5 | 166 |
| Rice pudding with raisins | 100 g | 146 | 3.6 | 3.1 | 2.0 | 1.0 | 11 | 26.7 | 71 |
| | 1 oz. | 42 | 1.0 | .9 | .6 | .3 | 3 | 7.6 | 20 |
| | 1 cup | 387 | 9.5 | 8.2 | 4.5 | 3.0 | 29 | 70.9 | 188 |
| Rolls, Danish pastry, plain without fruit or nuts | 100 g | 422 | 7.4 | 23.5 | 7.0 | 16.0 | — | 45.6 | 366 |
| | 1 oz. | 121 | 2.0 | 6.7 | 2.0 | 4.6 | — | 13.0 | 105 |
| | 1 roll | 274 | 4.8 | 15.2 | 4.5 | 9.9 | — | 29.6 | 238 |
| Sherbet, orange | 100 g | 134 | .9 | 1.2 | — | — | — | 30.8 | 10 |
| | 1 oz. | 38 | .3 | .3 | — | — | — | 8.8 | 3 |
| | 1 cup | 259 | 1.7 | 2.3 | — | — | — | 59.4 | 19 |
| Tapioca pudding | 100 g | 134 | 5.0 | 5.1 | 2.0 | 2.0 | — | 17.1 | 156 |
| | 1 oz. | 38 | 1.4 | 1.5 | .6 | .6 | — | 4.9 | 45 |
| | 1 cup | 221 | 8.3 | 8.4 | 3.9 | 3.5 | — | 59.0 | 197 |

**253**

| | Quantity or Amounts | Calories | Protein (g) | Total Fat (g) | Saturated Fat (g) | Unsaturated Fat (g) | Cholesterol (mg) | Carbohydrates (g) | Sodium (mg) |
|---|---|---|---|---|---|---|---|---|---|
| **Pies, all 9″ single crust, slice = ⅛ pie** | | | | | | | | | |
| Apple | 100 g | 256 | 2.2 | 11.1 | 3.0 | 8.0 | 0 | 35.0 | 301 |
| | 1 oz. | 73 | .6 | 3.1 | 1.0 | 2.3 | 0 | 10.0 | 86 |
| | 1 slice | 302 | 2.6 | 13.1 | 3.4 | 9.2 | 0 | 45.0 | 355 |
| Blueberry | 100 g | 242 | 2.4 | 10.8 | 3.0 | 8.0 | — | 34.9 | 268 |
| | 1 oz. | 69 | .7 | 3.1 | .9 | 2.3 | — | 10.0 | 77 |
| | 1 slice | 286 | 2.8 | 12.7 | 3.2 | 9.2 | — | 41.2 | 316 |
| Cherry | 100 g | 261 | 2.6 | 11.3 | 3.0 | 8.0 | — | 38.4 | 302 |
| | 1 oz. | 75 | .7 | 3.2 | .9 | 2.3 | — | 10.9 | 87 |
| | 1 slice | 308 | 3.1 | 13.3 | 3.5 | 9.4 | — | 45.3 | 359 |
| Chocolate meringue | 100 g | 252 | 4.8 | 12.0 | 3.0 | 8.0 | — | 33.5 | 256 |
| | 1 oz. | 72 | 1.4 | 3.4 | .9 | 2.3 | — | 9.6 | 73 |
| | 1 slice | 287 | 3.5 | 13.7 | 5.1 | 7.8 | — | 38.2 | 292 |
| Custard, plain | 100 g | 218 | 6.1 | 11.1 | 3.0 | 8.0 | 105 | 23.4 | 287 |
| | 1 oz. | 62 | 1.7 | 3.1 | .9 | 2.3 | 30 | 6.7 | 82 |
| | 1 slice | 248 | 7.0 | 12.7 | 4.3 | 7.4 | 120 | 26.7 | 327 |
| Lemon meringue | 100 g | 255 | 3.7 | 10.2 | 3.0 | 8.0 | 93 | 37.7 | 282 |
| | 1 oz. | 73 | 1.0 | 2.9 | .9 | 2.3 | 27 | 10.7 | 81 |
| | 1 slice | 268 | 3.9 | 10.7 | 3.2 | 6.8 | 98 | 39.6 | 296 |
| Mincemeat | 100 g | 271 | 2.5 | 11.5 | 3.0 | 8.0 | — | 41.2 | 448 |
| | 1 oz. | 77 | .7 | 3.3 | .9 | 2.3 | — | 11.7 | 128 |
| | 1 slice | 320 | 3.0 | 13.6 | 3.6 | 9.6 | — | 48.6 | 529 |
| Pecan | 100 g | 418 | 5.1 | 22.9 | 4.0 | 16.0 | — | 51.3 | 221 |
| | 1 oz. | 119 | 1.5 | 6.5 | 1.1 | 1.7 | — | 14.7 | 63 |
| | 1 slice | 431 | 5.3 | 23.6 | 3.3 | 18.3 | — | 52.8 | 228 |
| Pie crust, baked with vegetable shortening | 100 g | 500 | 6.1 | 33.4 | 7.0 | 21.0 | — | 43.8 | 611 |
| | 1 oz. | 143 | 1.7 | 9.5 | 2.0 | 6.0 | — | 12.5 | 175 |
| | 1 9″ shell | 900 | 11.0 | 60.1 | 14.9 | 43.3 | — | 78.8 | 1100 |
| Pumpkin | 100 g | 211 | 4.0 | 11.2 | 3.0 | 8.0 | 61 | 24.5 | 214 |
| | 1 oz. | 60 | 1.1 | 3.2 | .9 | 2.3 | 17 | 7.0 | 61 |
| | 1 slice | 241 | 4.6 | 12.8 | 4.5 | 6.4 | 70 | 27.9 | 182 |
| Strawberry | 100 g | 198 | 1.9 | 7.9 | 3.0 | 8.0 | — | 30.9 | 194 |
| | 1 oz. | 57 | .5 | 2.4 | .9 | 2.3 | — | 8.8 | 55 |
| | 1 slice | 184 | 1.8 | 7.3 | 1.8 | 5.4 | — | 28.7 | 180 |
| **Dairy Products** | | | | | | | | | |
| Butter | 100 g | 716 | .6 | 81.0 | 46.0 | 29.0 | 250 | .4 | 987 |
| | 1 oz. = 2 T. | 204 | .2 | 23.0 | 13.1 | 8.3 | 70 | .2 | 282 |
| | 1 pat | 36 | trace | 4.1 | 2.2 | 2.3 | 13 | .1 | 49 |
| | ½ cup | 812 | .7 | 91.9 | 50.5 | 33.1 | 282 | .5 | 1119 |

| | Quantity or Amounts | Calories | Protein (g) | Total Fat (g) | Saturated Fat (g) | Unsaturated Fat (g) | Cholesterol (mg) | Carbohydrates (g) | Sodium (mg) |
|---|---|---|---|---|---|---|---|---|---|
| Buttermilk made from | 100 g | 36 | 3.6 | .1 | — | — | 2 | 5.1 | 130 |
| skim milk | 1 oz. | 10 | 1.0 | — | — | — | 1 | 1.5 | 37 |
| | 1 cup | 88 | 8.8 | .2 | — | — | 5 | 12.5 | 319 |
| **Cheese** | | | | | | | | | |
| Blue or Roquefort | 100 g | 368 | 21.5 | 30.5 | 18.0 | 12.0 | 87 | 2.0 | — |
| | 1 oz. | 104 | 6.1 | 8.6 | 4.8 | 3.2 | 24 | .6 | — |
| Brick | 100 g | 370 | 21.5 | 30.5 | 18.0 | 12.0 | 90 | 1.9 | — |
| | 1 oz. | 105 | 6.3 | 8.6 | 4.8 | 3.2 | 25 | .5 | — |
| Camembert | 100 g | 299 | 17.5 | 24.7 | 15.0 | 10.0 | 92 | 1.8 | — |
| | 1 oz. | 85 | 5.0 | 7.0 | 3.8 | 2.5 | 26 | .5 | — |
| Cheddar | 100 g | 398 | 25.0 | 32.2 | 18.0 | 12.0 | 100 | 2.1 | 700 |
| | 1 oz. | 113 | 7.1 | 9.1 | 5.0 | 3.3 | 28 | .6 | 198 |
| Cottage cheese, | 100 g | 106 | 13.6 | 4.2 | 2.0 | 1.0 | 19 | 2.9 | 229 |
| creamed | 1 oz. | 30 | 3.9 | 1.2 | .7 | .4 | 5 | .9 | 65 |
| | 1 cup | 260 | 33.3 | 10.3 | 5.7 | 3.7 | 48 | 7.1 | 561 |
| Cottage cheese, | 100 g | 86 | 17.0 | .3 | .2 | .1 | 7 | 2.7 | 290 |
| uncreamed | 1 oz. | 24 | 4.8 | .1 | — | — | 2 | .8 | 82 |
| | 1 cup | 200 | 34.0 | .6 | — | — | 13 | 5.4 | 580 |
| Cream cheese | 100 g | 374 | 8.0 | 37.7 | 21.0 | 13.0 | 120 | 2.1 | 250 |
| | 1 oz. | 106 | 2.3 | 10.7 | 5.9 | 3.8 | 34 | .6 | 71 |
| Edam | 1 oz. | 105 | — | — | — | — | 29 | .3 | — |
| Monterey jack | 1 oz. | 103 | — | — | — | — | — | .4 | — |
| Mozzarella | 1 oz. | 96 | — | 4.7 | 2.3 | 2.3 | 18 | .8 | — |
| Muenster | 1 oz. | 102 | — | 8.5 | 4.2 | 4.2 | 25 | .6 | — |
| Neufchâtel | 1 oz. | 70 | — | — | — | — | 25 | .7 | — |
| Parmesan | 100 g | 393 | 36.0 | 26.0 | 15.0 | 10.0 | 95 | 2.9 | 734 |
| | 1 oz. | 132 | 12.1 | 8.7 | 4.8 | 3.2 | 27 | 1.0 | 247 |
| Pasteurized process | 100 g | 370 | 23.2 | 30.0 | 15.0 | 10.0 | 90 | 1.9 | 1136 |
| American cheese | 1 oz. slice | 105 | 6.6 | 8.5 | 4.7 | 2.8 | 25 | .5 | 322 |
| Ricotta | 1 oz. | 42 | — | 2.3 | 1.2 | 1.1 | 9 | 1.0 | — |
| Swiss | 100 g | 370 | 27.5 | 28.0 | 15.0 | 10.0 | 100 | 1.7 | 710 |
| | 1 oz. | 105 | 7.8 | 7.9 | 4.4 | 2.8 | 29 | .5 | 201 |
| **Cream** | | | | | | | | | |
| Half and half | 100 g | 134 | 3.2 | 11.7 | 6.0 | 4.0 | 43 | 4.5 | 46 |
| | 1 oz.=2 T. | 40 | 1.0 | 3.6 | 2.0 | 1.4 | 12 | 1.4 | 14 |
| Heavy whipping | 100 g | 352 | 2.2 | 37.6 | 21.0 | 12.0 | 85 | 3.1 | 32 |
| | 1 oz.=2 T. | 106 | .6 | 11.2 | 6.2 | 4.2 | 24 | 1.0 | 10 |

| | Quantity or Amounts | Calories | Protein (g) | Total Fat (g) | Saturated Fat (g) | Unsaturated Fat (g) | Cholesterol (mg) | Carbohydrates (g) | Sodium (mg) |
|---|---|---|---|---|---|---|---|---|---|
| Light table cream | 100 g | 211 | 3.0 | 20.6 | 11.0 | 7.0 | 35 | 4.3 | 43 |
| | 1 oz.=2 T. | 64 | 1.0 | 6.2 | 3.4 | 2.2 | 10 | 1.2 | 12 |
| Sour cream | 1 oz. | 50 | — | 4.0 | 2.0 | 2.0 | 16 | 1.0 | — |
| | 1 cup | 485 | — | 34.4 | 17.2 | 17.2 | 152 | 9.9 | — |
| Cream substitute, dry powder | 100 g | 509 | 13.9 | 27.7 | 15.0 | 9.0 | 11 | 53.2 | — |
| | 1 t. | 10 | .3 | .5 | .3 | .2 | .3 | 1.0 | — |
| Milk | | | | | | | | | |
| Whole | 100 g | 66 | 3.5 | 3.7 | 2.0 | 1.0 | 14 | 4.9 | 50 |
| | 1 oz. | 19 | 1.0 | 1.1 | .6 | .3 | 4 | 1.3 | 14 |
| | 1 cup | 159 | 8.5 | 8.5 | 4.7 | 3.0 | 34 | 12.0 | 122 |
| 2 percent | 100 g | 59 | 4.2 | 2.0 | 1.0 | 1.0 | 9 | 6.0 | 61 |
| | 1 oz. | 17 | 1.2 | .6 | .3 | .3 | 3 | 1.7 | 17 |
| | 1 cup | 145 | 10.3 | 4.9 | 2.7 | 1.7 | 22 | 14.8 | 150 |
| Skim | 100 g | 36 | 3.6 | .1 | — | — | 2 | 5.1 | 52 |
| | 1 oz. | 10 | 1.0 | — | — | — | .6 | 1.5 | 15 |
| | 1 cup | 88 | 8.8 | .2 | — | — | 5 | 12.5 | 127 |
| Evaporated | 100 g | 137 | 7.0 | 7.9 | 4.0 | 3.0 | 31 | 41.7 | 118 |
| | 1 oz. | 39 | 2.0 | 2.4 | 1.4 | .9 | 8 | 11.9 | 34 |
| Sweetened condensed | 100 g | 321 | 8.1 | 8.7 | 4.0 | 3.0 | 34 | 54.3 | 112 |
| | 1 oz. | 98 | 2.4 | 3.3 | 1.8 | 1.2 | 9 | 15.5 | 32 |
| Whole powder, dry | 100 g | 502 | 26.4 | 27.4 | 15.0 | 9.0 | 109 | 38.2 | 405 |
| | 1 oz. | 143 | 7.5 | 7.9 | 4.3 | 2.6 | 31 | 10.9 | 116 |
| Skim powder, dry | 100 g | 363 | 35.9 | .8 | — | — | 22 | 52.3 | 532 |
| | 1 oz. | 104 | 10.3 | .2 | — | — | 6 | 15.0 | 152 |
| 3.5 percent fat, chocolate flavored | 100 g | 85 | 3.4 | 3.4 | 1.0 | 1.0 | 13 | 11.0 | 47 |
| | 1 oz. | 25 | .9 | .9 | .3 | .3 | 4 | 3.1 | 13 |
| | 1 cup | 213 | 8.5 | 8.5 | 2.4 | 2.4 | 24 | 27.5 | 118 |
| Yogurt, low fat, plain | 100 g | 50 | 3.4 | 1.7 | 2.0 | 1.0 | 8 | 5.2 | 51 |
| | 1 oz. | 14 | 1.0 | .5 | .6 | .3 | 2 | 1.5 | 15 |

# Eggs

Eggs, raw, fresh

| | Quantity or Amounts | Calories | Protein (g) | Total Fat (g) | Saturated Fat (g) | Unsaturated Fat (g) | Cholesterol (mg) | Carbohydrates (g) | Sodium (mg) |
|---|---|---|---|---|---|---|---|---|---|
| Whole egg, large | 100 g | 163 | 12.9 | 11.5 | 4.0 | 5.0 | 504 | .9 | 122 |
| | 1 oz. | 47 | 3.7 | 3.3 | 1.1 | 1.4 | 157 | .2 | 35 |
| | 1 egg | 80 | 6.5 | 5.8 | 1.8 | 2.9 | 252 | .4 | 61 |
| White only | 100 g | 51 | 10.9 | trace | — | — | 0 | .8 | 146 |
| | 1 oz. | 15 | 3.1 | — | — | — | 0 | .2 | 42 |
| | 1 egg | 17 | 3.6 | — | — | — | 0 | .3 | 48 |
| Yolk only | 100 g | 348 | 16.0 | 30.6 | 10.0 | 13.0 | 1500 | .6 | 52 |

# Nutritional Guide

| Food | Quantity or Amounts | Calories | Protein (g) | Total Fat (g) | Saturated Fat (g) | Unsaturated Fat (g) | Cholesterol (mg) | Carbohydrates (g) | Sodium (mg) |
|---|---|---|---|---|---|---|---|---|---|
| | 1 oz. | 100 | 4.6 | 8.7 | 2.9 | 3.7 | 429 | .2 | 15 |
| | 1 egg | 59 | 2.7 | 5.2 | 1.7 | 2.7 | 252 | .1 | 9 |
| **Eggs, cooked** | | | | | | | | | |
| Fried in butter | 100 g | 216 | 13.8 | 17.2 | 6.0 | 7.0 | 411 | .3 | 338 |
| | 1 oz. | 62 | 3.9 | 4.9 | 1.7 | 2.0 | 117 | .1 | 97 |
| | 1 lg. egg | 99 | 6.3 | 7.9 | 2.9 | 3.8 | 263 | .1 | 155 |
| Hard-boiled or poached | 100 g | 163 | 12.9 | 11.5 | 4.0 | 5.0 | 504 | .9 | 122 |
| | 1 oz. | 47 | 3.7 | 3.3 | 1.1 | 1.4 | 144 | .3 | 34 |
| | 1 lg. egg | 80 | 6.5 | 5.8 | 1.8 | 2.9 | 252 | .4 | 61 |
| Omelet or scrambled | 100 g | 173 | 11.2 | 12.9 | 4.0 | 5.0 | 411 | 2.4 | 257 |
| with milk, cooked | 1 oz. | 49 | 3.2 | 3.7 | 1.1 | 1.4 | 117 | .7 | 73 |
| in fat | 1 lg. egg | 111 | 7.2 | 8.3 | 2.8 | 3.6 | 263 | 1.5 | 164 |

## Fish and Seafood

| Food | Quantity or Amounts | Calories | Protein (g) | Total Fat (g) | Saturated Fat (g) | Unsaturated Fat (g) | Cholesterol (mg) | Carbohydrates (g) | Sodium (mg) |
|---|---|---|---|---|---|---|---|---|---|
| Anchovy, pickled with oil, | 100 g | 176 | 19.2 | 10.3 | — | — | — | .3 | — |
| no salt | 1 oz. | 50 | 5.4 | 2.9 | — | — | — | .1 | — |
| Bass, baked | 100 g | 196 | 21.5 | 8.5 | 2.0 | 2.6 | — | 6.7 | — |
| | 1 oz. | 56 | 6.1 | 2.4 | — | — | — | 1.9 | — |
| Catfish, freshwater | 100 g | 103 | 17.6 | 3.1 | — | — | — | 0 | 60 |
| | 1 oz. | 29 | 5.0 | .8 | — | — | — | 0 | 17 |
| Caviar or roe | 100 g | 262 | 26.9 | 15.0 | — | — | 300 | 3.3 | 2200 |
| | 1 oz. | 74 | 7.6 | 4.3 | — | — | 86 | .9 | 624 |
| Clams, canned, drained | 100 g | 98 | 15.8 | 2.5 | .8 | 1.8 | 63 | 1.9 | — |
| | 1 oz. | 28 | 4.5 | .7 | .2 | .5 | 18 | .5 | — |
| Cod, broiled | 100 g | 170 | 28.5 | 5.3 | .1 | .4 | 50 | 0 | 110 |
| | 1 oz. | 48 | 8.1 | 1.5 | — | .1 | 14 | 0 | 31 |
| Crab, cooked meat | 100 g | 93 | 17.3 | 1.9 | .5 | 1.5 | 100 | .5 | — |
| | 1 oz. | 27 | 4.9 | .5 | .1 | .4 | 29 | .1 | — |
| Fish sticks, frozen, cooked | 100 g | 176 | 16.6 | 8.9 | — | — | — | 6.5 | — |
| | 1 stick | 50 | 4.7 | 2.5 | — | — | — | 1.8 | — |
| Flounder, baked | 100 g | 202 | 30.0 | 8.2 | — | — | 50 | 0 | 237 |
| | 1 oz. | 57 | 8.5 | 2.3 | — | — | 14 | 0 | 67 |
| Haddock, fried | 100 g | 165 | 19.6 | 6.4 | 1.0 | .3 | 60 | 5.8 | 177 |
| | 1 oz. | 47 | 5.6 | 1.8 | .3 | .1 | 17 | 1.6 | 50 |
| Halibut, broiled | 100 g | 171 | 24.2 | 7.0 | 1.4 | 4.2 | 60 | 0 | 134 |
| | 1 oz. | 48 | 7.1 | 2.0 | .4 | 1.2 | 17 | 0 | 38 |
| Herring, pickled | 100 g | 223 | 20.4 | 15.1 | 2.0 | 2.0 | 97 | 0 | — |
| | 1 oz. | 63 | 5.8 | 4.3 | .6 | .6 | 28 | 0 | — |
| Lake trout | 100 g | 168 | 18.3 | 10.0 | 2.0 | 6.0 | 55 | 0 | — |
| | 1 oz. | 48 | 5.2 | 2.9 | .6 | 1.7 | 16 | 0 | — |

# Nutritional Guide

| | Quantity or Amounts | Calories | Protein (g) | Total Fat (g) | Saturated Fat (g) | Unsaturated Fat (g) | Cholesterol (mg) | Carbohydrates (g) | Sodium (mg) |
|---|---|---|---|---|---|---|---|---|---|
| Lobster, cooked meat | 100 g | 95 | 18.7 | 1.5 | — | — | 85 | .3 | 210 |
| | 1 oz. | 27 | 5.3 | .4 | — | — | 24 | .1 | 60 |
| Mackerel, canned | 100 g | 183 | 19.3 | 11.1 | 3.0 | 6.5 | — | 0 | — |
| | 1 oz. | 52 | 5.5 | 3.1 | .9 | 1.9 | — | 0 | — |
| Mussels, canned | 100 g | 114 | 18.2 | 3.3 | — | — | 94 | 1.5 | — |
| | 1 oz. | 33 | 5.2 | .9 | — | — | 27 | .4 | — |
| Ocean perch, fried | 100 g | 227 | 19.0 | 13.3 | 1.6 | 7.0 | — | 6.8 | 153 |
| | 1 oz. | 64 | 5.4 | 3.8 | .5 | 2.0 | — | 1.9 | 43 |
| Oysters, raw | 100 g | 91 | 10.6 | 2.2 | 1.0 | 2.0 | 50 | 6.4 | — |
| | 1 oz. | 26 | 3.0 | .5 | .3 | .6 | 14 | 1.0 | — |
| Oysters, fried | 100 g | 239 | 8.6 | 13.9 | — | — | — | 18.6 | 206 |
| | 1 oz. | 68 | 2.4 | 3.9 | — | — | — | 5.3 | 58 |
| Red snapper | 100 g | 93 | 19.8 | .9 | .2 | .4 | — | 0 | 67 |
| | 1 oz. | 27 | 5.7 | .3 | — | .1 | — | 0 | 19 |
| Salmon, broiled with butter | 100 g | 217 | 22.5 | 13.4 | 4.0 | 4.0 | 47 | 0 | — |
| | 1 oz. | 52 | 7.7 | 2.1 | 1.1 | 1.1 | 13 | 0 | 33 |
| Salmon, canned, solids and liquid | 100 g | 171 | 20.3 | 9.3 | 3.0 | 3.0 | 40 | 0 | 522 |
| | 1 oz. | 49 | 5.8 | 2.7 | .9 | .9 | 11 | 0 | 149 |
| Sardines, canned in oil, drained | 100 g | 203 | 24.0 | 11.1 | — | — | 125 | 0 | 823 |
| | 1 oz. | 88 | 5.8 | 6.9 | — | — | 36 | 0 | 145 |
| Scallops, steamed | 100 g | 112 | 23.2 | 1.4 | .4 | .1 | 56 | 0 | 265 |
| | 1 oz. | 32 | 6.6 | .4 | .1 | — | 16 | 0 | 76 |
| Shrimp, boiled | 100 g | 91 | 18.1 | 1.2 | .2 | .8 | 150 | 1.5 | 140 |
| | 1 oz. | 33 | 6.9 | .4 | .1 | .2 | 43 | .2 | — |
| | 10 med. | 37 | 7.7 | .4 | .1 | .2 | 45 | .3 | — |
| Shrimp, fried in batter | 100 g | 225 | 20.3 | 10.8 | — | — | — | 10.0 | 186 |
| | 1 oz. | 64 | 5.8 | 3.1 | — | — | — | 2.8 | 53 |
| Sole, baked | 100 g | 202 | 30.0 | 8.2 | — | — | — | 0 | 237 |
| | 1 oz. | 58 | 8.6 | 2.3 | — | — | — | 0 | 68 |
| Tuna, fresh | 100 g | 145 | 25.2 | 4.1 | 1.0 | 1.0 | — | 0 | — |
| | 1 oz. | 41 | 7.2 | 1.1 | .3 | .3 | — | 0 | — |
| Tuna, canned in oil, drained | 100 g | 197 | 28.8 | 8.2 | 3.0 | 2.0 | 70 | 0 | — |
| | 1 oz. | 56 | 8.2 | 2.3 | .8 | .5 | 20 | 0 | — |
| Tuna, canned in water | 100 g | 127 | 28.0 | .8 | — | — | 63 | 0 | 41 |
| | 1 oz. | 36 | 8.0 | .2 | — | — | 18 | 0 | 12 |

## Fruit and Fruit Juices

| | | | | | | | | | |
|---|---|---|---|---|---|---|---|---|---|
| Apple, fresh with skin | 100 g | 59 | .2 | .6 | — | — | — | 14.5 | 1 |
| | 1 oz. | 17 | — | .1 | — | — | — | 4.1 | — |
| | 1 med. | 80 | .3 | .8 | — | — | — | 20.0 | 1 |

# Nutritional Guide

| | Quantity or Amounts | Calories | Protein (g) | Total Fat (g) | Saturated Fat (g) | Unsaturated Fat (g) | Cholesterol (mg) | Carbohydrates (g) | Sodium (mg) |
|---|---|---|---|---|---|---|---|---|---|
| Apple juice | 100 g | 47 | .1 | tr. | — | — | — | 11.9 | 2 |
| | 1 fl. oz. | 15 | — | — | — | — | — | 3.7 | — |
| Applesauce, sweetened | 100 g | 91 | .2 | .1 | — | — | — | 23.8 | 2 |
| | 1 oz. | 26 | .1 | — | — | — | — | 6.8 | — |
| | ½ cup | 116 | .3 | .1 | — | — | — | 30.5 | 1 |
| Apricots, fresh | 100 g | 51 | 1.0 | .2 | — | — | — | 12.8 | 1 |
| | 1 oz. | 15 | .3 | .1 | — | — | — | 3.7 | — |
| | 3 whole | 55 | 1.1 | .2 | — | — | — | 13.7 | 1 |
| Apricot halves, canned in heavy syrup | 100 g | 86 | .6 | .1 | — | — | — | 22.0 | 1 |
| | 1 oz. | 25 | .2 | — | — | — | — | 6.3 | — |
| | ½ cup | 108 | .7 | .1 | — | — | — | 27.7 | 1 |
| Apricots, uncooked, dehydrated | 100 g | 332 | 5.6 | 1.0 | — | — | — | 84.6 | 33 |
| | 1 oz. | 95 | 1.6 | 1.0 | — | — | — | 24.0 | 9 |
| | 10 med. | 91 | 1.8 | .2 | — | — | — | 23.3 | 9 |
| Avocado, fresh | 100 g | 167 | 2.1 | 16.4 | 3.0 | 7.0 | — | 6.3 | 4 |
| | 1 oz. | 48 | .6 | 4.7 | .9 | 2.0 | — | 1.8 | 1 |
| | ½ avocado | 188 | 2.4 | 18.5 | 3.0 | 7.0 | — | 7.1 | 4 |
| Banana | 100 g | 85 | 1.1 | .2 | — | — | — | 22.2 | 1 |
| | 1 oz. | 24 | .3 | — | — | — | — | 6.3 | — |
| | 1 med. | 100 | 1.3 | .2 | — | — | — | 26.4 | 1 |
| Blackberries, fresh | 100 g | 58 | 1.2 | .9 | — | — | — | 12.9 | 1 |
| | 1 oz. | 17 | .3 | .3 | — | — | — | 3.7 | — |
| | ½ cup | 42 | .9 | .6 | — | — | — | 9.4 | — |
| Blueberries, fresh | 100 g | 62 | .7 | .5 | — | — | — | 15.3 | 1 |
| | 1 oz. | 18 | .2 | .1 | — | — | — | 4.4 | — |
| | ½ cup | 45 | .5 | .3 | — | — | — | 11.2 | — |
| Cherries, sweet, fresh | 100 g | 70 | 1.3 | .3 | — | — | — | 17.4 | 4 |
| | 1 oz. | 20 | .4 | .1 | — | — | — | 4.9 | 1 |
| | ½ lb. | 143 | 2.6 | .6 | — | — | — | 36.0 | 4 |
| Cherries, pitted, canned in heavy syrup | 100 g | 81 | .9 | .2 | — | — | — | 20.5 | 1 |
| | 1 oz. | 23 | .3 | — | — | — | — | 5.9 | 1 |
| | ½ cup | 96 | 1.2 | — | — | — | — | 24.2 | 1 |
| Cranberries, fresh | 100 g | 46 | .4 | .7 | — | — | — | 10.8 | 2 |
| | 1 oz. | 13 | .1 | .2 | — | — | — | 3.1 | 1 |
| Cranberry sauce, canned | 100 g | 146 | .1 | .2 | — | — | — | 37.5 | 1 |
| | 1 oz. | 42 | — | .1 | — | — | — | 10.7 | — |
| | ½ cup | 199 | .1 | .3 | — | — | — | 51.0 | 1 |
| Cranberry juice | 100 g | 65 | .1 | .1 | — | — | — | 16.5 | 1 |
| | 1 fl. oz. | 19 | — | — | — | — | — | 4.7 | — |

| | Quantity or Amounts | Calories | Protein (g) | Total Fat (g) | Saturated Fat (g) | Unsaturated Fat (g) | Cholesterol (mg) | Carbohydrates (g) | Sodium (mg) |
|---|---|---|---|---|---|---|---|---|---|
| Dates, dried | 100 g | 274 | 2.2 | .5 | — | — | — | 72.9 | 1 |
| | 1 oz. | 78 | .6 | .2 | — | — | — | 20.8 | — |
| | 10 dates | 219 | 1.9 | .4 | — | — | — | 58.3 | — |
| Figs, fresh | 100 g | 80 | 1.2 | .3 | — | —→ | — | 20.3 | 1 |
| | 1 oz. | 23 | .3 | .1 | — | — | — | 5.8 | 2 |
| | 1 fig | 32 | .5 | .1 | — | — | — | 8.1 | 1 |
| Figs, canned in heavy syrup | 100 g | 84 | .5 | .2 | — | — | — | 21.8 | 1 |
| | 1 oz. | 24 | .1 | .1 | — | — | — | 6.2 | 2 |
| | ½ cup | 106 | .6 | .2 | — | — | — | 27.5 | 1 |
| Fruit cocktail, canned in heavy syrup | 100 g | 76 | .4 | .1 | — | — | — | 19.7 | 5 |
| | 1 oz. | 22 | .1 | — | — | — | — | 5.6 | 5 |
| | ½ cup | 97 | .5 | .1 | — | — | — | 25.2 | 1 |
| Grapefruit, fresh | 100 g | 41 | .5 | .1 | — | — | — | 10.6 | 6 |
| | 1 oz. | 12 | .1 | .1 | — | — | — | 3.0 | 1 |
| | ½ med. | 49 | .5 | .1 | — | — | — | 12.8 | — |
| Grapefruit juice, canned, sweetened | 100 g | 53 | .5 | .1 | — | — | — | 12.8 | 1 |
| | 1 fl. oz. | 17 | .1 | — | — | — | — | 3.7 | 1 |
| | ½ cup | 66 | .6 | .1 | — | — | — | 16.0 | — |
| Grapes, fresh | 100 g | 69 | 1.3 | 1.0 | — | — | — | 15.7 | 1 |
| | 1 oz. | 20 | .4 | .3 | — | — | — | 4.6 | 3 |
| | 20 grapes | 54 | 1.0 | 1.0 | — | — | — | 13.8 | 1 |
| Grape juice, canned or bottled | 100 g | 66 | .2 | — | — | — | — | 16.6 | 3 |
| | 1 fl. oz. | 21 | .1 | — | — | — | — | 5.2 | 2 |
| | ½ cup | 83 | .3 | — | — | — | — | 20.9 | 1 |
| Lemon juice | 100 g | 25 | .5 | .2 | — | — | — | 8.0 | 2 |
| | 1 oz.=2 T. | 7 | .2 | .1 | — | — | — | 2.3 | 1 |
| Lemonade with sugar, frozen, diluted | 100 g | 44 | .1 | — | — | — | — | 11.4 | — |
| | 1 fl. oz. | 13 | — | — | — | — | — | 3.3 | — |
| | 6 fl. oz. | 81 | .1 | — | — | — | — | 21.1 | — |
| Lime, fresh | 100 g | 28 | .7 | .2 | — | — | — | 9.5 | 1 |
| | 1 oz. | 8 | .2 | .1 | — | — | — | 2.7 | 2 |
| | 1 med. | 19 | .5 | .1 | — | — | — | 6.4 | 1 |
| Mango, fresh | 100 g | 66 | .7 | .4 | — | — | — | 16.8 | 1 |
| | 1 oz. | 19 | .2 | .1 | — | — | — | 4.8 | 7 |
| | 1 med. | 152 | 1.6 | .9 | — | — | — | 38.8 | 2 |
| Muskmelons Cantaloupe | 100 g | 30 | .7 | .1 | — | — | — | 7.5 | 16 |
| | 1 oz. | 9 | .2 | — | — | — | — | 2.1 | 12 |
| | 1 med. | 159 | 3.7 | .5 | — | — | — | 39.8 | 3 |
| Honeydew | 100 g | 33 | .8 | .3 | — | — | — | 7.7 | 64 |
| | 1 oz. | 9 | .2 | .1 | — | — | — | 2.2 | 12 |
| | 1 cup | 56 | 1.4 | .5 | — | — | — | 13.1 | 3 |

# Nutritional Guide

| | Quantity or Amounts | Calories | Protein (g) | Total Fat (g) | Saturated Fat (g) | Unsaturated Fat (g) | Cholesterol (mg) | Carbohydrates (g) | Sodium (mg) |
|---|---|---|---|---|---|---|---|---|---|
| Nectarines | 100 g | 64 | .6 | — | — | — | — | 17.1 | 6 |
| | 1 oz. | 18 | .2 | — | — | — | — | 4.9 | 2 |
| | 1 med. | 88 | .8 | — | — | — | — | 23.6 | 1 |
| Oranges, fresh | 100 g | 49 | 1.0 | .2 | — | — | — | 12.2 | 1 |
| | 1 oz. | 14 | .3 | .1 | — | — | — | 3.5 | 1 |
| | 1 med. | 64 | 1.3 | .3 | — | — | — | 16.0 | 1 |
| Orange juice, frozen, diluted | 100 g | 45 | .7 | .1 | — | — | — | 10.7 | 1 |
| | 1 oz. | 13 | .2 | — | — | — | — | 3.1 | 1 |
| | 6 fl. oz. | 92 | 1.3 | .2 | — | — | — | 21.7 | 2 |
| Papaya | 100 g | 39 | .6 | .1 | — | — | — | 10.0 | 3 |
| | 1 oz. | 11 | .2 | — | — | — | — | 2.9 | 1 |
| | 1 cup | 55 | .8 | .1 | — | — | — | 14.0 | 4 |
| Peaches, fresh | 100 g | 38 | .6 | .1 | — | — | — | 9.7 | 1 |
| | 1 oz. | 11 | .2 | — | — | — | — | 2.8 | — |
| | 1 med. | 38 | .6 | .1 | — | — | — | 9.7 | 1 |
| Peach slices, canned in heavy syrup | 100 g | 78 | .4 | .1 | — | — | — | 20.1 | 2 |
| | 1 oz. | 22 | .1 | — | — | — | — | 5.7 | 1 |
| | ½ cup | 98 | .5 | .2 | — | — | — | 25.3 | 2 |
| Pears, fresh | 100 g | 61 | .7 | .4 | — | — | — | 15.3 | 2 |
| | 1 oz. | 17 | .2 | .1 | — | — | — | 4.4 | 1 |
| | 1 med. | 101 | 1.1 | .7 | — | — | — | 25.4 | 3 |
| Pears, canned in heavy syrup | 100 g | 76 | .2 | .2 | — | — | — | 19.6 | 1 |
| | 1 oz. | 22 | .1 | .1 | — | — | — | 5.6 | 1 |
| | 1 cup | 194 | .5 | .5 | — | — | — | 50.0 | 3 |
| Persimmons, fresh | 100 g | 77 | .7 | .4 | — | — | — | 19.7 | 6 |
| | 1 oz. | 22 | .2 | .1 | — | — | — | 5.6 | 2 |
| | 1 med. | 129 | 1.2 | .7 | — | — | — | 33.1 | 10 |
| Pineapple, fresh | 100 g | 54 | .4 | .2 | — | — | — | 13.7 | 1 |
| | 1 oz. | 15 | .1 | .1 | — | — | — | 3.9 | 1 |
| | 1 cup | 81 | .6 | .3 | — | — | — | 21.2 | 2 |
| Pineapple slices, canned in heavy syrup | 100 g | 74 | .3 | .1 | — | — | — | 19.4 | 1 |
| | 1 oz. | 21 | .1 | — | — | — | — | 5.5 | — |
| | 1 cup | 189 | .8 | .3 | — | — | — | 49.5 | 3 |
| Pineapple juice, canned, unsweetened | 100 g | 55 | .4 | .1 | — | — | — | 13.5 | 1 |
| | 1 oz. | 17 | .1 | — | — | — | — | 4.2 | — |
| | 1 cup | 138 | 1.0 | .3 | — | — | — | 33.8 | 2 |
| Plums, fresh | 100 g | 48 | .5 | .2 | — | — | — | 12.3 | 1 |
| | 1 oz. | 14 | .1 | .1 | — | — | — | 3.5 | 1 |
| | 1 med. | 32 | .3 | .1 | — | — | — | 8.1 | 1 |
| Plums, canned in heavy syrup | 100 g | 83 | .4 | .1 | — | — | — | 21.6 | 1 |
| | 1 oz. | 24 | .1 | — | — | — | — | 6.1 | — |
| | ½ cup | 106 | .5 | .1 | — | — | — | 27.6 | 1 |

| | Quantity or Amounts | Calories | Protein (g) | Total Fat (g) | Saturated Fat (g) | Unsaturated Fat (g) | Cholesterol (mg) | Carbohydrates (g) | Sodium (m |
|---|---|---|---|---|---|---|---|---|---|
| Prunes, soft dried, uncooked | 100 g | 255 | 2.1 | .6 | — | — | — | 67.4 | 8 |
| | 1 oz. | 73 | .6 | .2 | — | — | — | 19.2 | 2 |
| | 10 prunes | 260 | 2.1 | .6 | — | — | — | 68.7 | 8 |
| Prune juice | 100 g | 77 | .4 | .1 | — | — | — | 19.0 | 2 |
| | 1 oz. | 22 | .1 | — | — | — | — | 5.4 | 1 |
| | ½ cup | 99 | .5 | .1 | — | — | — | 24.3 | 5 |
| Raisins, seedless, uncooked | 100 g | 289 | 2.5 | .2 | — | — | — | 77.4 | 27 |
| | 1 oz. | 82 | .7 | .1 | — | — | — | 21.9 | 8 |
| | ½ cup | 209 | 1.8 | .1 | — | — | — | 56.0 | 20 |
| Raspberries, red, fresh | 100 g | 57 | 1.2 | .5 | — | — | — | 13.6 | 1 |
| | 1 oz. | 16 | .3 | .1 | — | — | — | 3.9 | — |
| | 1 cup | 70 | 1.5 | .6 | — | — | — | 16.7 | 1 |
| Rhubarb, cooked, sweetened, solids and liquid | 100 g | 141 | .5 | .1 | — | — | — | 36.0 | 2 |
| | 1 oz. | 40 | .1 | — | — | — | — | 10.2 | 1 |
| | ½ cup | 190 | .7 | .1 | — | — | — | 48.6 | 3 |
| Strawberries, fresh | 100 g | 37 | .7 | .5 | — | — | — | 8.4 | 1 |
| | 1 oz. | 11 | .2 | .1 | — | — | — | 2.4 | — |
| | 1 cup | 55 | 1.0 | .7 | — | — | — | 12.5 | 1 |
| Tangerines | 100 g | 46 | .8 | .2 | — | — | — | 11.6 | 2 |
| | 1 oz. | 13 | .2 | .1 | — | — | — | 3.3 | 1 |
| | 1 med. | 39 | .7 | .2 | — | — | — | 10.0 | 2 |
| Tomatoes, canned, solids and liquid | 100 g | 21 | 1.0 | .2 | — | — | — | 4.3 | 130 |
| | 1 oz. | 6 | .3 | .1 | — | — | — | 1.2 | 37 |
| | 1 cup | 51 | 2.4 | .5 | — | — | — | 10.4 | 313 |
| Tomatoes, fresh, sliced | 100 g | 22 | 1.1 | .2 | — | — | — | 4.7 | 3 |
| | 1 oz. | 6 | .3 | .1 | — | — | — | 1.3 | 1 |
| | 1 med. | 40 | 2.0 | .4 | — | — | — | 8.6 | 5 |
| Tomato juice, canned with salt | 100 g | 19 | .9 | .1 | — | — | — | 4.3 | 200 |
| | 1 oz. | 5 | .2 | — | — | — | — | 1.2 | 57 |
| | 6 fl. oz. | 35 | 1.5 | .2 | — | — | — | 7.8 | 413 |
| Tomato paste | 100 g | 82 | 3.4 | .4 | — | — | — | 18.6 | 38 |
| | 1 oz. | 23 | .9 | .1 | — | — | — | 5.3 | 11 |
| | 6 oz. can | 139 | 5.8 | .7 | — | — | — | 31.6 | 65 |
| Tomato sauce | 100 g | — | — | — | — | — | — | — | — |
| | 1 oz. | — | — | — | — | — | — | — | — |
| | 1 cup | 80 | — | — | — | — | — | 16.8 | — |

**262**

| | Quantity or Amounts | Calories | Protein (g) | Total Fat (g) | Saturated Fat (g) | Unsaturated Fat (g) | Cholesterol (mg) | Carbohydrates (g) | Sodium (mg) |
|---|---|---|---|---|---|---|---|---|---|
| Watermelon | 100 g | 25 | .5 | .2 | — | — | — | 6.4 | 1 |
| | 1 oz. | 7 | .2 | .1 | — | — | — | 1.8 | — |
| | 1 cup | 42 | .8 | .3 | — | — | — | 10.2 | 2 |

## Jams, Jellies, Sugars, Syrups

| | Quantity or Amounts | Calories | Protein (g) | Total Fat (g) | Saturated Fat (g) | Unsaturated Fat (g) | Cholesterol (mg) | Carbohydrates (g) | Sodium (mg) |
|---|---|---|---|---|---|---|---|---|---|
| Honey | 100 g | 304 | .3 | 0 | — | — | — | 82.3 | 5 |
| | 1 oz. | 87 | .1 | 0 | — | — | — | 24.0 | 1 |
| | 1 T. | 61 | — | 0 | — | — | — | 17.0 | 1 |
| Jams and preserves | 100 g | 272 | .6 | .1 | — | — | — | 70.0 | 12 |
| | 1 oz. | 77 | .2 | — | — | — | — | 20.0 | 3 |
| | 1 T. | 54 | .1 | — | — | — | — | 14.0 | 2 |
| Jellies | 100 g | 273 | .1 | .1 | — | — | — | 70.6 | 17 |
| | 1 oz. | 78 | — | — | — | — | — | 20.0 | 5 |
| | 1 T. | 49 | — | — | — | — | — | 13.0 | 3 |
| Marmalade | 100 g | 257 | .5 | .1 | — | — | — | 70.1 | 14 |
| | 1 oz. | 73 | .1 | — | — | — | — | 20.0 | 4 |
| | 1 T. | 51 | — | — | — | — | — | 14.0 | 3 |
| Molasses, cane, light | 100 g | 252 | — | — | — | — | — | 65.0 | 15 |
| | 1 oz. | 72 | — | — | — | — | — | 19.0 | 4 |
| | 1 T. | 48 | — | — | — | — | — | 13.0 | 3 |
| Molasses, cane, medium | 100 g | 232 | — | — | — | — | — | 60.0 | 37 |
| | 1 oz. | 66 | — | — | — | — | — | 17.0 | 10 |
| | 1 T. | 46 | — | — | — | — | — | 12.0 | 7 |
| Molasses, cane, blackstrap | 100 g | 213 | — | — | — | — | — | 55.0 | 96 |
| | 1 oz. | 61 | — | — | — | — | — | 16.0 | 27 |
| | 1 T. | 43 | — | — | — | — | — | 11.0 | 19 |
| Sugar, beet or cane | | | | | | | | | |
| Brown | 100 g | 373 | 0 | 0 | — | — | — | 96.4 | 30 |
| | 1 oz. | 106 | 0 | 0 | — | — | — | 28.0 | 9 |
| | 1 cup | 791 | 0 | 0 | — | — | — | 210.0 | 64 |
| Granulated | 100 g | 385 | 0 | 0 | — | — | — | 99.5 | 1 |
| | 1 oz. | 110 | 0 | 0 | — | — | — | 28.4 | — |
| | 1 T. | 46 | 0 | 0 | — | — | — | 11.4 | — |
| | 1 t. | 15 | 0 | 0 | — | — | — | 4.0 | — |
| Powdered | 100 g | 385 | 0 | 0 | — | — | — | 99.5 | 1 |
| | 1 oz. | 110 | 0 | 0 | — | — | — | 28.4 | — |
| | 1 cup | 462 | 0 | 0 | — | — | — | 119.4 | 1 |
| | 1 T. | 31 | 0 | 0 | — | — | — | 8.0 | — |
| Sugar, maple | 100 g | 348 | — | — | — | — | — | 90.0 | — |
| | 1 oz. | 99 | — | — | — | — | — | 26.0 | — |

# Nutritional Guide

| | Quantity or Amounts | Calories | Protein (g) | Total Fat (g) | Saturated Fat (g) | Unsaturated Fat (g) | Cholesterol (mg) | Carbohydrates (g) | Sodium (mg) |
|---|---|---|---|---|---|---|---|---|---|
| **Syrups** | | | | | | | | | |
| Cane | 100 g | 263 | 0 | 0 | — | — | — | 68.0 | — |
| | 1 oz. | 75 | 0 | 0 | — | — | — | 19.0 | — |
| | 1 T. | 53 | 0 | 0 | — | — | — | 13.0 | — |
| Maple | 100 g | 252 | 0 | 0 | — | — | — | 65.0 | 10 |
| | 1 oz. | 72 | 0 | 0 | — | — | — | 19.0 | 3 |
| | 1 T. | 50 | 0 | 0 | — | — | — | 13.0 | 2 |
| Sorghum | 100 g | 257 | 0 | 0 | — | — | — | 68.0 | — |
| | 1 oz. | 73 | 0 | 0 | — | — | — | 19.0 | — |
| | 1 T. | 51 | 0 | 0 | — | — | — | 13.0 | — |

## Meats: Beef, Lamb, Organ, Pork, Veal, Venison

| | Quantity or Amounts | Calories | Protein (g) | Total Fat (g) | Saturated Fat (g) | Unsaturated Fat (g) | Cholesterol (mg) | Carbohydrates (g) | Sodium (mg) |
|---|---|---|---|---|---|---|---|---|---|
| Beef, corned, cooked | 100 g | 372 | 22.9 | 30.4 | 15.0 | 13.0 | — | 0 | 1740 |
| | 1 oz. | 106 | 6.5 | 8.7 | 4.3 | 3.7 | — | 0 | 497 |
| Beef, dried, chipped | 100 g | 203 | 34.3 | 6.3 | 3.0 | 3.0 | 27 | 0 | 4300 |
| | 1 oz. | 58 | 9.8 | 1.8 | .9 | .9 | 8 | 0 | 1229 |
| Beef, fresh, choice grade, retail cuts | | | | | | | | | |
| Hamburger, regular grind, cooked | 100 g | 286 | 24.2 | 20.3 | 10.0 | 9.0 | 95 | 0 | 47 |
| | 1 oz. | 82 | 6.9 | 5.8 | 3.0 | 3.0 | 27 | 0 | 13 |
| Hamburger, lean grind, cooked | 100 g | 219 | 27.4 | 11.3 | 6.0 | 5.0 | 95 | 0 | 48 |
| | 1 oz. | 63 | 7.8 | 3.2 | 2.0 | 1.0 | 27 | 0 | 14 |
| Roast, chuck (pot roast), cooked | 100 g | 327 | 26.0 | 23.9 | 10.0 | 10.0 | 95 | 0 | 60 |
| (81% lean, 19% fat) | 1 oz. | 93 | 7.4 | 6.8 | 3.0 | 3.0 | 27 | 0 | 17 |
| Roast, rib, cooked | 100 g | 440 | 19.9 | 39.4 | 19.0 | 18.0 | 95 | 0 | 60 |
| (64% lean, 36% fat) | 1 oz. | 126 | 5.7 | 11.3 | 5.0 | 5.0 | 27 | 0 | 17 |
| Roast, rump, cooked | 100 g | 347 | 23.6 | 27.3 | 13.0 | 13.0 | 95 | 0 | 197 |
| (75% lean, 25% fat) | 1 oz. | 99 | 6.7 | 7.8 | 4.0 | 4.0 | 27 | 0 | 56 |
| Steak | | | | | | | | | |
| Flank, braised | 100 g | 196 | 30.5 | 7.3 | — | — | 95 | 0 | 60 |
| (100% lean) | 1 oz. | 56 | 8.7 | 2.1 | — | — | 27 | 0 | 17 |
| Round, broiled | 100 g | 261 | 28.6 | 14.4 | 7.0 | 6.0 | 95 | 0 | 60 |
| (81% lean, 19% fat) | 1 oz. | 75 | 8.2 | 4.4 | 2.0 | 2.0 | 27 | 0 | 17 |
| Sirloin, broiled | 100 g | 408 | 22.2 | 34.7 | 15.0 | 15.0 | 95 | 0 | 60 |
| (66% lean, 34% fat) | 1 oz. | 117 | 6.3 | 9.9 | 4.3 | 4.3 | 27 | 0 | 17 |
| T-bone, broiled | 100 g | 473 | 19.5 | 43.2 | 18.0 | 22.7 | 95 | 0 | 60 |
| (56% lean, 44% fat) | 1 oz. | 135 | 5.6 | 12.2 | 5.1 | 6.5 | 27 | 0 | 17 |
| Lamb, choice grade, retail cuts | | | | | | | | | |
| Leg, roasted | 100 g | 279 | 25.3 | 18.9 | 8.9 | 8.9 | 98 | 0 | 70 |

**264**

# Nutritional Guide

| | Quantity or Amounts | Calories | Protein (g) | Total Fat (g) | Saturated Fat (g) | Unsaturated Fat (g) | Cholesterol (mg) | Carbohydrates (g) | Sodium (mg) |
|---|---|---|---|---|---|---|---|---|---|
| (83% lean, 17% fat) | 1 oz. | 80 | 7.2 | 5.4 | 2.0 | 2.0 | 28 | 0 | 20 |
| Loin chops, broiled | 100 g | 359 | 22.0 | 29.4 | — | — | 98 | 0 | 70 |
| (66% lean, 34% fat) | 1 oz. | 103 | 6.3 | 8.4 | — | — | 28 | 0 | 20 |
| Shoulder roast | 100 g | 338 | 21.7 | 27.2 | 12.8 | 12.9 | 98 | 0 | 70 |
| (74% lean, 26% fat) | 1 oz. | 97 | 6.2 | 7.8 | 4.0 | 4.0 | 28 | 0 | 20 |
| **Organ meats** | | | | | | | | | |
| Brains, beef, calf, | 100 g | 125 | 10.4 | 8.6 | — | — | 2000 | .8 | 125 |
| hog, raw | 1 oz. | 36 | 2.9 | 2.5 | — | — | 572 | .2 | 36 |
| Heart, beef, braised | 100 g | 372 | 25.8 | 29.0 | — | — | 274 | .1 | — |
| | 1 oz. | 106 | 7.4 | 8.3 | — | — | 78 | — | — |
| Heart, chicken, | 100 g | 173 | 25.3 | 7.2 | — | — | 231 | .1 | 69 |
| simmered | 1 oz. | 49 | 7.2 | 2.1 | — | — | 66 | — | 20 |
| Heart, hog, braised | 100 g | 195 | 30.8 | 6.9 | — | — | — | .3 | 65 |
| | 1 oz. | 56 | 8.8 | 1.9 | — | — | — | — | 19 |
| Kidneys, beef, braised | 100 g | 252 | 33.0 | 12.0 | — | — | 375 | .8 | 253 |
| | 1 oz. | 72 | 9.4 | 3.4 | — | — | 107 | .2 | 72 |
| Liver, beef, fried | 100 g | 229 | 26.4 | 10.6 | — | — | 438 | 5.3 | 184 |
| | 1 oz. | 65 | 7.5 | 3.0 | — | — | 125 | 1.5 | 53 |
| Liver, calf, fried | 100 g | 261 | 29.5 | 13.2 | — | — | 438 | 4.0 | 118 |
| | 1 oz. | 75 | 8.4 | 3.8 | — | — | 125 | 1.1 | 34 |
| Liver, chicken, | 100 g | 165 | 26.5 | 4.4 | — | — | 746 | 3.1 | 61 |
| simmered | 1 oz. | 47 | 7.9 | 1.3 | — | — | 213 | .9 | 17 |
| Liver, hog, fried | 100 g | 241 | 29.9 | 11.5 | 3.0 | 5.0 | — | 2.5 | 111 |
| | 1 oz. | 69 | 8.5 | 3.3 | .9 | 1.4 | — | .7 | 32 |
| Sweetbreads, | 100 g | 320 | 25.9 | 23.2 | — | — | 466 | 0 | 116 |
| beef, braised | 1 oz. | 91 | 7.4 | 6.6 | — | — | 133 | 0 | 33 |
| Tongue, beef, cooked | 100 g | 244 | 21.5 | 16.7 | — | — | — | .4 | 61 |
| | 1 oz. | 70 | 6.1 | 4.8 | — | — | — | .1 | 17 |
| Tripe, beef, cooked | 100 g | 100 | 19.1 | 2.0 | — | — | — | 0 | 72 |
| | 1 oz. | 29 | 5.5 | .6 | — | — | — | 0 | 21 |
| **Pork, cured** | | | | | | | | | |
| Bacon, Canadian, | 100 g | 277 | 27.6 | 17.5 | 5.0 | 7.0 | 216 | .3 | 2555 |
| fried, drained | 1 oz. | 79 | 7.9 | 5.0 | 1.4 | 2.0 | 62 | .1 | 730 |
| Bacon, thick sliced, | 100 g | 611 | 30.4 | 52.0 | 17.0 | 30.0 | — | 3.2 | 1021 |
| fried, drained | 1 oz. | 175 | 8.7 | 14.8 | 4.8 | 8.6 | — | .9 | 292 |
| | 2 slices | 143 | 6.4 | 12.5 | 4.3 | 7.5 | — | .8 | 245 |
| Ham, country style, | 100 g | 389 | 16.9 | 35.0 | 13.0 | 18.0 | — | .3 | — |
| long, dry cure | 1 oz. | 111 | 4.8 | 10.0 | 3.7 | 5.0 | — | .1 | — |
| Ham, canned | 100 g | 193 | 18.3 | 12.3 | 4.0 | 6.0 | — | 0 | 1100 |
| | 1 oz. | 55 | 5.2 | 3.4 | 1.1 | 1.7 | — | 0 | 314 |

| | Quantity or Amounts | Calories | Protein (g) | Total Fat (g) | Saturated Fat (g) | Unsaturated Fat (g) | Cholesterol (mg) | Carbohydrates (g) | Sodium (mg) |
|---|---|---|---|---|---|---|---|---|---|
| Ham, light cure, baked | 100 g | 289 | 20.9 | 22.1 | 8.0 | 12.0 | — | 0 | — |
| | 1 oz. | 83 | 6.0 | 6.3 | 2.3 | 3.4 | — | 0 | — |
| **Pork, fresh,** | | | | | | | | | |
| trimmed for retail cuts | | | | | | | | | |
| Boston butt, roasted | 100 g | 353 | 22.5 | 28.5 | 10.0 | 13.0 | 89 | 0 | 65 |
| (79% lean, 21% fat) | 1 oz. | 101 | 6.4 | 8.1 | 2.8 | 3.8 | 25 | 0 | 19 |
| Ham, roasted | 100 g | 374 | 23.0 | 30.6 | 11.0 | 12.0 | 89 | 0 | 65 |
| (74% lean, 26% fat) | 1 oz. | 107 | 6.6 | 8.7 | 3.0 | 3.4 | 25 | 0 | 19 |
| Loin chops, broiled | 100 g | 391 | 24.7 | 31.7 | 10.0 | 13.0 | 89 | 0 | 65 |
| (72% lean, 28% fat) | 1 oz. | 112 | 7.1 | 9.1 | 2.8 | 3.7 | 25 | 0 | 19 |
| Spareribs, braised | 100 g | 440 | 20.8 | 38.9 | 14.0 | 19.0 | 89 | 0 | 65 |
| | 1 oz. | 126 | 5.9 | 11.1 | 4.0 | 5.4 | 25 | 0 | 19 |
| **Veal steak or cutlet,** | | | | | | | | | |
| broiled | 100 g | 216 | 27.1 | 11.1 | 6.0 | 5.0 | 101 | 0 | 80 |
| (79% lean, 21% fat) | 1 oz. | 62 | 7.7 | 3.2 | 1.7 | 1.4 | 29 | 0 | 23 |
| Venison, lean meat, raw | 100 g | 126 | 21.0 | 4.0 | 3.0 | 1.0 | — | 0 | — |
| | 1 oz. | 36 | 6.0 | 1.1 | .9 | .3 | — | 0 | — |

## Meats: Cold Cuts, Luncheon, Sausages

| | Quantity or Amounts | Calories | Protein (g) | Total Fat (g) | Saturated Fat (g) | Unsaturated Fat (g) | Cholesterol (mg) | Carbohydrates (g) | Sodium (mg) |
|---|---|---|---|---|---|---|---|---|---|
| Boiled ham | 100 g | 234 | 19.0 | 17.0 | 6.0 | 9.0 | — | 0 | — |
| | 1 oz. | 66 | 5.4 | 4.8 | 1.7 | 2.6 | — | 0 | — |
| Bologna, all meat | 100 g | 277 | 13.3 | 22.8 | — | — | — | 3.7 | 230 |
| | 1 oz. | 86 | 3.4 | 7.8 | — | — | — | .3 | 66 |
| | 1 slice | 73 | 2.7 | 6.2 | — | — | — | .2 | 53 |
| Braunschweiger | 100 g | 319 | 14.8 | 27.4 | 10.0 | 14.0 | — | 2.3 | — |
| | 1 oz. | 91 | 4.2 | 7.8 | 2.9 | 4.0 | — | .7 | — |
| Brockwurst | 100 g | 264 | 11.3 | 23.7 | — | — | — | .6 | — |
| | 1 oz. | 75 | 3.2 | 6.8 | — | — | — | .2 | — |
| Brown and serve sausage, | 100 g | 422 | 16.5 | 37.8 | — | — | — | 2.8 | — |
| browned | 1 oz. | 111 | 3.8 | 10.2 | — | — | — | .8 | — |
| | 1 link | 72 | 2.8 | 6.4 | — | — | — | .5 | — |
| Country style | 100 g | 345 | 15.1 | 31.9 | 11.0 | 16.0 | — | 0 | — |
| smoked sausage | 1 oz. | 99 | 4.3 | 8.9 | 3.0 | 4.6 | — | 0 | — |
| Deviled ham, canned | 100 g | 351 | 13.9 | 32.3 | 12.0 | 17.0 | — | 0 | — |
| | 1 oz. | 100 | 3.9 | 9.2 | 3.4 | 4.9 | — | 0 | — |
| Frankfurters, raw, | 100 g | 309 | 12.5 | 27.6 | — | — | — | 1.8 | 1100 |
| all samples | 1 oz. | 88 | 3.6 | 7.9 | — | — | — | .5 | 314 |
| All beef | 1 frank | 143 | — | — | — | — | — | 1.4 | — |

# Nutritional Guide

| | Quantity or Amounts | Calories | Protein (g) | Total Fat (g) | Saturated Fat (g) | Unsaturated Fat (g) | Cholesterol (mg) | Carbohydrates (g) | Sodium (mg) |
|---|---|---|---|---|---|---|---|---|---|
| All meat | 1 frank | 134 | 5.9 | 11.5 | — | — | 62 | 1.1 | — |
| With cereal | 1 frank | 112 | 6.5 | 9.3 | — | — | — | — | — |
| With nonfat dry milk | 1 frank | 136 | 5.9 | 11.5 | — | — | — | 1.5 | — |
| Liverwurst | 100 g | 307 | 16.2 | 25.6 | — | — | — | 1.8 | — |
| | 1 oz. | 88 | 4.5 | 7.3 | — | — | — | .5 | — |
| Meat, potted | 100 g | 248 | 17.5 | 19.2 | — | — | — | 0 | — |
| (beef, chicken, turkey) | 1 oz. | 70 | 5.0 | 5.4 | — | — | — | 0 | — |
| Polish style sausage | 100 g | 304 | 15.7 | 25.8 | — | — | — | 0 | — |
| | 1 oz. | 87 | 4.5 | 7.4 | — | — | — | 0 | — |
| Pork, chopped, spiced | 100 g | 294 | 15.0 | 24.9 | 9.0 | 13.0 | — | 1.3 | 1234 |
| or unspiced Spam | 1 oz. | 83 | 4.3 | 7.1 | 2.6 | 3.7 | — | .4 | 350 |
| Pork sausage, fresh, | 100 g | 476 | 18.1 | 44.2 | 16.0 | 23.0 | — | — | 958 |
| bulk or links, cooked | 1 oz. | 129 | 4.9 | 11.9 | 4.6 | 6.6 | — | — | 259 |
| Salami, cooked | 100 g | 311 | 17.5 | 25.6 | — | — | — | 1.4 | — |
| | 1 oz. | 88 | 5.0 | 7.3 | — | — | — | .4 | — |
| Salami, dry | 100 g | 450 | 23.8 | 38.1 | — | — | — | 1.2 | — |
| | 1 oz. | 128 | 6.7 | 10.8 | — | — | — | .3 | — |
| Thuringer | 100 g | 307 | 18.6 | 24.5 | — | — | — | 1.6 | — |
| (summer sausage) | 1 oz. | 87 | 5.3 | 6.9 | — | — | — | .5 | — |
| Vienna sausage, canned | 100 g | 240 | 14.0 | 19.8 | — | — | — | .3 | — |
| | 1 oz. = 2 | 69 | 4.0 | 5.7 | — | — | — | .1 | — |

## Nuts, Nut Products, Relishes, Snacks

Nuts and nut products

| | Quantity or Amounts | Calories | Protein (g) | Total Fat (g) | Saturated Fat (g) | Unsaturated Fat (g) | Cholesterol (mg) | Carbohydrates (g) | Sodium (mg) |
|---|---|---|---|---|---|---|---|---|---|
| Almonds, shelled, fresh | 100 g. | 598 | 18.6 | 54.2 | 4.0 | 47.0 | — | 19.5 | 4 |
| | 1 oz. | 170 | 5.3 | 15.4 | 1.0 | 13.0 | — | 5.5 | 1 |
| Almonds, shelled, | 100 g | 627 | 18.6 | 57.7 | 5.0 | 51.0 | — | 19.5 | 198 |
| roasted in oil | 1 oz. = 22 | 178 | 5.3 | 16.4 | 1.4 | 15.0 | — | 5.5 | 56 |
| Cashews, roasted in oil | 100 g | 561 | 17.2 | 45.7 | 9.2 | 33.8 | — | 29.3 | 15 |
| | 1 oz. = 18 | 159 | 4.9 | 13.0 | 2.6 | 9.7 | — | 8.3 | 4 |
| Coconut, fresh | 100 g | 346 | 3.5 | 35.3 | 30.0 | 2.0 | — | 9.4 | 23 |
| | 1 oz. | 99 | 1.0 | 10.0 | 8.6 | .6 | — | 2.7 | 7 |
| Coconut, dried, | 100 g | 548 | 3.6 | 39.1 | 34.0 | 3.0 | — | 53.2 | — |
| shredded, sweetened | 1 oz. | 157 | 1.0 | 11.0 | 9.7 | .9 | — | 15.2 | — |
| | ½ cup | 252 | 1.6 | 16.0 | 15.5 | 1.4 | — | 24.3 | — |
| Coconut water (liquid | 100 g | 22 | .3 | .2 | — | — | — | 4.7 | 25 |
| from coconut) | 1 oz. | 6 | .1 | .1 | — | — | — | 1.3 | 7 |
| Peanuts, shelled, | 100 g | 585 | 26.0 | 48.7 | 11.0 | 35.0 | — | 18.8 | 418 |
| roasted, salted | 1 oz. | 166 | 7.4 | 14.1 | 3.0 | 10.0 | — | 5.3 | 119 |
| | ½ cup | 421 | 19.0 | 36.0 | — | — | — | 14.0 | 301 |

**267**

| | Quantity or Amounts | Calories | Protein (g) | Total Fat (g) | Saturated Fat (g) | Unsaturated Fat (g) | Cholesterol (mg) | Carbohydrates (g) | Sodium (m |
|---|---|---|---|---|---|---|---|---|---|
| Peanut butter with | 100 g | 589 | 25.2 | 50.6 | 9.0 | 39.0 | — | 18.8 | 627 |
| moderate amts. of oil, | 1 oz. | 168 | 7.2 | 14.5 | 2.6 | 11.0 | — | 5.4 | 179 |
| salt, and sugar | 1 T. | 94 | 4.0 | 8.1 | — | — | — | 3.0 | 97 |
| Pecans, shelled | 100 g | 687 | 9.2 | 71.2 | 5.0 | 59.0 | — | 14.6 | — |
| | 1 oz. | 195 | 2.6 | 20.2 | 1.4 | 17.0 | — | 4.1 | — |
| Pistachio nuts | 100 g | 594 | 19.3 | 53.7 | 5.0 | 45.0 | — | 19.0 | — |
| | 1 oz. | 170 | 5.5 | 15.3 | 1.4 | 12.9 | — | 5.4 | — |
| Sunflower, pumpkin | 100 g | 560 | 24.0 | 47.3 | 6.0 | 39.0 | — | 19.9 | 920 |
| seeds, hulled | 1 oz. | 160 | 6.9 | 13.5 | 1.7 | 11.0 | — | 5.7 | 263 |
| Walnuts, black, shelled | 100 g | 628 | 20.5 | 59.3 | 4.0 | 49.0 | — | 14.8 | 3 |
| | 1 oz. | 178 | 5.8 | 16.8 | 1.1 | 14.0 | — | 4.2 | 1 |
| Walnuts, English, | 100 g | 651 | 14.8 | 64.0 | 4.0 | 50.0 | — | 15.8 | 2 |
| shelled | 1 oz. | 185 | 4.2 | 18.1 | 1.1 | 14.2 | — | 4.5 | 1 |
| | 1 cup | 781 | 17.8 | 76.8 | — | — | — | 19.0 | 2 |
| | | | | | | | | | |
| **Relishes** | | | | | | | | | |
| Olives, green, large | 100 g | 116 | 1.4 | 12.7 | — | — | — | 1.3 | 2400 |
| | 1 oz. | 33 | .4 | 3.6 | — | — | — | .4 | 685 |
| | 10 olives | 45 | .5 | 4.9 | — | — | — | .5 | 926 |
| Olives, ripe, large | 100 g | 184 | 1.2 | 20.1 | 2.0 | 16.0 | — | 3.2 | 750 |
| | 1 oz. | 52 | .3 | 5.7 | .6 | 4.6 | — | .9 | 214 |
| | 10 olives | 73 | .5 | 8.0 | — | — | — | 1.3 | 297 |
| | | | | | | | | | |
| **Pickles** | | | | | | | | | |
| Dill, whole, 4″ | 100 g | 11 | .7 | .2 | — | — | — | 2.2 | 1428 |
| | 1 oz. | 3 | .2 | .1 | — | — | — | .6 | 408 |
| | 1 pickle | 7 | .5 | .1 | — | — | — | 1.4 | 928 |
| Fresh, bread and butter | 100 g | 73 | .9 | .2 | — | — | — | 17.9 | 673 |
| | 1 oz. | 21 | .3 | .1 | — | — | — | 5.1 | 192 |
| Sour, whole, large | 100 g | 10 | .5 | .2 | — | — | — | 2.0 | 1353 |
| | 1 oz. | 3 | .1 | .1 | — | — | — | .6 | 387 |
| | 1 pickle | 14 | .7 | .3 | — | — | — | 2.7 | 1827 |
| Sweet gherkins, | 100 g | 146 | .7 | .4 | — | — | — | 36.5 | — |
| whole, 3″ | 1 oz. | 42 | .2 | .1 | — | — | — | 10.4 | — |
| | 1 pickle | 51 | .2 | .1 | — | — | — | 12.8 | — |
| Sweet pickle relish | 1 T. | 21 | .1 | .1 | — | — | — | 5.1 | 107 |
| | | | | | | | | | |
| **Snacks** | | | | | | | | | |
| Corn chips | 1 oz. | 159 | — | — | — | — | — | 14.8 | — |

| | Quantity or Amounts | Calories | Protein (g) | Total Fat (g) | Saturated Fat (g) | Unsaturated Fat (g) | Cholesterol (mg) | Carbohydrates (g) | Sodium (mg) |
|---|---|---|---|---|---|---|---|---|---|
| **Crackers** | | | | | | | | | |
| Cheese flavored | 100 g | 479 | 11.2 | 21.3 | 8.0 | 11.0 | — | 60.4 | 1039 |
| | 1 oz. | 136 | 3.2 | 6.1 | 2.3 | 3.0 | — | 17.1 | 290 |
| | 10 crackers | 165 | 3.9 | 7.3 | — | — | — | 20.8 | 357 |
| Club crackers (butter) | 100 g | 458 | 7.0 | 17.8 | — | — | — | 67.3 | 1092 |
| | 1 oz. | 131 | 2.0 | 5.1 | — | — | — | 19.2 | 312 |
| | 10 crackers | 151 | 2.3 | 5.9 | — | — | — | 22.2 | 360 |
| Graham, plain | 100 g | 384 | 8.0 | 9.4 | — | — | — | 73.3 | 670 |
| | 1 oz. | 110 | 2.3 | 2.7 | — | — | — | 20.9 | 191 |
| | 1 $(5 \times 2\frac{1}{2})$ | 55 | 1.1 | 1.3 | — | — | — | 10.4 | 95 |
| Oyster | 100 g | 439 | 9.2 | 13.1 | — | — | — | 70.6 | 1100 |
| | 1 oz. | 125 | 2.6 | 3.7 | — | — | — | 20.1 | 312 |
| | 10 crackers | 33 | .7 | 1.0 | — | — | — | 5.3 | 83 |
| Ritz | 1 cracker | 16 | — | — | — | — | — | 2.1 | — |
| Ry-Krisp | 1 cracker | 27 | — | — | — | — | — | 4.5 | — |
| Saltines | 100 g | 433 | 9.0 | 12.0 | 3.0 | 8.0 | — | 71.5 | 1100 |
| | 1 oz.=10 | 123 | 2.6 | 3.4 | .8 | 2.3 | — | 20.3 | 312 |
| Soda | 100 g | 439 | 9.2 | 13.1 | — | — | — | 70.4 | 1100 |
| | 1 oz.=10 | 125 | 2.6 | 3.7 | — | — | — | 20.1 | 312 |
| Triscuit | 1 cracker | 21 | — | — | — | — | — | 3.0 | — |
| Wheat thins | 100 g | 403 | 8.4 | 13.8 | — | — | — | 68.2 | 547 |
| | 1 cracker | 9 | .1 | .2 | — | — | — | 1.2 | 10 |
| Popcorn, plain | 100 g | 386 | 12.7 | 5.0 | 1.0 | 4.0 | — | 76.7 | 3 |
| | 1 oz.=$4\frac{1}{2}$ c. | 109 | 3.6 | 1.4 | .3 | 1.1 | — | 21.7 | 1 |
| Popcorn, butter and salt | 100 g | 456 | 9.8 | 21.8 | 10.0 | 10.0 | — | 59.1 | 1940 |
| | 1 oz.=3 c. | 129 | 2.8 | 6.2 | 2.9 | 2.9 | — | 16.8 | 554 |
| Popcorn, sugar-coated | 100 g | 383 | 6.1 | 3.5 | 1.0 | 2.0 | — | 85.4 | 1 |
| | 1 oz.=$\frac{3}{4}$ c. | 109 | 1.7 | 1.0 | .3 | .6 | — | 24.2 | 1 |
| Potato chips | 100 g | 568 | 5.3 | 39.8 | 10.0 | 28.0 | — | 50.0 | 1000 |
| | 1 oz. | 162 | 1.5 | 11.3 | 2.9 | 8.0 | — | 14.3 | 285 |
| | 10 chips | 114 | 1.1 | 8.0 | — | — | — | 10.0 | — |
| Pretzels | 100 g | 390 | 9.8 | 4.5 | — | — | — | 75.9 | 1680 |
| | 1 oz. | 112 | 2.8 | 1.3 | — | — | — | 21.7 | 480 |
| | 10 sticks | 23 | .6 | .3 | — | — | — | 4.6 | 101 |
| | 10 twists | 117 | 2.9 | 1.4 | — | — | — | 22.8 | 504 |

## Poultry: Chicken, Duck, Goose, Turkey

| | Quantity or Amounts | Calories | Protein (g) | Total Fat (g) | Saturated Fat (g) | Unsaturated Fat (g) | Cholesterol (mg) | Carbohydrates (g) | Sodium (mg) |
|---|---|---|---|---|---|---|---|---|---|
| Chicken, light meat, cooked | 100g | 166 | 31.6 | 3.4 | — | — | 80 | 0 | 64 |
| | 1 oz. | 47 | 9.0 | .9 | — | — | 23 | 0 | 18 |
| | $\frac{1}{2}$ breast | 160 | 25.7 | 5.1 | — | — | — | — | — |

# Nutritional Guide

| | Quantity or Amounts | Calories | Protein (g) | Total Fat (g) | Saturated Fat (g) | Unsaturated Fat (g) | Cholesterol (mg) | Carbohydrates (g) | Sodium (mg) |
|---|---|---|---|---|---|---|---|---|---|
| Chicken, dark meat, cooked | 100 g | 176 | 28.0 | 6.3 | 2.0 | 3.0 | 91 | 0 | 86 |
| | 1 oz. | 50 | 8.0 | 1.8 | 1.0 | 1.0 | 26 | 0 | 25 |
| | 1 thigh | 122 | 15.0 | 5.9 | — | — | — | — | — |
| Chicken, broiled, meat and skin | 100 g | 136 | 23.8 | 3.8 | — | — | — | 0 | 66 |
| | 1 oz. | 39 | 6.8 | 1.1 | — | — | — | 0 | 19 |
| Chicken, fried, meat and skin | 100 g | 250 | 30.6 | 11.9 | — | — | — | 2.8 | — |
| | 1 oz. | 71 | 8.7 | 3.4 | — | — | — | .8 | — |
| Chicken, roasted, meat and skin | 100 g | 248 | 27.1 | 14.7 | — | — | — | 0 | — |
| | 1 oz. | 70 | 7.7 | 4.2 | — | — | — | 0 | — |
| Chicken, stewed, meat and skin | 100 g | 317 | 26.1 | 22.8 | — | — | — | 0 | — |
| | 1 oz. | 91 | 7.4 | 6.5 | — | — | — | 0 | — |
| Duck, domestic, raw meat only | 100 g | 165 | 21.4 | 8.2 | — | — | — | 0 | 74 |
| | 1 oz. | 47 | 6.1 | 2.3 | — | — | — | 0 | 21 |
| Duck, wild, raw meat only | 100 g | 138 | 21.3 | 5.2 | — | — | — | 0 | 82 |
| | 1 oz. | 39 | 6.1 | 1.5 | — | — | — | 0 | 23 |
| Goose, domestic, roasted | 100 g | 441 | 22.9 | 38.1 | — | — | — | 0 | — |
| | 1 oz. | 126 | 6.5 | 10.8 | — | — | — | 0 | — |
| Turkey, roasted, meat and skin | 100 g | 223 | 31.9 | 9.6 | 3.0 | 8.0 | 77 | 0 | — |
| | 1 oz. | 64 | 9.1 | 2.7 | 1.0 | 2.0 | 22 | 0 | — |
| Turkey, giblets, simmered | 100 g | 233 | 20.6 | 15.4 | — | — | 229 | 1.6 | — |
| | 1 oz. | 67 | 5.9 | 4.4 | — | — | 65 | .4 | — |

## Miscellaneous Prepared Dishes

| | Quantity or Amounts | Calories | Protein (g) | Total Fat (g) | Saturated Fat (g) | Unsaturated Fat (g) | Cholesterol (mg) | Carbohydrates (g) | Sodium (mg) |
|---|---|---|---|---|---|---|---|---|---|
| Beans and franks | 1 cup | 367 | 19.4 | 18.1 | — | — | — | 32.1 | 1374 |
| Beef and vegetable stew, home recipe | 1 cup | 218 | 15.7 | 10.5 | 4.9 | 4.7 | 63 | 15.2 | 91 |
| Beef pot pie ($\frac{1}{3}$ of 9″ pie) | 1 piece | 517 | 21.2 | 30.5 | 8.4 | 20.9 | 44 | 39.5 | 596 |
| Bread stuffing, moist | 1 cup | 416 | 8.8 | 25.6 | 13.1 | 10.2 | — | 39.4 | 1008 |
| Cheese soufflé, home recipe | $\frac{1}{4}$ of 7″ | 240 | 10.9 | 18.8 | 9.5 | 7.3 | 184 | 6.8 | 400 |
| Chicken a la king, home recipe | 1 cup | 468 | 27.4 | 34.3 | 12.7 | 17.6 | 185 | 12.3 | 760 |
| Chicken pot pie ($\frac{1}{3}$ of 9″ pie) | 1 piece | 545 | 23.4 | 31.3 | 10.9 | 18.2 | 71 | 42.5 | 594 |
| Chicken with noodles | 1 cup | 367 | 22.3 | 18.5 | 5.9 | 10.6 | 96 | 25.7 | 600 |
| Chili con carne, canned | 1 cup | 339 | 19.1 | 15.6 | 7.5 | 7.1 | — | 31.1 | 1354 |
| Chop suey with meat, no noodles | 1 cup | 300 | 26.0 | 17.0 | 8.5 | 6.9 | 64 | 12.8 | 1053 |
| Chow mein with chicken, no noodles | 1 cup | 255 | 31.0 | 10.0 | 2.4 | 6.5 | 77 | 10.0 | 718 |

| | Quantity or Amounts | Calories | Protein (g) | Total Fat (g) | Saturated Fat (g) | Unsaturated Fat (g) | Cholesterol (mg) | Carbohydrates (g) | Sodium (mg) |
|---|---|---|---|---|---|---|---|---|---|
| Crab, deviled | 1 cup | 451 | 27.4 | 22.6 | — | — | 244 | 31.9 | 2081 |
| Ham croquette | 1×3 | 163 | 10.6 | 9.8 | 3.9 | 5.0 | — | 7.6 | 222 |
| Lobster Newburg | 1 cup | 485 | 46.3 | 26.5 | — | — | 456 | 12.8 | 573 |
| Macaroni and cheese | 1 cup | 430 | 16.8 | 22.2 | 11.9 | 8.3 | 42 | 22.2 | 1086 |
| Oyster stew | 1 cup | 233 | 12.5 | 15.4 | — | — | 63 | 10.8 | 814 |
| Pizza, 14", cheese, home recipe | $\frac{1}{8}$ of 14" | 153 | 7.8 | 5.4 | 2.1 | 2.8 | — | 18.4 | 456 |
| Pizza, 14", sausage, home recipe | $\frac{1}{8}$ of 14" | 157 | 5.2 | 6.2 | 1.8 | 3.7 | — | 19.8 | 488 |
| Soup, canned, diluted | | | | | | | | | |
|   Asparagus, cream of | 1 cup | 147 | 6.9 | 5.9 | — | — | — | 16.7 | 1068 |
|   Bean with pork | 1 cup | 168 | 8.0 | 5.8 | 1.3 | 3.9 | — | 21.8 | 1008 |
|   Beef broth | 1 cup | 31 | 5.0 | 0 | — | — | — | 2.6 | 782 |
|   Chicken noodle | 1 cup | 130 | 6.9 | 3.9 | — | — | — | 16.2 | 1999 |
|   Clam chowder, Manhattan style | 1 cup | 81 | 2.2 | 2.5 | — | — | — | 12.3 | 938 |
|   Minestrone | 1 cup | 105 | 4.9 | 3.4 | — | — | — | 14.2 | 995 |
|   Mushroom, cream of, with milk | 1 cup | 216 | 6.9 | 14.2 | 4.0 | 8.9 | — | 16.2 | 1039 |
|   Split pea | 1 cup | 145 | 8.6 | 3.2 | 1.0 | 1.8 | — | 20.6 | 941 |
|   Tomato, with milk | 1 cup | 173 | 6.5 | 7.0 | 2.9 | 3.4 | — | 22.5 | 1055 |
|   Vegetable beef | 1 cup | 78 | 5.1 | 2.2 | — | — | — | 9.6 | 1046 |
| Spaghetti with meatballs, sauce | 1 cup | 332 | 18.6 | 11.7 | 3.3 | 7.2 | 75 | 38.7 | 1009 |
| Stuffed pepper with meat and bread crumbs | 1 pepper | 314 | 24.1 | 10.2 | 4.8 | 4.6 | 56 | 31.1 | 581 |
| Tuna salad | 1 cup | 349 | 29.9 | 21.5 | 5.0 | 12.5 | — | 7.2 | — |
| Welsh rarebit | 1 cup | 415 | 18.8 | 31.6 | 17.3 | 11.4 | 71 | 14.6 | 770 |

## Salad Dressings, Sauces, Spreads, Fats, Oils

| | Quantity or Amounts | Calories | Protein (g) | Total Fat (g) | Saturated Fat (g) | Unsaturated Fat (g) | Cholesterol (mg) | Carbohydrates (g) | Sodium (mg) |
|---|---|---|---|---|---|---|---|---|---|
| Fat, cooking, lard | 100 g | 902 | 0 | 100.0 | 17.5 | 24.5 | 95 | 0 | 0 |
| | 1 oz. | 115 | 0 | 13.0 | 5.0 | 7.0 | 13 | 0 | 0 |
| Fat, cooking, vegetable, Crisco | 100 g | 884 | 0 | 100.0 | 43.0 | 52.0 | 0 | 0 | 0 |
| | 1 oz. = 1 T. | 110 | 0 | 13.0 | 3.0 | 9.0 | 0 | 0 | 0 |
| | 1 cup | 1768 | 0 | 200.0 | 49.9 | | 0 | 0 | 0 |
| Oils, salad and cooking | 100 g | 884 | 0 | 100.0 | 18.0 | 76.0 | 0 | 0 | 0 |
| | 1 oz. = 1 T. | 120 | 0 | 14.0 | 3.0 | 9.0 | 0 | 0 | 0 |
| | 1 cup | 1972 | 0 | 218.0 | 38.9 | 164.0 | 0 | 0 | 0 |
| Salad dressings | | | | | | | | | |
|   Blue cheese | 100 g | 504 | 4.8 | 52.3 | 11.0 | 36.0 | — | 7.4 | 1094 |
| | 1 oz. = 2 T. | 152 | 1.4 | 15.6 | 3.2 | 10.1 | — | 2.2 | 238 |

| | Quantity or Amounts | Calories | Protein (g) | Total Fat (g) | Saturated Fat (g) | Unsaturated Fat (g) | Cholesterol (mg) | Carbohydrates (g) | Sodium (mg) |
|---|---|---|---|---|---|---|---|---|---|
| French | 100 g | 410 | .6 | 38.9 | 7.0 | 28.0 | — | 17.5 | 1370 |
| | 1 oz.=2 T. | 132 | .2 | 12.4 | 2.2 | 9.0 | — | 5.6 | 438 |
| Italian | 100 g | 552 | .2 | 60.0 | 10.0 | 44.0 | — | 6.0 | 2092 |
| | 1 oz.=2 T. | 166 | .1 | 18.0 | 3.2 | 13.2 | — | 2.0 | 628 |
| Russian | 100 g | 494 | 1.6 | 50.8 | 9.0 | 37.0 | — | 10.4 | 868 |
| | 1 oz.=2 T. | 148 | .4 | 14.2 | 2.8 | 11.0 | — | 1.6 | 130 |
| Thousand Island | 100 g | 502 | .8 | 50.2 | 9.0 | 36.0 | — | 15.4 | 700 |
| | 1 oz.=2 T. | 160 | .2 | 16.0 | 2.8 | 11.4 | — | 5.0 | 224 |
| Salad dressings, dietetic, low calorie | | | | | | | | | |
| Blue cheese | 100 g | 76 | 3.0 | 5.9 | 3.0 | 2.0 | — | 4.1 | 1108 |
| | 1 oz.=2 T. | 6 | .4 | 1.8 | .5 | .3 | — | .4 | 340 |
| French | 100 g | 96 | .4 | 4.3 | 1.0 | 3.0 | — | 15.6 | 787 |
| | 1 oz.=2 T. | 30 | .2 | 1.5 | .2 | 1.0 | — | 5.0 | 225 |
| Thousand Island | 100 g | 180 | .9 | 13.7 | 2.0 | 10.0 | — | 15.6 | 700 |
| | 1 oz.=2 T. | 54 | .2 | 4.2 | .8 | 1.0 | — | 5.0 | 210 |
| Sauces | | | | | | | | | |
| Barbecue sauce | 100 g | 91 | 1.5 | 6.9 | — | — | — | 8.0 | 815 |
| | 1 oz.=2 T. | 26 | .4 | 1.9 | — | — | — | 2.3 | 232 |
| Catsup | 100 g | 106 | 2.0 | .4 | — | — | — | 25.4 | 1042 |
| | 1 T. | 18 | .4 | .1 | — | — | — | 4.6 | 178 |
| Chili sauce | 100 g | 104 | 2.5 | .3 | — | — | — | 24.8 | 1338 |
| | 1 oz.=2 T. | 29 | .7 | .1 | — | — | — | 8.0 | 297 |
| Mustard, prepared, yellow and brown | 100 g | 75 | 4.7 | 4.4 | — | — | — | 6.4 | 1252 |
| | 1 t. | 8 | — | — | — | — | — | .5 | — |
| Seafood cocktail | 1 oz.=2 T. | 22 | — | — | — | — | — | 4.9 | — |
| Soy sauce | 100 g | 68 | 5.6 | 1.3 | — | — | — | 9.5 | 7325 |
| | 1 oz.=2 T. | 19 | 1.6 | .4 | — | — | — | 2.7 | 2093 |
| Steak sauce | 1 T. | 18 | — | — | — | — | — | 4.8 | — |
| Tartar sauce | 100 g | 531 | 1.4 | 57.8 | — | — | 51 | 4.2 | 707 |
| | 1 oz.=2 T. | 151 | .4 | 16.5 | — | — | 14 | 1.2 | 202 |
| White sauce, medium | 100 g | 162 | 3.9 | 12.5 | 7.0 | 4.0 | 13 | 8.8 | 379 |
| | 1 oz.=2 T. | 46 | 1.1 | 3.6 | 2.0 | 1.0 | 4 | 2.5 | 108 |
| Worcestershire sauce | 1 oz.=2 T. | 15 | — | — | — | — | — | 3.6 | — |
| Spreads | | | | | | | | | |
| Butter | 100 g | 716 | .6 | 81.0 | 46.0 | 29.0 | 250 | .4 | 987 |
| | 1 oz. | 200 | .2 | 23.0 | 12.6 | 8.2 | 71 | .2 | 280 |

# Nutritional Guide

| | Quantity or Amounts | Calories | Protein (g) | Total Fat (g) | Saturated Fat (g) | Unsaturated Fat (g) | Cholesterol (mg) | Carbohydrates (g) | Sodium (mg) |
|---|---|---|---|---|---|---|---|---|---|
| | 1 pat | 36 | — | 4.1 | 2.2 | 1.4 | 13 | .1 | 49 |
| | ½ cup | 812 | .7 | 91.9 | 50.5 | 33.1 | 265 | .5 | 1119 |
| Margarine, ⅔ animal, | 100 g | 720 | .6 | 81.0 | 18.0 | 61.0 | 65 | .4 | 987 |
| ⅓ vegetable fat | 1 oz. | 204 | .2 | 22.4 | 4.8 | 16.4 | 14 | .1 | 282 |
| | 1 pat | 36 | — | 4.1 | .7 | 3.2 | — | — | 49 |
| Margarine, corn oil | 1 oz.=2 T. | 200 | — | 22.4 | 4.2 | 17.4 | 0 | — | — |
| Margarine, diet | 1 oz.=2 T. | 122 | — | 11.0 | 2.0 | 8.6 | 0 | — | — |
| Mayonnaise | 100 g | 718 | 1.1 | 79.9 | 14.0 | 57.0 | 70 | 14.4 | 597 |
| | 1 oz.=1 T. | 101 | .2 | 11.2 | 2.0 | 8.0 | 20 | .3 | 84 |
| | 1 cup | 1587 | 2.4 | 175.8 | 31.3 | 126.7 | 154 | 4.9 | 1313 |
| Sandwich spread with | 100 g | 379 | .7 | 36.2 | — | — | — | 15.9 | 626 |
| chopped pickle | 1 oz.=2 T. | 114 | .2 | 10.8 | — | — | — | 5.0 | 188 |

## Vegetables and Salads

| | Quantity or Amounts | Calories | Protein (g) | Total Fat (g) | Saturated Fat (g) | Unsaturated Fat (g) | Cholesterol (mg) | Carbohydrates (g) | Sodium (mg) |
|---|---|---|---|---|---|---|---|---|---|
| Artichokes, boiled, | 100 g | 8–44 | 2.8 | .2 | — | — | — | 9.9 | 30.0 |
| drained | 1 oz. | 3–13 | .8 | .1 | — | — | — | 2.8 | 9.0 |
| | 1 med. | 10–53 | 3.4 | .2 | — | — | — | 11.9 | 36.0 |
| Asparagus, boiled, | 100 g | 20 | 2.2 | .2 | — | — | — | 3.6 | 1.0 |
| drained | 1 oz. | 6 | .6 | .1 | — | — | — | 1.0 | 1.0 |
| | 4 spears | 12 | 1.3 | .1 | — | — | — | 2.2 | 1.0 |
| Beans, baby lima, | 100 g | 111 | 7.6 | .5 | — | — | — | 19.8 | 1.0 |
| fresh, cooked | 1 oz. | 32 | 2.2 | .1 | — | — | — | 5.6 | 1.0 |
| | ½ cup | 94 | 6.3 | .5 | — | — | — | 16.8 | 2.0 |
| Beans, baked with | | | | | | | | | |
| brown sugar | 1 cup | 310 | — | — | — | — | — | 48.1 | — |
| Beans, green, boiled, | 100 g | 25 | 1.6 | .2 | — | — | — | 5.4 | 4.0 |
| drained | 1 oz. | 7 | .5 | .1 | — | — | — | 1.5 | 1.0 |
| | ½ cup | 17 | 1.0 | .1 | — | — | — | 3.7 | 3.0 |
| Beans, pinto, dry, | 100 g | 349 | 22.9 | 1.2 | — | — | — | 63.7 | 10.0 |
| uncooked | 1 oz. | 100 | 6.5 | .3 | — | — | — | 18.2 | 3.0 |
| | ½ cup | 331 | 21.9 | 1.1 | — | — | — | 61.2 | 9.0 |
| Beans, refried, canned | 100 g | — | — | — | — | — | — | — | — |
| | 1 oz. | — | — | — | — | — | — | — | — |
| | ½ cup | 120 | — | — | — | — | — | — | — |
| Bean sprouts, raw | 100 g | 35 | 3.8 | .2 | — | — | — | 6.6 | 5.0 |
| | 1 oz. | 10 | 1.1 | .1 | — | — | — | 1.9 | 1.0 |
| | ½ cup | 16 | 2.0 | .1 | — | — | — | 3.0 | 3.0 |
| Beets, canned, diced | 100 g | 37 | 1.0 | .1 | — | — | — | 8.8 | 236.0 |
| solids, salt added | 1 oz. | 11 | .3 | — | — | — | — | 2.5 | 67.0 |
| | ½ cup | 31 | .9 | .1 | — | — | — | 7.2 | 200.0 |

| | Quantity or Amounts | Calories | Protein (g) | Total Fat (g) | Saturated Fat (g) | Unsaturated Fat (g) | Cholesterol (mg) | Carbohydrates (g) | Sodium (mg) |
|---|---|---|---|---|---|---|---|---|---|
| Broccoli spears, frozen, boiled | 100 g | 26 | 3.1 | .2 | — | — | — | 4.7 | 12.0 |
| | 1 oz. | 7 | .9 | .1 | — | — | — | 1.3 | 3.0 |
| | 1 cup | 48 | 5.4 | .6 | — | — | — | 8.5 | 28.0 |
| Brussels sprouts, boiled, drained | 100 g | 36 | 4.2 | .4 | — | — | — | 6.4 | 10.0 |
| | 1 oz. | 10 | 1.2 | .1 | — | — | — | 1.8 | 3.0 |
| | 7–8 sprouts | 51 | 5.0 | .3 | — | — | — | 10.1 | 22.0 |
| Cabbage, white, raw | 100 g | 24 | 1.3 | .2 | — | — | — | 5.4 | 20.0 |
| | 1 oz. | 7 | .4 | .1 | — | — | — | 1.5 | 6.0 |
| | 1 cup | 22 | 1.2 | .2 | — | — | — | 4.9 | 18.0 |
| Carrot, raw | 100 g | 42 | 1.1 | .2 | — | — | — | 9.7 | 47.0 |
| | 1 oz. | 12 | .3 | .1 | — | — | — | 2.8 | 13.0 |
| | 1 med. | 30 | .8 | .1 | — | — | — | 7.0 | 34.0 |
| Cauliflower, fresh, boiled | 100 g | 22 | 2.3 | .2 | — | — | — | 4.1 | 9.0 |
| | 1 oz. | 6 | .7 | .1 | — | — | — | 1.2 | 3.0 |
| | 1 cup | 28 | 2.9 | .3 | — | — | — | 5.1 | 11.0 |
| Celery, raw | 100 g | 17 | .9 | .1 | — | — | — | 3.9 | 126.0 |
| | 1 oz. | 5 | .3 | — | — | — | — | 1.1 | 36.0 |
| | 3 stalks | 8 | .4 | — | — | — | — | 2.0 | 50.0 |
| Coleslaw with mayonnaise | 100 g | 144 | 1.3 | 14.0 | 2.0 | 10.0 | — | 4.8 | 120.0 |
| | 1 oz. | 41 | .4 | 4.0 | .6 | 2.9 | — | 1.4 | 34.0 |
| | 1 cup | 173 | 1.6 | 16.8 | — | — | — | 5.8 | 144.0 |
| Corn, canned, drained, whole kernel | 100 g | 84 | 2.6 | .8 | — | — | — | 19.8 | 236.0 |
| | 1 oz. | 24 | .7 | .2 | — | — | — | 5.7 | 67.0 |
| | ½ cup | 88 | 2.5 | .5 | — | — | — | 21.7 | 243.0 |
| Corn, sweet, fresh, boiled on cob | 100 g | 91 | 3.3 | 1.0 | — | — | — | 21.0 | 196.0 |
| | 1 oz. | 26 | .9 | .3 | — | — | — | 6.0 | 56.0 |
| | 1 ear | 70 | 2.5 | .8 | — | — | — | 16.2 | — |
| Cucumber, fresh, pared | 100 g | 15 | .9 | .1 | — | — | — | 3.4 | 6.0 |
| | 1 oz. | 4 | .3 | — | — | — | — | .9 | 2.0 |
| | ½ cup | 10 | .4 | .1 | — | — | — | 2.3 | 4.0 |
| Eggplant, boiled, diced, drained | 100 g | 19 | 1.0 | .2 | — | — | — | 4.1 | 1.0 |
| | 1 oz. | 5 | .3 | .1 | — | — | — | 1.1 | .3 |
| | 1 cup | 38 | 2.0 | .4 | — | — | — | 8.2 | 2.0 |
| Leeks | 100 g | 52 | 2.2 | .3 | — | — | — | 11.2 | 5.0 |
| | 1 oz. | 15 | .6 | .1 | — | — | — | 3.2 | 1.4 |
| Lentils, cooked and drained | 100 g | 106 | 7.8 | — | — | — | — | 19.3 | — |
| | 1 oz. | 30 | 2.2 | — | — | — | — | 5.5 | — |
| | ½ cup | 107 | 7.0 | — | — | — | — | 19.5 | — |
| Lettuce, iceberg chunks | 100 g | 13 | .9 | .1 | — | — | — | 2.9 | 9.0 |
| | 1 oz. | 4 | .3 | — | — | — | — | .8 | 3.0 |
| | 1 cup | 10 | .7 | .1 | — | — | — | 2.2 | 7.0 |

| | Quantity or Amounts | Calories | Protein (g) | Total Fat (g) | Saturated Fat (g) | Unsaturated Fat (g) | Cholesterol (mg) | Carbohydrates (g) | Sodium (mg) |
|---|---|---|---|---|---|---|---|---|---|
| Mushrooms, raw, | 100 g | 28 | 2.7 | .3 | — | — | — | 4.4 | 15.0 |
| trimmed, sliced | 1 oz. | 8 | .8 | .1 | — | — | — | 1.3 | 4.0 |
| | ½ cup | 10 | 1.0 | .1 | — | — | — | 1.5 | 11.0 |
| Mustard greens, boiled, | 100 g | 23 | 2.2 | .4 | — | — | — | 4.0 | 18.0 |
| drained | 1 oz. | 7 | .6 | .1 | — | — | — | 1.1 | 5.0 |
| | 1 cup | 32 | 3.1 | .6 | — | — | — | 5.6 | 25.0 |
| Okra, frozen, cut, | 100 g | 29 | 2.0 | .3 | — | — | — | 6.0 | 2.0 |
| boiled, drained | 1 oz. | 8 | .6 | .1 | — | — | — | 1.7 | 1.0 |
| | ½ cup | 35 | 2.0 | .1 | — | — | — | 8.1 | 3.0 |
| Onion, green, raw, | 100 g | 45 | 1.1 | .2 | — | — | — | 10.5 | 5.0 |
| trimmed | 1 oz. | 13 | .3 | .1 | — | — | — | 3.0 | 1.4 |
| | 3 | 14 | .3 | .1 | — | — | — | 3.2 | 2.0 |
| Onion, raw, chopped | 100 g | 38 | 1.5 | .1 | — | — | — | 8.7 | 10.0 |
| | 1 oz. | 11 | .4 | — | — | — | — | 2.5 | 3.0 |
| | ½ cup | 33 | 1.3 | .1 | — | — | — | 7.5 | 8.0 |
| Parsnips, boiled, drained, | 100 g | 66 | 1.5 | .5 | — | — | — | 14.9 | 8.0 |
| pieces | 1 oz. | 19 | .4 | .1 | — | — | — | 4.3 | 2.3 |
| | 1 cup | 102 | 2.3 | .8 | — | — | — | 23.1 | 12.0 |
| Peas, green, shelled, | 100 g | 71 | 5.4 | .4 | — | — | — | 12.1 | 1.0 |
| boiled | 1 oz. | 20 | 1.5 | .1 | — | — | — | 3.5 | .3 |
| | ½ cup | 58 | 4.3 | .3 | — | — | — | 9.9 | 1.0 |
| Pea pods, boiled, drained | 100 g | 43 | 2.9 | .2 | — | — | — | 9.5 | — |
| | 1 oz. | 13 | .8 | .1 | — | — | — | 2.7 | — |
| | 1 cup | 49 | 3.2 | .4 | — | — | — | 10.8 | — |
| Peas, split, dried, cooked, | 100 g | 115 | 8.0 | .3 | — | — | — | 20.8 | 13.0 |
| drained | 1 oz. | 33 | 2.3 | .1 | — | — | — | 5.9 | 4.0 |
| | ½ cup | 115 | 8.0 | .3 | — | — | — | 20.2 | 13.0 |
| Peppers, sweet green, | 100 g | 22 | 1.2 | .2 | — | — | — | 4.8 | 13.0 |
| raw, chopped | 1 oz. | 6 | .3 | .1 | — | — | — | 1.4 | 4.0 |
| | ½ cup | 16 | .9 | .1 | — | — | — | 3,6 | 10.0 |
| Pimientos, canned, | 100 g | 27 | .9 | .5 | — | — | — | 5.8 | — |
| drained | 1 oz. | 8 | .3 | .1 | — | — | — | 1.6 | — |
| | ¼ cup | 15 | .5 | .3 | — | — | — | 3.3 | — |
| Potatoes au gratin | 100.g | 145 | 5.3 | 7.9 | 4.0 | 3.0 | — | 13.6 | 447.0 |
| | 1 oz. | 41 | 1.5 | 2.3 | 1.1 | .1 | — | 3.9 | 128.0 |
| | ½ cup | 177 | 6.0 | 9.7 | 5.0 | 4.0 | — | 16.6 | 545.0 |
| Potatoes, baked, with | 100 g | 93 | 2.6 | .1 | — | — | — | 21.1 | 4.0 |
| peel | 1 oz. | 27 | .7 | — | — | — | — | 6.0 | 1.0 |
| | 1 med. | 104 | 2.9 | .1 | — | — | — | 23.3 | 4.0 |

# Nutritional Guide

| | Quantity or Amounts | Calories | Protein (g) | Total Fat (g) | Saturated Fat (g) | Unsaturated Fat (g) | Cholesterol (mg) | Carbohydrates (g) | Sodium (mg) |
|---|---|---|---|---|---|---|---|---|---|
| Potatoes, french fried, $2 \times \frac{1}{2} \times \frac{1}{2}$ | 100 g | 274 | 4.3 | 13.2 | 3.0 | 10.0 | — | 36.0 | 6.0 |
| | 1 oz. | 78 | 1.2 | 3.7 | .9 | 2.8 | — | 10.2 | 1.7 |
| | 10 pieces | 137 | 2.2 | 6.6 | 1.0 | 5.0 | — | 18.0 | 3.0 |
| Potatoes, hash browned, fried from raw | 100 g | 268 | 4.0 | 14.2 | 3.0 | 10.0 | — | 32.6 | 223.0 |
| | 1 oz. | 77 | 1.1 | 4.0 | .9 | 2.9 | — | 9.3 | 64.0 |
| | $\frac{1}{2}$ cup | 223 | 3.4 | 12.0 | 3.0 | 10.0 | — | 28.0 | 189.0 |
| Potatoes, mashed, with milk and butter | 100 g | 94 | 2.1 | 4.3 | 2.0 | 1.0 | — | 12.3 | 331.0 |
| | 1 oz. | 27 | .6 | 1.2 | 1.0 | — | — | 3.5 | 95.0 |
| | 1 cup | 197 | 4.4 | 9.0 | — | — | — | 25.8 | 695.0 |
| Potatoes, peeled, boiled, diced | 100 g | 65 | 1.9 | .1 | — | — | — | 14.5 | 2.0 |
| | 1 oz. | 19 | .5 | — | — | — | — | 4.1 | 1.0 |
| | $\frac{1}{2}$ cup | 51 | 1.5 | .1 | — | — | — | 11.3 | 1.0 |
| Potato salad, with mayo., eggs, and seasonings | 100 g | 145 | 3.0 | 9.2 | 2.0 | 6.0 | — | 13.4 | 480.0 |
| | 1 oz. | 41 | .9 | 2.6 | .6 | 1.7 | — | 3.8 | 137.0 |
| | 1 cup | 363 | 7.5 | 23.0 | 5.0 | 13.0 | — | 33.5 | 1200.0 |
| Pumpkin, canned | 100 g | 33 | 1.0 | .3 | — | — | — | 7.9 | 2.0 |
| | 1 oz. | 9 | .3 | .1 | — | — | — | 2.3 | .6 |
| | $\frac{1}{2}$ cup | 40 | 1.2 | .3 | — | — | — | 9.6 | 2.0 |
| Radish, raw, trimmed, whole | 100 g | 17 | 1.0 | .1 | — | — | — | 3.6 | 18.0 |
| | 1 oz. | 5 | .3 | — | — | — | — | 1.0 | 5.0 |
| | 10 med. | 8 | .5 | — | — | — | — | 1.6 | 8.0 |
| Rutabaga, boiled, diced, drained | 100 g | 35 | .9 | .1 | — | — | — | 8.2 | 4.0 |
| | 1 oz. | 10 | .3 | — | — | — | — | 2.3 | 1.0 |
| | $\frac{1}{2}$ cup | 30 | .7 | .1 | — | — | — | 7.1 | .3 |
| Sauerkraut, canned, drained | 100 g | 18 | 1.0 | .2 | — | — | — | 4.0 | 747.0 |
| | 1 oz. | 5 | .3 | .1 | — | — | — | 1.1 | 213.0 |
| | 1 cup | 42 | 2.4 | .5 | — | — | — | 9.4 | 1755.0 |
| Soybean, dried, cooked | 100 g | 130 | 11.0 | 5.7 | 1.0 | 4.0 | — | 10.8 | 2.0 |
| | 1 oz. | 37 | 3.1 | 1.6 | .3 | 1.0 | — | 3.1 | 1.0 |
| | 1 cup | 234 | 19.8 | 10.3 | — | — | — | 19.4 | 4.0 |
| Spinach, chopped, boiled, drained | 100 g | 23 | 3.0 | .3 | — | — | — | 3.6 | 50.0 |
| | 1 oz. | 7 | .9 | .1 | — | — | — | 1.0 | 14.0 |
| | 1 cup | 41 | 5.4 | .5 | — | — | — | 6.5 | 90.0 |
| Spinach, leaves, raw, trimmed | 100 g | 26 | 3.2 | .3 | — | — | — | 4.3 | 71.0 |
| | 1 oz. | 7 | .9 | .1 | — | — | — | 1.2 | 20.0 |
| | 1 cup | 14 | 1.8 | .2 | — | — | — | 2.4 | 39.0 |
| Squash, summer, boiled, drained slices | 100 g | 14 | .9 | .1 | — | — | — | 3.1 | 1.0 |
| | 1 oz. | 4 | .3 | — | — | — | — | .8 | .3 |
| | $\frac{1}{2}$ cup | 13 | .7 | .1 | — | — | — | 2.7 | 1.0 |

# Nutritional Guide

| | Quantity or Amounts | Calories | Protein (g) | Total Fat (g) | Saturated Fat (g) | Unsaturated Fat (g) | Cholesterol (mg) | Carbohydrates (g) | Sodium (mg) |
|---|---|---|---|---|---|---|---|---|---|
| Squash, winter, baked, | 100 g | 63 | 1.8 | .4 | — | — | — | 15.4 | 1.0 |
| meat only | 1 oz. | 18 | .5 | .1 | — | — | — | 4.4 | .3 |
| Acorn, $\frac{1}{2}$ squash | 4 oz. | 97 | 3.3 | .2 | — | — | — | 24.6 | 1.0 |
| Sweet potato, baked | 100 g | 141 | 2.1 | .5 | — | — | — | 32.5 | 12.0 |
| | 1 oz. | 40 | .6 | .1 | — | — | — | 9.3 | 3.4 |
| | 5×2 | 161 | 2.4 | .6 | — | — | — | 37.0 | 14.0 |
| Sweet potato, candied, | 100 g | 168 | 1.3 | 3.3 | 2.0 | 1.0 | — | 34.2 | — |
| home recipe | 1 oz. | 48 | .4 | .9 | 1.0 | — | — | 9.8 | — |
| | $\frac{1}{2}$ potato | 176 | 1.4 | 3.5 | — | — | — | 35.9 | 44.0 |
| Turnips, boiled, drained, | 100 g | 23 | .8 | .2 | — | — | — | 4.9 | 34.0 |
| mashed | 1 oz. | 7 | .2 | .1 | — | — | — | 1.4 | 10.0 |
| | $\frac{1}{2}$ cup | 26 | .9 | .3 | — | — | — | 5.6 | 36.0 |
| Vegetable juice, cocktail | 100 g | 17 | .9 | .1 | — | — | — | 3.6 | 200.0 |
| | 1 fl. oz. | 5 | .3 | — | — | — | — | 1.1 | 61.0 |
| | $\frac{1}{2}$ cup | 19 | 1.1 | .1 | — | — | — | 4.1 | 242.0 |

**277**

# Nutritional Analyses of Fast Foods

*Through the courtesy of Ross Laboratories*
*(Dashes indicate information not provided by sources.)*

| | Weight (g) | Calories | Protein (g) | Carbohydrate (g) | Fat (g) | Cholesterol (mg) |
|---|---|---|---|---|---|---|
| **Burger Chef[1]** | | | | | | |
| Big Shef | 186 | 542 | 23 | 35 | 34 | — |
| Cheeseburger | 104 | 304 | 14 | 24 | 17 | — |
| Double Cheeseburger | 145 | 434 | 24 | 24 | 26 | — |
| French Fries | 68 | 187 | 3 | 25 | 9 | — |
| Hamburger, Regular | 91 | 258 | 11 | 24 | 13 | — |
| Mariner Platter | 373 | 680 | 32 | 85 | 24 | — |
| Rancher Platter | 316 | 640 | 30 | 44 | 38 | — |
| Shake | 305 | 326 | 11 | 47 | 11 | — |
| Skipper's Treat | 179 | 604 | 21 | 47 | 37 | — |
| Super Shef | 252 | 600 | 29 | 39 | 37 | — |
| **Burger King[2]** | | | | | | |
| Cheeseburger | — | 305 | 17 | 29 | 13 | — |
| Hamburger | — | 252 | 14 | 29 | 9 | — |
| Whopper | — | 606 | 29 | 51 | 32 | — |
| French Fries | — | 214 | 3 | 28 | 10 | — |
| Vanilla Shake | — | 332 | 11 | 50 | 11 | — |
| Whaler | — | 486 | 18 | 64 | 46 | — |
| Hot Dog | — | 291 | 11 | 23 | 17 | — |
| **Dairy Queen[3]** | | | | | | |
| Big Brazier Deluxe | 213 | 470 | 28 | 36 | 24 | — |
| Big Brazier Regular | 184 | 457 | 27 | 37 | 23 | — |
| Big Brazier w/Cheese | 213 | 553 | 32 | 38 | 30 | — |
| Brazier w/Cheese | 121 | 318 | 18 | 30 | 14 | — |
| Brazier Cheese Dog | 113 | 330 | 15 | 24 | 19 | — |
| Brazier Chili Dog | 128 | 330 | 13 | 25 | 20 | — |
| Brazier Dog | 99 | 273 | 11 | 23 | 15 | — |
| Brazier French Fries, 2.5 oz. | 71 | 200 | 2 | 25 | 10 | — |
| Brazier French Fries, 4.0 oz. | 113 | 320 | 3 | 40 | 16 | — |

| | Weight (g) | Calories | Protein (g) | Carbohydrate (g) | Fat (g) | Cholesterol (mg) |
|---|---|---|---|---|---|---|
| Brazier Onion Rings | 85 | 300 | 6 | 33 | 17 | — |
| Brazier Regular | 106 | 260 | 13 | 28 | 9 | — |
| Fish Sandwich | 170 | 400 | 20 | 41 | 17 | — |
| Fish Sandwich w/Cheese | 177 | 440 | 24 | 39 | 21 | — |
| Super Brazier | 298 | 783 | 53 | 35 | 48 | — |
| Super Brazier Dog | 182 | 518 | 20 | 41 | 30 | — |
| Super Brazier Dog w/Cheese | 203 | 593 | 26 | 43 | 36 | — |
| Super Brazier Chili Dog | 210 | 555 | 23 | 42 | 33 | — |
| Banana Split | 383 | 540 | 10 | 91 | 15 | — |
| Buster Bar | 149 | 390 | 10 | 37 | 22 | — |
| DQ Chocolate Dipped Cone, sm. | 78 | 150 | 3 | 20 | 7 | — |
| DQ Chocolate Dipped Cone, med. | 156 | 300 | 7 | 40 | 13 | — |
| DQ Chocolate Dipped Cone, lg. | 234 | 450 | 10 | 58 | 20 | — |
| DQ Chocolate Malt, sm. | 241 | 340 | 10 | 51 | 11 | — |
| DQ Chocolate Malt, med. | 418 | 600 | 15 | 89 | 20 | — |
| DQ Chocolate Malt, lg. | 588 | 840 | 22 | 125 | 28 | — |
| DQ Chocolate Sundae, sm. | 106 | 170 | 4 | 30 | 4 | — |
| DQ Chocolate Sundae, med. | 184 | 300 | 6 | 53 | 7 | — |
| DQ Chocolate Sundae, lg. | 248 | 400 | 9 | 71 | 9 | — |
| DQ Cone, sm. | 71 | 110 | 3 | 18 | 3 | — |
| DQ Cone, med. | 142 | 230 | 6 | 35 | 7 | — |
| DQ Cone, lg. | 213 | 340 | 10 | 52 | 10 | — |
| Dairy Queen Parfait | 284 | 460 | 10 | 81 | 11 | — |
| Dilly Bar | 85 | 240 | 4 | 22 | 15 | — |
| DQ Float | 397 | 330 | 6 | 59 | 8 | — |
| DQ Freeze | 397 | 520 | 11 | 89 | 13 | — |
| DQ Sandwich | 60 | 140 | 3 | 24 | 4 | — |
| Fiesta Sundae | 269 | 570 | 9 | 84 | 22 | — |
| Hot Fudge Brownie Delight | 266 | 570 | 11 | 83 | 22 | — |
| Mr. Misty Float | 404 | 440 | 6 | 85 | 8 | — |

| | Weight (g) | Calories | Protein (g) | Carbohydrate (g) | Fat (g) | Cholesterol (mg) |
|---|---|---|---|---|---|---|
| Mr. Misty Freeze | 411 | 500 | 10 | 87 | 12 | — |

## Kentucky Fried Chicken[4]

| | Weight (g) | Calories | Protein (g) | Carbohydrate (g) | Fat (g) | Cholesterol (mg) |
|---|---|---|---|---|---|---|
| Original Recipe Dinner* | 425 | 830 | 52 | 56 | 46 | 285 |
| Extra Crispy Dinner** | 437 | 950 | 52 | 63 | 54 | 265 |
| Individual Pieces*** | | | | | | |
| (Original Recipe) | | | | | | |
| Drumstick | 54 | 136 | 14 | 2 | 8 | 73 |
| Keel | 96 | 283 | 25 | 6 | 13 | 90 |
| Rib | 82 | 241 | 19 | 8 | 15 | 97 |
| Thigh | 97 | 276 | 20 | 12 | 19 | 147 |
| Wing | 45 | 151 | 11 | 4 | 10 | 70 |
| 9 Pieces | 652 | 1892 | 152 | 59 | 116 | 864 |

## Long John Silver's[5]

| | Weight (g) | Calories | Protein (g) | Carbohydrate (g) | Fat (g) | Cholesterol (mg) |
|---|---|---|---|---|---|---|
| Breaded Oysters, 6 pc. | — | 460 | 14 | 58 | 19 | — |
| Breaded Clams, 5 oz. | — | 465 | 13 | 46 | 25 | — |
| Chicken Planks, 4 pc. | — | 458 | 27 | 35 | 23 | — |
| Cole Slaw, 4 oz. | — | 138 | 1 | 16 | 8 | — |
| Corn on Cob, 1 pc. | — | 174 | 5 | 29 | 4 | — |
| Fish w/Batter, 2 pc. | — | 318 | 19 | 19 | 19 | — |
| Fish w/Batter, 3 pc. | — | 477 | 28 | 28 | 28 | — |
| Fryes, 3 oz. | — | 275 | 4 | 32 | 15 | — |
| Hush Puppies, 3 pc. | — | 153 | 1 | 20 | 7 | — |
| Ocean Scallops, 6 pc. | — | 257 | 10 | 27 | 12 | — |
| Peg Leg w/Batter, 5 pc. | — | 514 | 25 | 30 | 33 | — |
| Shrimp w/Batter, 6 pc. | — | 269 | 9 | 31 | 13 | — |
| Treasure Chest 2 pc. fish, 2 Peg Legs | — | 467 | 25 | 27 | 29 | — |

## McDonald's[6]

| | Weight (g) | Calories | Protein (g) | Carbohydrate (g) | Fat (g) | Cholesterol (mg) |
|---|---|---|---|---|---|---|
| Egg McMuffin | 132 | 352 | 18 | 26 | 20 | 192 |

* Dinner comprises mashed potatoes and gravy, cole slaw, roll, and three pieces of chicken: either (1) wing, rib, and thigh; (2) wing, drumstick, and thigh; or (3) wing, drumstick, and keel.
** Edible portion of chicken.
*** Calculated from percentage of U.S. RDA.

| | Weight (g) | Calories | Protein (g) | Carbohydrate (g) | Fat (g) | Cholesterol (mg) |
|---|---|---|---|---|---|---|
| English Muffin, Buttered | 62 | 186 | 6 | 28 | 6 | 12 |
| Hot Cakes, w/Butter and Syrup | 206 | 472 | 8 | 89 | 9 | 36 |
| Sausage (Pork) | 48 | 184 | 9 | tr | 17 | 43 |
| Scrambled Eggs | 77 | 162 | 12 | 2 | 12 | 301 |
| Big Mac | 187 | 541 | 26 | 39 | 31 | 75 |
| Cheeseburger | 114 | 306 | 16 | 31 | 13 | 41 |
| Filet o' Fish | 131 | 402 | 15 | 34 | 23 | 43 |
| French Fries | 69 | 211 | 3 | 26 | 11 | 10 |
| Hamburger | 99 | 257 | 13 | 30 | 9 | 26 |
| Quarter Pounder | 164 | 418 | 26 | 33 | 21 | 69 |
| Quarter Pounder w/Cheese | 193 | 518 | 31 | 34 | 29 | 96 |
| Apple Pie | 91 | 300 | 2 | 31 | 19 | 14 |
| Cherry Pie | 92 | 298 | 2 | 33 | 18 | 14 |
| McDonaldland Cookies | 63 | 294 | 4 | 45 | 11 | 9 |
| Chocolate Shake | 289 | 364 | 11 | 60 | 9 | 29 |
| Strawberry Shake | 293 | 345 | 10 | 57 | 9 | 30 |
| Vanilla Shake | 289 | 323 | 10 | 52 | 8 | 29 |

**Pizza Hut[7] †**

| | Weight (g) | Calories | Protein (g) | Carbohydrate (g) | Fat (g) | Cholesterol (mg) |
|---|---|---|---|---|---|---|
| **Thin'N Crispy** | | | | | | |
| Beef†† | — | 490 | 29 | 51 | 19 | — |
| Pork†† | — | 520 | 27 | 51 | 23 | — |
| Cheese | — | 450 | 25 | 54 | 15 | — |
| Pepperoni | — | 430 | 23 | 45 | 17 | — |
| Supreme | — | 510 | 27 | 51 | 21 | — |
| **Thick'N Chewy** | | | | | | |
| Beef†† | — | 620 | 38 | 73 | 20 | — |
| Pork†† | — | 640 | 36 | 71 | 23 | — |
| Cheese | — | 560 | 34 | 71 | 14 | — |
| Pepperoni | — | 560 | 31 | 68 | 18 | — |
| Supreme | — | 640 | 36 | 74 | 22 | — |

† Based on a serving size of one-half of a 10″ pizza (3 slices).
†† Ingredients of topping mixture.

| | Weight (g) | Calories | Protein (g) | Carbohydrate (g) | Fat (g) | Cholesterol (mg) |
|---|---|---|---|---|---|---|
| **Taco Bell[8]** | | | | | | |
| Bean Burrito | 166 | 343 | 11 | 48 | 12 | — |
| Beef Burrito | 184 | 466 | 30 | 37 | 21 | — |
| Beefy Tostada | 184 | 291 | 19 | 21 | 15 | — |
| Bellbeefer | 123 | 221 | 15 | 23 | 7 | — |
| Bellbeefer w/Cheese | 137 | 278 | 19 | 23 | 12 | — |
| Burrito Supreme | 225 | 457 | 21 | 43 | 22 | — |
| Combination Burrito | 175 | 404 | 21 | 43 | 16 | — |
| Enchirito | 207 | 454 | 25 | 42 | 21 | — |
| Pintos'N Cheese | 158 | 168 | 11 | 21 | 5 | — |
| Taco | 83 | 186 | 15 | 14 | 8 | — |
| Tostada | 138 | 179 | 9 | 25 | 6 | — |
| **Beverages[9]** | | | | | | |
| Coffee, 6 oz. | 180 | 2 | tr | tr | tr | — |
| Tea, 6 oz. | 180 | 2 | tr | — | tr | — |
| Orange Juice, 6 oz. | 183 | 82 | 1 | 20 | tr | — |
| Chocolate Milk, 8 oz. | 250 | 213 | 9 | 28 | 9 | — |
| Skim Milk, 8 oz. | 245 | 88 | 9 | 13 | tr | — |
| Whole Milk, 8 oz. | 244 | 159 | 9 | 12 | 9 | 27 |
| Coca-Cola, 8 oz. | 246 | 96 | 0 | 24 | 0 | — |
| Fanta Ginger Ale, 8 oz. | 244 | 84 | 0 | 21 | 0 | — |
| Fanta Grape, 8 oz. | 247 | 114 | 0 | 29 | 0 | — |
| Fanta Orange, 8 oz. | 248 | 117 | 0 | 30 | 0 | — |
| Fanta Root Beer, 8 oz. | 246 | 103 | 0 | 27 | 0 | — |
| Mr. Pibb, 8 oz. | 245 | 93 | 0 | 25 | 0 | — |
| Mr. Pibb without Sugar, 8 oz. | 237 | 1 | 0 | tr | 0 | — |
| Sprite, 8 oz. | 245 | 95 | 0 | 24 | 0 | — |
| Sprite without Sugar, 8 oz. | 237 | 3 | 0 | 0 | 0 | — |
| Tab, 8 oz. | 237 | tr | 0 | tr | 0 | — |
| Fresca, 8 oz. | 237 | 2 | 0 | 0 | 0 | — |

**282**

[1]Source: Burger Chef Systems, Inc., Indianapolis, Ind., 1978 (analyses obtained from USDA Handbook No. 8).

[2]Source: Chart House, Inc., Oak Brook, Ill., 1978.

[3]Source: International Dairy Queen, Inc., Minneapolis, Minn., 1978. Dairy Queen stores in Texas do not conform to Dairy Queen–approved products. Any nutritional information shown does not necessarily pertain to their products.

[4]Source: Nutritional Content of Average Serving, Heublein Food Service and Franchising Group, June 1976.

[5] Source: Long John Silver's Seafood Shoppes, Jan. 8, 1978 (nutritional analysis information furnished in study conducted by Department of Nutrition and Food Science, University of Kentucky).

[6] Source: "Nutritional analysis of food served at McDonald's restaurants," WARF Institute, Inc., Madison, Wisconsin, June 1977.

[7] Source: Research 900 and Pizza Hut, Inc., Wichita, Kan.

[8] Sources: Menu Item Portions, July 1976. Taco Bell Co., San Antonio, Tex.
Adams, C.F.: Nutritive Value of American Foods in Common Units. USDA Agricultural Research Service, Agricultural Handbook No. 456, November 1975.
Church, C.F. and Church, H.N.: Food Values of Portions Commonly Used, ed. 12. Philadelphia: J.B. Lippincott Co., 1975.
Valley Baptist Medical Center, Food Service Department: Descriptions of Mexican-American Foods, NASCO, Fort Atkinson, Wisconsin.

[9] Sources: Adams, C.F.: Nutritive Value of American Foods in Common Units. USDA Agricultural Research Service, Agricultural Handbook No. 456, November 1975.
Coca-Cola Company, Atlanta, Ga., January 1977.
American Hospital Formulary Service. Washington, D.C., American Society of Hospital Pharmacists, Section 28:20, March 1978.

NOTE: Sodium content reflects sodium content of bottling water; average sodium content, 12 mg/8 oz. Caffeine content depends on strength.

# Percentile Standards for Growth

*Boys: Birth to 24 Months*
*(Adapted from NCHS Growth Charts, 1976)*

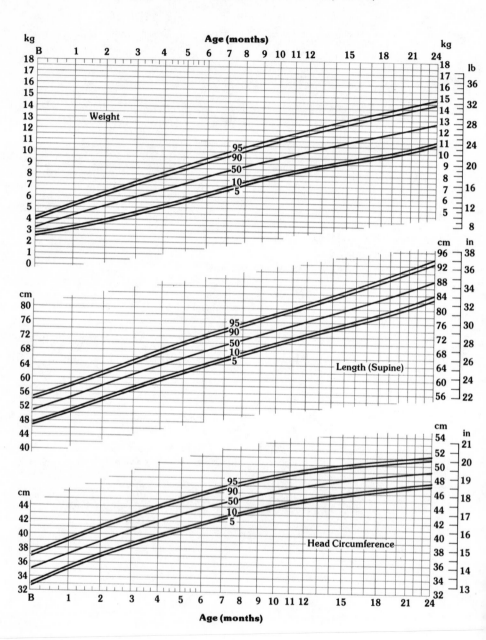

# Percentile Standards for Growth

*Boys: 2 to 18 Years*

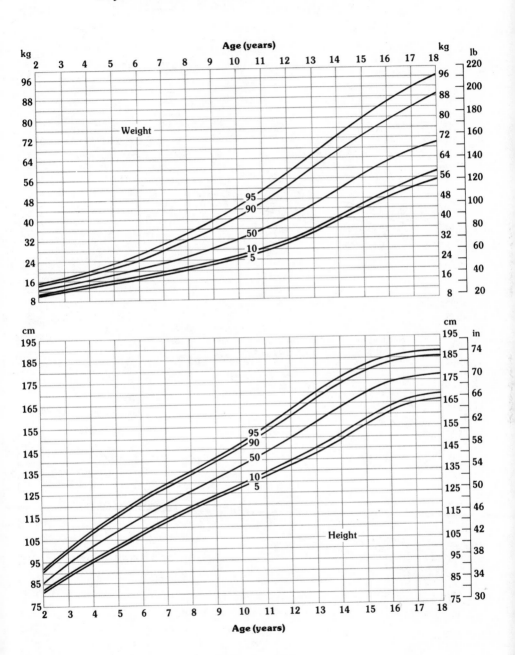

# Percentile Standards for Growth

*Girls: Birth to 24 Months*
*(Adapted from NCHS Growth Charts, 1976)*

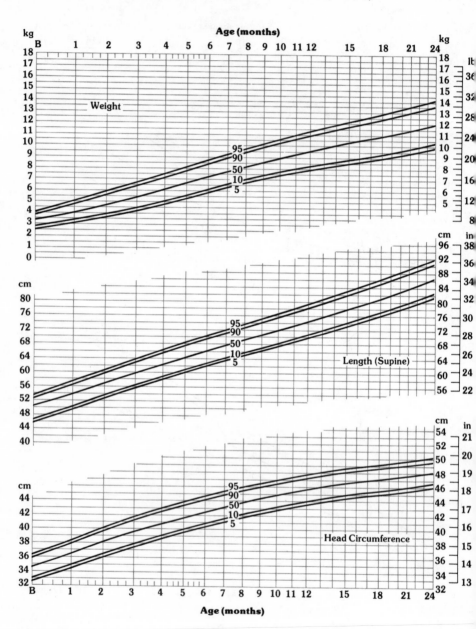

# Percentile Standards for Growth

*Girls: 2 to 18 Years*

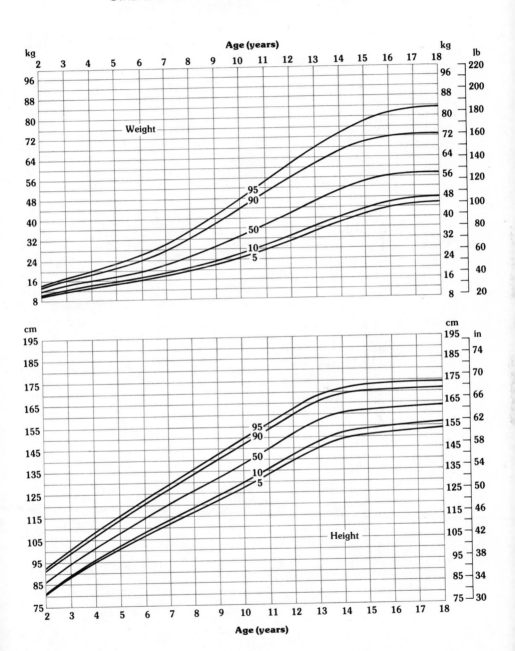

# Calories Burned Up During Ten Minutes of Continuous Activity for Body Weight of 150–200 Pounds

| Activity | Calories Burned |
| --- | --- |
| Sleeping and sitting | 12 to 16 |
| Standing | 15 to 20 |
| Walking, 2 mph | 35 to 40 |
| Walking, 4.5 mph | 65 to 85 |
| Walking upstairs | 175 to 225 |
| Walking downstairs | 64 to 90 |
| Running, 6 mph | 120 to 180 |
| Bicycling, 12 mph | 100 to 140 |
| Office work | 20 to 40 |
| Housework | 40 to 55 |
| Gardening | 50 to 75 |
| Light work in shop or factory | 30 to 50 |
| Heavy work | |
| Shoveling snow | 75 to 100 |
| Chopping wood | 70 to 95 |
| Recreational activity | |
| Volleyball | 50 to 75 |
| Baseball | 45 to 60 |
| Basketball | 70 to 95 |
| Dancing | 45 to 75 |
| Golf | 40 to 55 |
| Skiing (alpine) | 95 to 125 |
| Skiing (cross country) | 120 to 160 |
| Swimming, vigorous | 80 to 100 |
| Tennis | 60 to 90 |

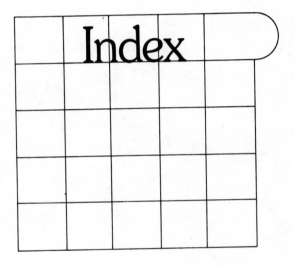

Index

Accidents, 1,9
Addiction to nicotine, 112–13, 117
  see also Smoking
Adenosine triphosphate (ATP), 175,
  177
Advertising by tobacco industry, 37,
  105, 111, 113
Aerobic conditioning, see Exercise,
  aerobic
Air pollution, 141, 157
Alcoholic beverages, 61
Alcoholics Anonymous, 43, 62, 120
American Cancer Society, 118
American College of Cardiology, 15

American Heart Association, 92, 120,
  226
Anaerobic energy system, 175
Angina, 110, 226, 234, 335
Animal fats, 89, 90
Animal homologies, 129
Anxiety, eating in response to, 59
  see also Stress
Aorta, 109, 125, 207, 225
Appetite, increased, 112
Arm circles, 162
Arm hangs, 205, 206
Arm wraps with arm flings, 162
Arnold, Matthew, 13–14, 224

Mineral(s): *(cont'd)*
supplements, 52
Minority groups, smoking and, 106
Miscarriages, 108
Multifactorial inheritance, 22
*see also* Heredity
Mid-term exam, 27
Mormons, 38
Multiple Risk Factor Intervention Trial (MRFIT), 119

Nasal irritation from cigarette smoke, 110
National Academy of Sciences, 129
National Clearing House for Smoking and Health, Public Health Service, 115
National Institute of Health, 14
National Heart, Lung, and Blood Institute, 92
Nausea, 112
Nicotine:
addiction model, 112–13, 117
in sidestream smoke, 111
*see also* Smoking
Nitroglycerin, 224–25, 227, 234, 335
Notebook to record food intake, 55, 56, 59
Nutrition:
basic balanced daily food plan, 58–59, 81
sample menu patterns using, 82–84, 323, 325
nutritional values on packages, 57
tables, 50–51, 242–77
for fast food, 278–82
for food diary, 278–82
*see also* Diet; Weight control
Nuts, 91

Obesity, 13, 46–47, 48, 200
in children, 203
family habits and, 49–50
hypertension and, 131, 133, 207
*see also* Overweight; Weight control

Oils:
in basic balanced daily food plan, 81
cooking, 89
Oral contraceptives, 106, 109, 221
hypertension and, 131–33
Oranges, 131
Osler, Sir William, 14
Overweight, 47–50, 88
defining, 47–49
family habits and, 49–50
hypertension and, 131, 133
*see also* Obesity; Weight control
Oxygen debt, 175, 176

Parties, dieting and eating at, 58, 59, 61
Pavlov, Ivan, 113
PC, *see* Phosphocreatine
Personality type, 43–44
*see also* Type A behavior; Type B behavior
Phosphocreatine (PC), 175, 177
Physical condition:
evaluating your basic, 16–19
aerobic exercise, 19, 32
height, 17
measurements, 17–19, 32
pulse, 16–17
stage of entry into conditioning, 171–72, 181
charts, 189–94
Physician(s), 133, 200, 234, 335
consulting your, 10, 86, 91, 93, 203, 224, 226
before starting aerobic exercise program, 179, 181, 224
identifying children at risk of early heart attack, 210–12, 214
Pickles, 130, 131
Pill, the, 106, 109, 221
hypertension and, 131–33
"Pinch test," 18–19, 48, 60, 223
Pipe smoking, 188
*see also* Smoking
Platelets, 220, 227
Pole-climbs, 205

tear - out

# Appendix

TABLE
**2–1**

# Basic Measurements

| | | | | | | |
|---|---|---|---|---|---|---|
| Pulse rate | | | | | | |
| Height | | | | | | |
| Chest (bust) | | | | | | |
| Waist | | | | | | |
| Hips (women) | | | | | | |
| Weight | | | | | | |
| Pinch tests | | | | | | |
| Belly | | | | | | |
| Upper arm | | | | | | |
| Thigh | | | | | | |
| Chest | | | | | | |
| Love-handles | | | | | | |
| Aerobic exercise | | | | | | |

Figure 2-3: Sample pedigree to practice drawing your family tree.

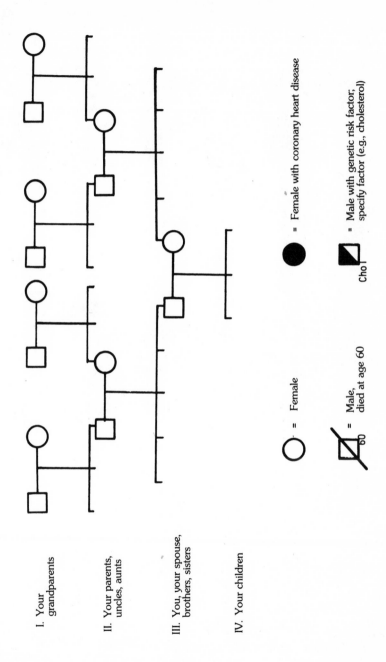

I. Your
   grandparents

II. Your parents,
    uncles, aunts

III. You, your spouse,
     brothers, sisters

IV. Your children

○ = Female

◉ = Female with coronary heart disease

⬕ = Male,
     died at age 60

◪ = Male with genetic risk factor;
Chol   specify factor (e.g., cholesterol)

TABLE
2-2

# First Mid-Term Examination:
## Risk Factor Questionnaire

1   Has a first-degree relative (parent, sibling, child) had a heart attack or developed coronary heart disease before age 55?

2   Has a first-degree relative (parent, sibling, child) had a heart attack or developed coronary heart disease before age 65?

3   Has a second-degree relative (grandparent, uncle, aunt) had a heart attack or developed coronary heart disease before age 65?

4   Has a first-degree relative had a stroke before age 55?

5   Has a first-degree relative had a stroke before age 65?

6   Is your blood cholesterol greater than 270?

7   Is your blood cholesterol greater than 240?

8   Is your blood cholesterol greater than 220?

9   Is your level of triglycerides greater than 200?

10  Do you smoke more than half a pack of cigarettes per day?

11  Do you have diabetes?

12  Does a first-degree relative have diabetes that started before adulthood and requires the use of insulin?

13  Do you get regular aerobic exercise, sustain an exercise heart rate greater than 150 for at least 10 consecutive minutes, with no more than two days between exercise periods, and totaling a minimum of 60 minutes per week?

14  Is your blood pressure greater than 140/90 without treatment? (Note: either a systolic, upper reading, of 140 or a diastolic, lower reading, of 90 is sufficient.)

15  Is your relative weight greater than 1.20? That is, are you more than 20 percent overweight? (See page 47 for method of calculating relative weight.)

16  Do you get 14 or more points on the Type A behavior scale? (See page 148.)

TABLE
**3-1**

# Whole Heart Program

## STANDARD CONTRACT

### (Sample)

Because I'm concerned about my health, I hereby commit myself to participate in the Whole Heart Program as an act of free will.

1   My entire program is based first on the understanding that I am a mature person capable of making a decision to change my life-style to one that promotes good health. This new life-style is inner controlled and will become an integral part of my personal value system.

2   I will practice meditation for no less than 10 minutes a day, but preferably for 20 minutes once or twice daily.

3   If I have been a smoker, I have now abrogated the habit and will continue my resolve not to return to smoking.

4   If I require weight reduction, I will follow my systematic program, one step at a time, until I reach my ideal weight. I will then maintain my ideal weight.

5   As a second dietary commitment, I will follow a prudent diet or a more strict special diet, if indicated.

6   I will faithfully follow my personal exercise prescription (which in most cases will require at least 30 minutes a day, six days a week).

7   At bedtime each night I will review and record my progress and outline my program for the next day for as long a period as required (generally at least four months).

This contract is binding on the signatories for the period specified. It is the obligation of the signatories to help each other and assume responsibility for the success of the program for all participants.

The contract is considered binding and in force during the following dates:


_____          _____
*Dates*                                *Signatories*


_____          _____
*Dates*                                *Signatories*


_____          _____
*Dates*                                *Signatories*

TABLE
**3–1**

# Whole Heart Program

## STANDARD CONTRACT

### (Sample)

Because I'm concerned about my health, I hereby commit myself to participate in the Whole Heart Program as an act of free will.

1    My entire program is based first on the understanding that I am a mature person capable of making a decision to change my life-style to one that promotes good health. This new life-style is inner controlled and will become an integral part of my personal value system.

2    I will practice meditation for no less than 10 minutes a day, but preferably for 20 minutes once or twice daily.

3    If I have been a smoker, I have now abrogated the habit and will continue my resolve not to return to smoking.

4    If I require weight reduction, I will follow my systematic program, one step at a time, until I reach my ideal weight. I will then maintain my ideal weight.

5    As a second dietary commitment, I will follow a prudent diet or a more strict special diet, if indicated.

6    I will faithfully follow my personal exercise prescription (which in most cases will require at least 30 minutes a day, six days a week).

7    At bedtime each night I will review and record my progress and outline my program for the next day for as long a period as required (generally at least four months).

This contract is binding on the signatories for the period specified. It is the obligation of the signatories to help each other and assume responsibility for the success of the program for all participants.

The contract is considered binding and in force during the following dates:


_Dates_                _Signatories_


_Dates_                _Signatories_


_Dates_                _Signatories_

TABLE
**4-5**

**Weight Loss Chart**

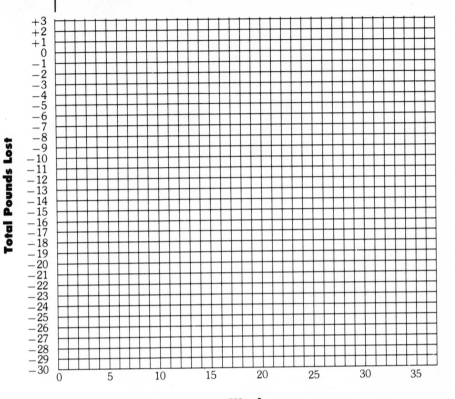

Total Pounds Lost

Weeks

**Beginning Weight** _____

| Date | Week | Weight | Total Lbs. Lost |
|------|------|--------|-----------------|
|      | 0    |        |                 |
|      | 1    |        |                 |
|      | 2    |        |                 |
|      | 3    |        |                 |
|      | 4    |        |                 |
|      | 5    |        |                 |
|      | 6    |        |                 |
|      | 7    |        |                 |
|      | 8    |        |                 |
|      | 9    |        |                 |
|      | 10   |        |                 |
|      | 11   |        |                 |
|      | 12   |        |                 |
|      | 13   |        |                 |
|      | 14   |        |                 |
|      | 15   |        |                 |
|      | 16   |        |                 |
|      | 17   |        |                 |
|      | 18   |        |                 |
|      | 19   |        |                 |
|      | 20   |        |                 |
|      | 21   |        |                 |
|      | 22   |        |                 |
|      | 23   |        |                 |
|      | 24   |        |                 |
|      | 25   |        |                 |
|      | 26   |        |                 |
|      | 27   |        |                 |
|      | 28   |        |                 |
|      | 29   |        |                 |
|      | 30   |        |                 |

**Goal Weight** _____

TABLE
**4-8**

**Daily Food Diary**

| | Calories | Protein (g) |
|---|---|---|
| **Breakfast** | | |
| **Morning Snack** | | |
| **Lunch** | | |
| **Afternoon Snack** | | |
| **Dinner** | | |
| **Bedtime Snack** | | |
| **TOTALS** | | |

TABLE
4–8

# Daily Food Diary

|  | Calories | Protein (g) |
|---|---|---|
| **Breakfast** | | |
| **Morning Snack** | | |
| **Lunch** | | |
| **Afternoon Snack** | | |
| **Dinner** | | |
| **Bedtime Snack** | | |
| **TOTALS** | | |

TABLE
4-11

# Weight Reduction Plan, _____ calories

## Daily Food Plan

___ Servings (3 ounces each) poultry, fish, or lean trimmed meat, or appropriate substitute
___ Servings fruits and vegetables
___ Servings bread or cereal
___ Servings (8 ounces each) skim milk
___ Servings (1 teaspoon each) allowed fat (i.e., vegetable oil or polyunsaturated margarine)

### Morning Snack:

___ _____

___ _____

___ _____

### Afternoon Snack:

___ _____

___ _____

___ _____

### Bedtime Snack:

___ _____

___ _____

___ _____

## Sample Menu Pattern

### Breakfast:
___ Serving citrus fruit or juice
___ Serving cereal or toast
___ Servings allowed fat
___ Serving skim milk

### Lunch:
___ Serving poultry, fish, or lean trimmed meat
___ Serving potato, rice, or substitute
___ Servings vegetable
___ Serving bread
___ Servings allowed fat
___ Serving fruit
___ Serving skim milk

### Dinner:
___ Serving poultry, fish, or lean trimmed meat
___ Serving potato, rice, or substitute
___ Servings vegetable
___ Servings bread
___ Servings allowed fat
___ Serving fruit
___ Serving skim milk

TABLE
**4-12**

# Maintenance Diet

## Daily Food Plan

___ Servings (3 ounces each) poultry, fish, or lean trimmed meat, or appropriate substitute
___ Servings fruits and vegetables
___ Servings bread or cereal
___ Servings (8 ounces each) skim milk
___ Servings (1 teaspoon each) allowed fat (i.e., vegetable oil or polyunsaturated margarine)

### Morning Snack:

___ _____

___ _____

___ _____

### Afternoon Snack:

___ _____

___ _____

___ _____

### Bedtime Snack:

___ _____

___ _____

___ _____

## Sample Menu Pattern

### Breakfast:
___ Serving citrus fruit or juice
___ Serving cereal or toast
___ Servings allowed fat
___ Serving skim milk

### Lunch:
___ Serving poultry, fish, or lean trimmed meat
___ Serving potato, rice, or substitute
___ Servings vegetable
___ Serving bread
___ Servings allowed fat
___ Serving fruit
___ Serving skim milk

### Dinner:
___ Serving poultry, fish, or lean trimmed meat
___ Serving potato, rice, or substitute
___ Servings vegetable
___ Servings bread
___ Servings allowed fat
___ Serving fruit
___ Serving skim milk

TABLE
6-1

# Why Do You Smoke?

Here are some statements made by people to describe what they get out of smoking cigarettes. HOW OFTEN do you feel this way when smoking them? Circle one number for each statement. It's necessary that you answer every question.

| | | Always | Frequently | Occasionally | Seldom | Never |
|---|---|---|---|---|---|---|
| **A** | I smoke cigarettes in order to keep myself from slowing down. | 4 | 3 | 2 | 1 | 0 |
| **B** | Handling a cigarette is part of the enjoyment of smoking it. | 4 | 3 | 2 | 1 | 0 |
| **C** | Smoking cigarettes is pleasant and relaxing. | 4 | 3 | 2 | 1 | 0 |
| **D** | I light up a cigarette when I feel angry about something. | 4 | 3 | 2 | 1 | 0 |
| **E** | When I have run out of cigarettes I find it almost unbearable until I can get them. | 4 | 3 | 2 | 1 | 0 |
| **F** | I smoke cigarettes automatically without even being aware of it. | 4 | 3 | 2 | 1 | 0 |
| **G** | I smoke cigarettes to stimulate me, to perk myself up. | 4 | 3 | 2 | 1 | 0 |
| **H** | Part of the enjoyment of smoking a cigarette comes from the steps to take to light up. | 4 | 3 | 2 | 1 | 0 |
| **I** | I find cigarettes pleasurable. | 4 | 3 | 2 | 1 | 0 |
| **J** | When I feel uncomfortable or upset about something, I light up a cigarette. | 4 | 3 | 2 | 1 | 0 |
| **K** | I am very much aware of the fact when I am smoking a cigarette. | 4 | 3 | 2 | 1 | 0 |
| **L** | I light up a cigarette without realizing I still have one burning in the ashtray. | 4 | 3 | 2 | 1 | 0 |
| **M** | I smoke cigarettes to give me a "lift." | 4 | 3 | 2 | 1 | 0 |
| **N** | When I smoke a cigarette, part of the enjoyment is watching the smoke as I exhale it. | 4 | 3 | 2 | 1 | 0 |
| **O** | I want a cigarette most when I am comfortable and relaxed. | 4 | 3 | 2 | 1 | 0 |

**P** When I feel "blue" or want to take my mind off cares and worries, I smoke cigarettes.

    4   3   2   1   0

**Q** I get a real gnawing hunger for a cigarette when I haven't smoked for a while.

    4   3   2   1   0

**R** I've found a cigarette in my mouth and didn't remember putting it there.

    4   3   2   1   0

## Score Card

When you have completed the test, score yourself:

**1** Take the numbers on the first line and add across; that is, add the numbers for A, G, and M and put the total in the last column.

**2** Follow the same procedure for each line.

Scores can vary from 0 to 12. Any score 8 and above is high; any score 4 and below is low.

___ + ___ + ___ = _____
 A     G     M           Stimulation

___ + ___ + ___ = _____
 B     H     N           Handling

___ + ___ + ___ = _____
 C     I     O           Pleasurable Relaxation

___ + ___ + ___ = _____
 D     J     P           Crutch: Tension Reduction

___ + ___ + ___ = _____
 E     K     Q           Craving: Addiction

___ + ___ + ___ = _____
 F     L     R           Habit

TABLE
8-1

# Type A Personality Questionnaire

PLEASE TAKE YOUR TIME ANSWERING THESE QUESTIONS. It is important to give as frank an answer as possible. Feel free to ask your spouse or friends how you should answer the question. Some of these items, such as the way you talk, may not be apparent to you, but would be to those who know you well.

**1** Do you feel there are not enough hours in the day to do all the things you must do?

( ) yes ( ) no

**2** Do you always move, walk, and eat rapidly?

( ) yes ( ) no

**3** Do you feel an impatience with the rate at which most events take place?

( ) yes ( ) no

**4** Do you say, "Uh-huh, uh-huh," or "yes, yes, yes, yes," to someone who is talking, unconsciously urging him to "get on with it" or hasten his rate of speaking? Do you have a tendency to finish the sentences of others for them?

( ) yes ( ) no

**5** Do you become unduly irritated or even enraged when a car ahead of you in your lane runs at a pace you consider too slow? Do you find it anguishing to wait in line or to wait your turn to be seated at a restaurant?

( ) yes ( ) no

**6** Do you find it intolerable to watch others perform tasks you know you can do faster?

( ) yes ( ) no

**7** Do you become impatient with yourself as you are obliged to perform repetitious duties (making out bank deposit slips, writing checks, washing and cleaning dishes, and so on), which are necessary but take you away from doing things you really have an interest in doing?

( ) yes ( ) no

**8** Do you find yourself hurrying your own reading or always attempting to obtain condensations or summaries of truly interesting and worthwhile literature?

( ) yes ( ) no

**9** Do you strive to think of or do two or more things simultaneously? For example, while trying to listen to another person's speech, do you persist in continuing to think about an irrelevant subject?

( ) yes ( ) no

**10** While engaged in recreation, do you continue to ponder your business, home, or professional problems?

( ) yes ( ) no

**11** Do you have (a) a habit of explosively accentuating various key words in your ordinary speech even when there is no real need for such accentuation, and (b) a tendency to utter

**329**

the last few words of your sentences far more rapidly than the opening words?

( ) yes    ( ) no

**12** Do you find it difficult to refrain from talking about or bringing the theme of any conversation around to those subjects that especially interest and intrigue you, and when unable to accomplish this maneuver, do you pretend to listen but really remain preoccupied with your own thoughts?

( ) yes    ( ) no

**13** Do you almost always feel vaguely guilty when you relax and do absolutely nothing for several hours to several days?

( ) yes    ( ) no

**14** Do you attempt to schedule more and more in less and less time, and in doing so make fewer and fewer allowances for unforeseen contingencies?

( ) yes    ( ) no

**15** In conversation, do you frequently clench your fist or bang your hand upon a table or pound one fist into the palm of your hand in order to emphasize a conversational point?

( ) yes    ( ) no

**16** If employed, does your job include frequent deadlines that are difficult to meet?

( ) yes    ( ) no

**17** Do you frequently clench your jaw, or even grind your teeth?

( ) yes    ( ) no

**18** Do you frequently bring your work or study material (related to your job, not to school) home with you at night?

( ) yes    ( ) no

**19** Do you find yourself evaluating not only your own but also the activities of others in terms of numbers?

( ) yes    ( ) no

**20** Are you dissatisfied with your present work?

( ) yes    ( ) no

### Score Card

| | | |
|---|---|---|
| 4+ | = | 14 or more points |
| 3+ | = | 9–13 points |
| 2+ | = | 4–8 points |
| 1+ | = | 3 or fewer points |

TABLE
**12–3**

# Risk Index for Early-Onset Coronary Heart Disease

*(Maximum Score = 10)*

| Circle and Add Your Points | **Family History** *(Select the single highest value. The maximum score for this section is 3.)* |
|:---:|:---|
| 3.0 | Coronary disease in first-degree relative before age 55. |
| 2.5 | Coronary disease in first-degree relative before age 65. |
| 1.0 | Coronary disease in second-degree relative before age 65. |
| 1.0 | Stroke in first-degree relative before age 55. |
| 0.5 | Stroke in second-degree relative before age 65. |

| | **Cholesterol and Triglycerides** *(Select the single highest cholesterol value. Select the triglyceride value—if elevated. The maximum score for this section is 2.)* |
|:---:|:---|
| 2.0 | Cholesterol greater than 270. |
| 1.0 | Cholesterol greater than 240. |
| 0.5 | Cholesterol greater than 220. |
| 0.5 | Triglycerides greater than 200. |

| | **Other Risks** *(Add all values. The maximum score for this section is 5.)* |
|:---:|:---|
| 1.5 | Smoking—more than $1/2$ pack per day. |
| 1.0 | Diabetes in patient or juvenile diabetes in first-degree relative. |
| 1.0 | No regular aerobic exercise. |
| 0.5 | Blood pressure greater than 140/90. |
| 0.5 | Relative weight greater than 1.20. |
| 0.5 | Type A. |

## Risk Scores and Increased
## Risks of Early-onset Coronary Heart Disease

| Risk Score | Increased Risk |
|:---:|:---:|
| 3 | 2× |
| 3.5 | 3× |
| 4 | 5× |
| 4.5 | 6× |
| 5 | 15× |
| 5.5 | not calculable by present methods |

TABLE
**12-4**

# Risk Index for Children and Adolescents*

| Circle and Add Your Points | **Family History** *(Same as for adults—single highest value.)* |
|---|---|
| 3.0 | Coronary disease in first-degree relative before age 55. |
| 2.5 | Coronary disease in first-degree relative before age 65. |
| 1.0 | Coronary disease in second-degree relative before age 55. |
| 1.0 | Stroke in first-degree relative before age 55. |
| 0.5 | Stroke in second-degree relative before age 65. |
|  | **Cholesterol and Triglycerides** *(Score as for adults. Maximum score is 2.)* |
| 2.0 | Cholesterol greater than 220. |
| 1.0 | Cholesterol greater than 190. |
| 0.5 | Triglycerides greater than 120. |
|  | **Other Risks** *(Add all values.)* |
| 1.5 | Smoking regularly. |
| 1.0 | Diabetes in patient or juvenile diabetes in first-degree relative. |
| 1.0 | No regular aerobic exercise. |
| 0.5 | Blood pressure greater than 140/90, or systolic (upper number) or diastolic (lower number) pressure greater than ninety-fifth percentile. |
| 0.5 | Relative weight greater than 1.20 ( > 20 percent overweight). |
| 0.5 | Type A. |

*See Risk Scores and Increased Risks, Table 12–3.*

TABLE
12–5

# Heart Attack

## Some Signals

1   Pressure, squeezing, fullness, or pain in the center of the chest behind the breastbone, which may spread to the shoulders, upper abdomen, neck, jaws, back, or arms (more often to the left shoulder and arm, but either or both sides may be involved).

2   The pain may *not* be severe *or* it may be crushing.

3   Shortness of breath.

4   Feeling of weakness.

5   Sweating.

6   Nausea.

## Actions for Survival

1   Recognize the signals (as described above).

2   Stop activity and sit down or lie down.

3   If pain lasts for more than two minutes call your mobile coronary care unit or emergency rescue service or go to the nearest hospital emergency room with 24-hour service.

4   For those under a doctor's care:

    a   If the doctor has prescribed nitroglycerin, place a tablet under the tongue. If the pain is typical angina it should disappear within three minutes. If it is "prolonged ischemia" or a heart attack (or some other condition), it is not as likely to "respond" to nitroglycerin within three minutes.

    b   If a physician has suggested a propranolol-type drug, swallow a tablet with a sip of water if nitroglycerin has not relieved the pain within three minutes.

    c   Immediately follow through with emergency rescue service or hospital emergency room.

    d   Have a family member or co-worker notify physician of where patient will be.